1/8/06

CORE TOPICS IN PAIN

Core Topics in Pain *provides a comprehensive, easy-to-read introduction to this multi-faceted topic. It covers a wide range of issues from the underlying neurobiology, through pain assessment in animals and humans, diagnostic strategies, clinical presentations, pain syndromes, to the many treatment options (for example, physical therapies, drug therapies, psychosocial care) and the evidence base for each of these. Written and edited by experts of international renown, the many concise but comprehensive chapters provide the reader with an up-to-date guide to all aspects of pain.*

It is an essential book for anaesthetic trainees and is also an invaluable first reference for surgical and nursing staff, ICU professionals, operating department practitioners, physiotherapists, psychologists, healthcare managers and researchers with a need for an overview of the key aspects of the topic.

CORE TOPICS IN PAIN

Edited by

Anita Holdcroft
Department of Anaesthetics and Intensive Care
Imperial College London
Chelsea and Westminster Campus
Fulham Road
London SW10 9NH, UK

Siân Jaggar
The Royal Brompton Hospital
Sydney Street
London SW3 6NP, UK

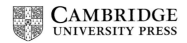
CAMBRIDGE
UNIVERSITY PRESS

PUBLISHED BY THE PRESS SYNDICATE OF THE UNIVERSITY OF CAMBRIDGE
The Pitt Building, Trumpington Street, Cambridge, United Kingdom

CAMBRIDGE UNIVERSITY PRESS
The Edinburgh Building, Cambridge CB2 2RU, UK
40 West 20th Street, New York, NY 10011-4211, USA
477 Williamstown Road, Port Melbourne, VIC 3207, Australia
Ruiz de Alarcón 13, 28014 Madrid, Spain
Dock House, The Waterfront, Cape Town 8001, South Africa

http://www.cambridge.org

First published 2005

Printed in the United Kingdom at the University Press, Cambridge

Typeface: Ehrhardt 10/11pt   System: QuarkXpress®

A catalog record for this book is available from the British Library

Library of Congress Cataloging in Publication data

ISBN 0 521 85778 3 hardback

The publisher has used its best endeavors to ensure that the URLs
for external websites referred to in this book are correct and
active at the time of going to press. However, the publisher has
no responsibility for the websites and can make no guarantee
that a site will remain live or that the content is or will
remain appropriate.

Every effort has been made in preparing this book to provide accurate and
up-to-date information that is in accord with accepted standards and
practice at the time of publication. Nevertheless, the authors, editors and
publisher can make no warranties that the information contained herein is
totally free from error, not least because clinical standards are constantly
changing through research and regulation. The authors, editors and
publisher therefore disclaim all liability for direct or consequential
damages resulting from the use of material contained in this book. Readers
are strongly advised to pay careful attention to information provided by the
manufacturer of any drugs or equipment that they plan to use.

CONTENTS

CONTRIBUTORS

Baranowski P. Andrew
Bennett Dave
Berkley J. Karen
Biasi Giovanni
Bromley Lesley
Cafferty Will
Carli Giancarlo
Carpenter Kate
Cashman Jeremy
Collett J. Beverly
Cox Sarah
Dickenson Anthony
Farquhar-Smith W. Paul
Fillingim B. Roger
Filshie Jacqueline
Finnerup B. Nanna
Gifford Louis
Gourlay Doug
Hanna Magdi
Hartle Andrew
Holdcroft Anita
Howard F. Richard
Howarth Amanda
Jaggar I Sian
Jensen S. Troels
Johnson E. Emma
Kent Alixe

Keogh Edmund
Kerr J. Bradley
Kirwan Trottie
Lund Samantha
Lambert G. David
Maze Mervyn
McQuay J. Henry
Macrae A. William
Miles B. John
Newton-John Toby
Patterson H. Paul
Pither Charles
Platt Michael
Price Cathy
Riley Julia
Schreyer T.
Serpell G. Mick
Skoglund Lassa
Stannard Cathy
Thacker Mick
Tyrer Stephen
Waheed Umeer
Welsh Ken
Wigham Ann
Wilder-Smith Oliver Hamilton Gottwaldt
Zarnegar Roxaneh

PREFACE

The driving force for this book comes from our patients, rarely those who complied with our therapies, but particularly those who only partly responded, those who received complete pain relief as a marvel, and those who were so consumed with anger that major barriers had to be broken down before healing could begin. In practicing pain therapy questions inevitably arise for which we have no easy answers, but over time it is possible to plan research to investigate and test theories. This book is written not to extol the science *per se* but rather to seek to identify where further exploration is warranted, because we have no simple answers and the breadth of factors that influence pain sensations and therapies is great.

The original publishers with whom we entered into a contract were Greenwich Medical, well known for their concise cutting edge anaesthesia textbooks. We concurred with this format, expecting a low cost no frills approach. Nevertheless we have attempted to provide the information needed to reach a postgraduate diploma standard. We hope that the breadth of subjects distilled into this small volume will be a treasured resource for pain management teams.

As far as possible we have attempted to format each chapter into an overall style. Some authors have resisted, you the readers are our judges. Since writing or editing a book offers little recompense to those involved we hope that the rewards are felt by your patients.

Anita Holdcroft and Siân Jaggar

ACKNOWLEDGEMENTS

We are indebted to Gavin Smith and Geoff Nuttall at Greenwich Medical for developing the ideas that we had for this book and for almost publishing it. We are also grateful to our teachers and collaborators, many of whom have distilled their expertise into this book. Of those we miss, Dr Frank Kurer and Professor Pat Wall are perhaps the most recent but there are also the patients and experimental subjects who have taught us to ask questions and seek answers.

FOREWARD

An understanding of pain management should be an essential component of the training for all healthcare professionals who deal with patients, irrespective of specialty. This includes doctors, nurses, dentists, physiotherapists and psychologists. All of them can contribute to a better outcome for patients who suffer pain.

There has been a huge explosion in our understanding of the basic mechanisms of pain and this is demonstrated in the first few chapters of this book. Despite these advances in physiology, pharmacology, psychology and related subjects, surveys repeatedly reveal that unrelieved pain remains a widespread problem. The challenges of pain management encompass more than just postoperative pain and includes other types of acute pain (e.g. trauma, burns, acute pancreatitis) as well as chronic pain and pain in patients with cancer. The range of topics dealt with in this book bear testament to the ubiquity of pain and the way in which pain impinges itself into virtually every realm of medical practice.

The cost of unrelieved pain can be measured in psychological, physiological and socio-economic terms. Governments around the world are developing awareness that pain and disability can be very expensive and that pain management strategies are sometimes very cost-effective. Despite this growing awareness there is a wide variation in provision of pain management services even in countries with developed health services such as the United Kingdom. The picture in parts of the developing world is sometimes much less rosy.

The advances in our understanding of pain mechanisms has lead to improved methods of management, either by introducing new treatments or by allowing more efficient usage of older therapies. The multidisciplinary approach remains a fundamental concept in the delivery of effective pain management.

Books such as this will be useful for trainees from many areas of medical practice. The Royal College of Anaesthetists has defined competency-based outcomes for pain management at all levels of the anaesthetic training programme and there is provision for up to 12 months of full-time advanced training in pain management. Many other professional groups are developing curricula for training in pain management. The International Association for the Study of Pain (IASP) has been at the forefront in promoting education in pain management. If you are interested in pain then please join IASP and also join the British Pain Society, a Chapter of IASP.

The provision of effective pain relief for all patients should be a prime objective of any healthcare service. This book provides a comprehensive introduction to the ways of delivering that effective pain relief.

Dr Douglas Justins MB BS FRCA
Consultant in Pain Management and Anaesthesia

GENERAL ABBREVIATIONS

AA	Acupuncture analgesia
ACR	American College of Rheumatology
AHCPR	US Agency for Health Care Policy and Research
BMA	British Medical Association
BPI	Brief pain inventory
CBT	Cognitive behavioural therapy
CEBM	Centre for evidence-based medicine (Oxford)
CER	Control event rate
CNS	Central nervous system
CNCP	Chronic non-cancer pain
COX	Cyclo-oxygenase – there are at least two different isoforms
CRF	Case report form
CRPS	Complex regional pain syndrome
DCN	Dorsal column nuclei
DDS	Descriptor differential scales
DNIC	Diffuse noxious inhibitor control
DREZ	Dorsal root entry zone
DSM	Diagnostic and statistical manual for mental disorders
EA	Electroacupuncture
EER	Experimental event rate
EMG	Electromyogram
FMS	Fibromyalgia syndrome
GP	General practitioner
HIV	Human immunodeficiency virus
IASP	International Association for the Study of Pain
ICU	Intensive care unit
IV	Intravenous
JCAHO	Joint Commission on Accreditation of Healthcare Organisations
LA	Local anaesthetic
MA	Manual acupuncture
MAOI	Monoamine oxidase inhibitor
MDT	Multidisciplinary teams
MPQ	McGill pain questionnaire
MRI	Magnetic resonance imaging
NCHSPCS	National Council for Hospice and Specialist Palliative Care Services
NHMRC	Australian National Health and Medical Research Council
NHS	National Health Service
NHSE	National Health Service Executive
NICE	National Institute for Clinical Excellence
NNT	Number needed to treat
NNH	Number needed to harm
NSAID	Non-steroidal anti-inflammatory drug
NCA	Nurse controlled analgesia
NO	Nitric oxide
NRS	Numerical rating scale
OR	Odds ratio

PCA	Patient controlled analgesia
PDN	Peripheral diabetic neuropathy
PET	Positron emission tomography
PG	Prostaglandin
PHN	Post-herpetic neuralgia
PMP	Pain management programme
RCS	Royal College of Surgeons
RCT	Randomised controlled trial
RSD	Reflex sympathetic dystrophy
SC	Spinal cord
SIP	Sympathetic independent pain
SMP	Sympathetic mediated pain
SN	Solitary nucleus
SOP	Special operating procedure
SR	Systematic review
SSRI	Selective serotonin reuptake inhibitors
TCA	Tricyclic agents (*note*: two uses – see below)
TCA	Traditional Chinese acupuncture (*note*: two uses – see above)
TENS	Transcutaneous electrical nerve stimulation
TGN	Trigeminal neuralgia
TP	Trigger point
TeP	Tender point
VAS	Visual analogue scale
VRS	Verbal rating scale
WHO	World Health Organisation

BASIC SCIENCE ABBREVIATIONS

5-HT	5-hydroxytryptamine (serotonin)
Δ^9-THC	Δ^9-tetrahydrocannabinol
A_2	Adenosine type two receptors
AA	Arachidonic acid
AC	Adenylyl cyclase
AEA	Anandamide/arachidonylethanolamide
AMPA	Alpha-amino-3-hydroxy-5-methyl-4-isoxazolepropionic acid
ASIC	Acid-sensing ion channels (numbered 1–3) – a family of pH sensors
ATP	Adenosine triphosphate
BDNF	Brain derived neurotrophic factor
BK	Bradykinin – peptide known to be algogenic
Ca^{2+}	Calcium ions
cAMP	Cyclic adenosine monophosphate – important intracellular messenger
CB_1	Cannabinoid receptor type 1
CB_2	Cannabinoid receptor type 2
cGMP	Cyclic guanosine monophosphate – important intracellular messenger
CGRP	Calcitonin gene related peptide
COX	Cyclo-oxygenase – there are at least two different isoforms
CRPS	Complex regional pain syndrome
DAG	Diacyl glycerol – important intracellular messenger
DCN	Dorsal column nucleus
DH	Dorsal horn
DOP	Delta opioid receptor
DRG	Dorsal root ganglion
EP_{1-4}	Prostanoid receptor – a family
GABA	Gamma amino butyric acid
GC	Guanylyl cyclase
GDP	Guanosine diphosphate
GDNF	Glial derived nerve growth factor
Gs	G-protein – through which many receptors link to intracellular events
GTP	Guanosine triphosphate
H^+	Hydrogen ions – important inflammatory mediator
H_1	Histamine receptor type 1
H_2	Histamine receptor type 2
IL-1β	Interleukin 1β
IL-2	Interleukin 2
IP_3	Inositol triphosphate – important intracellular messenger
$Ins(1,4,5)P_3$	Inositol (1,4,5) triphosphate
IUPHAR	International Union of Pharmacology
KOP	Kappa opioid receptor
LA	Local anaesthetic
LOX	Lipoxygenase
LTB_4	Leucotriene B_4
MOP	Mu opioid receptor
NE	Norepinephrine/Noradrenaline
NEP	Neutral endopeptidase

NGF	Nerve growth factor
NK1	Neurokinin 1
NK2	Neurokinin 2 – receptor for neurokinin A
NK3	Neurokinin 3 – receptor for neurokinin B
NKA	Neurokinin A – peptide related to substance P
NKB	Neurokinin B – peptide related to substance P
NMDA	N-methyl-D-aspartate
NO	Nitric oxide
N/OFQ	Nociceptin – also known as orphanin FQ
NOP	Nociceptin receptor
NOS	Nitric oxide synthase – enzyme that produces NO
NR1	Subunit of NMDA receptor – essential for activity
NSAID	Non-steroidal anti-inflammatory drug
NT-3	Neurotrophic factor 3
NTF	Neurotrophic factor
P_2X_3	Purine channel – responds to the algogen ATP
PAG	Periaqueductal grey
PEA	Palmitoylethanolamide
PET	Positron emission tomography
PGE_2	Prostaglandin E_2 – main pain producing prostanoid
PLA_2	Phospholipase A_2 – important intracellular messenger
PKA	Protein kinase A – important intracellular messenger
PKC	Protein kinase C
PLC	Phospholipase C – important intracellular messenger
PLA_2	Phospholipase A_2
PN3	Another name for SNS (also known as Nav 1.8)
RVM	Rostroventral medulla
SIP	Sympathetic independent pain
SMP	Sympathetic mediated pain
SNS	Sensory nerve-specific sodium channel – member of TTX-R
SN	Solitary nucleus – parasympathetic
SP	Substance P
Src	Serine receptor coupled (type of tyrosine kinase)
TNFα	Tumour necrosis factor α
TrKA	Tyrosine kinase A
TrKB	Tyrosine kinase B – receptor for NGF
TrKC	Tyrosine kinase C – receptor for NT-3
TRP	Transient receptor potential – superfamily of ligand-gated ion channels
TRPV1	Transient receptor potential vanilloid (alternative name for VR1)
TTX	Tetrodotoxin
TTX-R	TTX-resistant sodium channels
Vd	Volume of distribution
VPL	Ventroposterolateral (nucleus of thalamus)
VR1	Vanilloid receptor – sensor for heat, responsive to capsaicin
VRL	Vanilloid receptor like
VSCC	Voltage-sensitive calcium channels

OVERVIEW OF PAIN PATHWAYS

1

S.I. Jaggar

A major barrier to appropriate pain management is a general misperception that pain and nociception are interchangeable terms. This encourages the belief that every individual will experience the same sensation given the same stimulus. This is analogous to suggesting that all individuals will grow to the same height given the same nourishment – a situation that all would agree is unlikely!

Nociception is the neural mechanism by which an individual detects the presence of a potentially tissue-harming stimulus. There is no implication of (or requirement for) awareness of this stimulus.

Pain is 'an unpleasant sensory and emotional experience associated with actual or potential tissue damage, or described in terms of such damage'. Thus, perception of sensory events is a requirement, but actual tissue damage is not.

The nociceptive mechanism (prior to the perceptive event) consists of a multitude of events as follows:

- *Transduction*:
  This is the conversion of one form of energy to another. It occurs at a variety of stages along the nociceptive pathway from:
  - Stimulus events to chemical tissue events.
  - Chemical tissue and synaptic cleft events to electrical events in neurones.
  - Electrical events in neurones to chemical events at synapses.
- *Transmission*:
  Electrical events are transmitted along neuronal pathways, while molecules in the synaptic cleft transmit information from one cell surface to another.
- *Modulation*:
  The adjustment of events, by up- or downregulation. This can occur at all levels of the nociceptive pathway, from tissue, through primary (1°) afferent neurone and dorsal horn, to higher brain centres.

Thus, the pain pathway as described by Descartes has had to be adapted with time (see Figure 1.1).

The chapters that follow address the pathophysiological events occurring along the 'pain pathway'. It is important to recognise that all the anatomical structures and chemical compounds described are genetically coded. Therefore, to suggest that all individuals

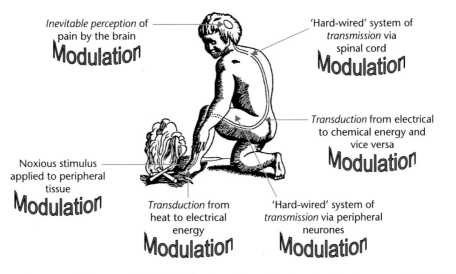

Figure 1.1 Development of the original 'hard-wired' pain pathway first described by Descartes in 1664 showing sites where modulation occurs.

ve pain in the same way (and if they do not fault) is unsustainable.

iple, we would not suggest that eye colour is something over which people have total control – we accept that this is genetically determined. Yet, we suggest that an individual who is unfortunate enough to suffer severe pain (perhaps consequent upon the expression of particular populations of receptors responding to nociceptive chemicals) is somehow 'over-reacting' to a stimulus. Moreover, we understand that the presence of male pattern baldness requires not only the presence of a gene, but also a particular hormonal environment (high testosterone levels). Why should we be surprised, therefore, that a particular stimulus may be perceived differently in individuals with varying hormonal make-up?

This is not to suggest that all pain is entirely genetically determined, but rather it is not 'all in the mind' – a phrase often used with negative connotations in regard to pain patients. Previous experience of pain can undoubtedly alter perceptions, but this should not suggest any 'unreality'. The presence of lung cancer is frequently consequent upon prior experience – in this case, of smoking. Similarly, prior experience of pain may facilitate activity, in particular neuronal pathways, leading to a reduction in pain threshold at a later date.

A variety of tissue-damaging stimuli leads to the production of a 'chemical or inflammatory soup'. This consists of a wide variety of substances, knowledge of which is continually being expanded. Whatever the composition of this soup, pain events are generated by chemical binding with receptors on 1° afferent neurones. Such receptors consists of three major groupings: excitatory, sensitising and inhibitory. It is the

balance of outcomes of these events that determines whether an action potential is generated in the neurone (Figure 1.2).

Once electrical activity is generated within the 1° afferent neurone, information is transmitted to the dorsal horn of the spinal cord. Activity is induced in the second-order neurone in a similar fashion. Quantal release of neurotransmitters from the 1° afferent neurone is dependent upon: (a) activity within the neurone, (b) external events affecting alterations in neuronal activity, for example, inhibitory and excitatory inputs upon pre-synaptic terminal. Activity in the second-order neurone is again dependent upon the balance of inputs upon it (Figure 1.3). These may arise from the 1° afferent neurone, inter-neurones or descending neurones from the brain stem and cortex.

The majority of second-order nociceptive neurones within the spinal cord cross to the contralateral side, where they synapse upon neurones in the antero-lateral aspect of the cord. Again modulation of transduction events will occur, prior to transmission in spino-thalamic pathways towards the cortical sensory centres.

While we have long considered neurological pathways to be hard wired, it is becoming increasingly clear that this is not the case. Indeed, the brain and spinal cord are able to learn and facilitate activity in commonly utilised pathways. This occurs not merely as regards useful details (e.g. how to drive a car), but also in relation to innocuous (e.g. what the blue colour looks like) and unpleasant (e.g. presence of ongoing pain in a now amputated limb) information. Thus, we should not be surprised that previous experiences can and do alter later pain perceptions. Plasticity of neuronal activity is the norm.

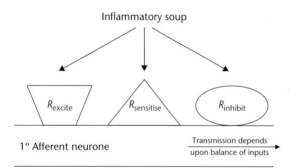

Figure 1.2 Tissue-damaging stimuli produce an 'inflammatory soup' which acts upon a variety of receptors. Onward transmission depends upon the balance of inputs affecting the 1° afferent neurone.

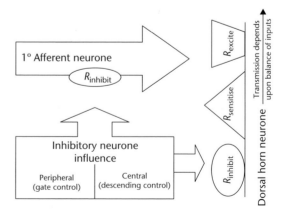

Figure 1.3 Onward transmission of information to higher centres, from the spinal cord, depends upon the balance of inputs effecting activity in the dorsal horn neurone.

The genetic basis of pain (using human and animal data to demonstrate the concepts) will be considered specifically in Chapter 4. However, when reading Chapters 2 and 3 on the peripheral and central mechanisms of pain, you should remember that the chemicals and structures described are genetically encoded, as are the receptors discussed in Chapter 8. Chapters 5–7 will deal in detail with the ways in which previous activity within the nociceptive pathways may alter current activity (and thus pain perception).

The psychological processing and consequences are central to all our human experience. Specific focus is placed on these in Chapters 13 and 47. The challenge now is to unite psychological and chemical (and thus genetic) events in an appropriate fashion when considering the problems faced by patients in pain.

PERIPHERAL MECHANISMS

2

W. Cafferty

Overview

Sensory systems are the nexus between the external world and the central nervous system (CNS). *Afferent* neurones of the somatosensory system continuously 'taste their environment' (Koltzenburg, 1999). They respond in a co-ordinated fashion, in order to instruct an integrated *efferent* response, which will retain the *homeostatic* integrity of the organism and curtail any tissue-damaging stimuli. This chapter will consider the peripheral apparatus that responds (and in some cases adapts) to a potentially injurious or noxious stimuli. Nociception forms an integral part of the somatosensory nervous system, whose main purpose can be described by *exteroceptive, proprioceptive* and *interoceptive functions.*

Exteroceptive functions include *mechanoreception, thermoception* and *nociception.* Proprioceptive functions provide information on the relative position of the body and limbs that arise from input from joints, muscles and tendons. Interoceptive information details the status and well-being of the viscera. These broad sensory modalities can be further subdivided in order to integrate more subtle stimuli (e.g. difference between flutter and vibration). In order to cope with the immense variety and magnitude of stimuli that impinge upon the CNS; sensory neurones are vastly heterogeneous and exquisitely specialized.

Heterogeneity of sensory neurones

Primary sensory neurones, whose cell bodies reside in the dorsal root ganglia (DRG), can be classified according to their cell body size, axon diameters, conduction velocity, neurochemistry, degree of myelination and ability to respond to neurotrophic factors (NTFs) (see Figure 2.1 and Table 2.1 for overview of classification). Early evidence for functional differences between populations of sensory neurones came from Erlander and Gasser who classified populations of afferents according to their conduction velocities.

Classification by size

A-fibres

A-fibres are myelinated, have large cell body diameters and can be subdivided into three further groups: Aα-, Aβ- and Aδ-fibres. Aα-fibres innervate *muscle spindles* and *Golgi tendon organs*, and determine proprioceptive function. Aβ-fibres are low-threshold, cutaneous, slowly or rapidly adapting mechanoreceptors and do not contribute to pain. Aδ-fibres are mechanical and thermal nociceptors. A-fibres generally terminate in laminae I and III–V of the dorsal horn (DH) of the spinal cord with some projection in lamina II inner (lamina IIi, see figure 2.2). They can be identified histologically by virtue of their expression of heavy neurofilament.

C-fibres

C-fibres, which constitute 65–70% of afferents entering the spinal cord, are characterized as being thinly myelinated or unmyelinated, with small diameter somata (10–25 μm), and are mainly nociceptive in function. These fibres terminate in laminae I and II, with lamina II outer (lamina IIo see figure 2.2) receiving C-fibre terminals exclusively. Afferent terminals are highly specific, both dorso-ventrally and medio-laterally. However, DH neurones can receive input from different laminae owing to their highly elaborate dendrites, spanning hundreds of microns in the dorso-ventral plane.

Neurochemical classification of sensory neurones

Sensory neurones can also be classified according to their neurochemistry, C-fibres in particular are classified as either peptidergic or non-peptidergic. Half of the c-fibre population expresses neuropeptides, such as calcitonin gene-related peptide (CGRP), substance P (SP), somatostatin (SOM), vasoactive intestinal peptide (VIP) and galanin. The remaining unmyelinated afferents can be identified by virtue of the fact that they express cell surface glycoconjugates that bind the lectin IB4. This population also expresses the purinoceptor P_2X_3 (purine channel – responds to

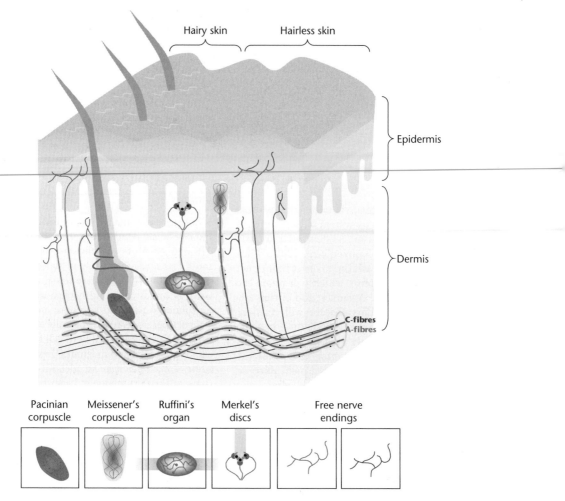

Figure 2.1 *Morphology of sensory receptors.* Receptors are found within the superficial epidermal and deeper dermal layers. Superficial receptor distribution varies between glabrous (hairless) and hairy skin. Glabrous skin presents Meissener's corpuscles, Merkel's discs and free nerve endings, while the dermal papillae of hairy skin include only Merkel's discs and free nerve endings. Subcutaneous receptors common to both glabrous and hairy skin include the Pacinian and Ruffini's corpuscles. *Meissener's corpuscles* are pressure mechanoreceptors, located on the epidermis–dermis boundary – especially on the fingertips, palm, sole of the foot and nipple. They are oval in shape and consist of many stacked, flattened Schwann cells. The nerve fibres enter the deep end of the corpuscle and are generally associated with Aβ-fibres. *Merkel's discs* are touch receptors, located in the dermis, especially of the thick skin over the palms of the hands and soles of the feet. The Merkel's discs consist of two components, the specialized Merkel's cell and a nerve ending that loses its myelination as it penetrates the epidermal basal layer. The free nerve ending forms a disc which contacts the Merkel's cell with a junction similar to a synapse. Merkel's discs are also associated with Aβ-fibres. *Pacinian corpuscles* are highly sensitive pressure receptors – approximately 2 mm × 0.5 mm located deep in the dermis, joint capsules and mesenteries. They cover nerve endings with flat fibroblast-like cells to produce sheets of 'lamellae', which contain fluid. As the Pacinian corpuscles are pressed, the fluid in the lamellae redistributes and the lamellae act as energy filters. Pacinian corpuscles are associated with Aβ nerve fibres. *Ruffini's endings* respond to tension and stretch in the skin. They are found deep in the dermis of the skin and have a thin capsule surrounding a fluid-filled cavity. This cavity contains a collagen mesh that penetrates the capsule to anchor it to the surrounding tissue. The nerve ending loses its myelination as it enters, leaving branches weaving around the collagen fibres and responding to movements of the surrounding tissue. The Ruffini's endings are associated with Aβ-fibres. *Free nerve endings* are widely distributed throughout the body, and are found as branches of unmyelinated, or lightly myelinated fibres, fasciculated beneath the epithelium. Branches of one nerve may cover a wide area and overlap the territories of others. The free nerve endings detect pain, touch, pressure and temperature, and are associated with c-fibres.

Table 2.1 Summary of receptor types

	Aβ-fibres	Aδ-fibres	C-fibres
Threshold	Low	Medium	High
Axon diameter	6–14 μm	1–6 μm	0.2–1 μm
Myelination	Yes	Thinly	No
Velocity	36–90 m/s	5–36 m/s	0.2–1 m/s
Receptor types	Mechano-receptor	Mechano/nociceptor	Nociceptor
Receptive field	Small	Small	Large
Quality	Touch	Sharp/first pain	Dull/second pain

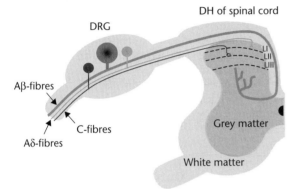

Figure 2.2 *Organization of the DH.* The central terminal projections of primary afferents are highly organized with different sub types of neurones terminating within cytoarchitectonically specific laminae. Table 2.1 above summarizes the function and properties of the three main groups. Aβ-fibres project to laminae III–IV, Aδ-fibres terminate in lamina I and c-fibres terminate in lamina in lamina II. Table 2.1 summarizes sensory neurone phenotype.

the algogen ATP) and enzyme activity of thiamine monophosphatase (TMP).

Classification by response to growth factors

Prior to propagating action potentials relating to tissue-damaging stimuli, sensory neurones have to make appropriate connections with their specific targets in the periphery, the DH of the spinal cord (Figure 2.2) and dorsal column nuclei of the brain stem. Primary sensory neurones (which are of neural crest origin) are induced shortly after the folding of the neural tube. Migration of boundary cap cells to the presumptive dorsal root entry zone (DREZ) triggers the penetration of growing sensory axons through the neuroepithelium. Large diameter axons penetrate before smaller cells.

Peripheral targets innervation depends on the availability of limited amounts of NTFs. The neurotrophic hypothesis (first proposed by Levi-Montalcini) details that survival of developing sensory neurones depends largely on factors released from their targets (Cowan, 2001). Many developing axons compete for limited quantities of targets-derived NTFs for successful development and survival. A limited number of growing fibres will receive and internalize this retrogradely supplied support. This selection process ensures appropriate targets innervation and the elimination of inaccurate projections. Thus, it is accepted that cell death is normal in the process of the development of the nervous system.

Sub-populations of sensory neurones have exquisite sensitivity to trophic factors, owing to a differential expression of high-affinity NTF receptors. The small diameter peptidergic c-fibre population expresses the high-affinity nerve growth factor (NGF) receptor tyrosine kinase A (TrkA). The non-peptidergic fibres express receptor components for another family of NTFs, namely the glial cell line-derived NTF (GDNF) receptor GFRα1–4 and their cognate signalling kinase domain c-ret. The large diameter A-fibres express the high-affinity receptor for neurotrophin-3 (NT3), TrkC. Sensory neurones retain their ability to respond to NTFs during adulthood, where they mediate:

* Homoeostatic functions under physiological conditions.
* Sensitization after injury or inflammation (see Chapter 6).

Properties of peripheral receptors

Mechanoreceptors

Mechanoreceptors, which respond to tactile non-painful stimuli, can be assessed psychophysically by the ability of a human subject to discriminate whether application of a two blunt-point stimuli is perceived as one or two points (by varying the distance between the points). These receptors are divided into two functional groups (rapidly or slowly adapting) depending on their response during stimuli. Rapidly adapting mechanoreceptors respond at the onset and offset of the stimuli, while slowly adapting mechanoreceptors respond throughout the stimuli duration. Mechanoreceptors (see Figure 2.1) can be divided into those expressed in:

* Hairy skin (hair follicle receptors):
  – Low threshold, rapidly adapting.
  – Three major subtypes: 'down', 'guard', tylotrich'.

- Glabrous (hairless) skin:
  - Small receptive fields.
  - Two major subtypes: 'Meissener's capsule' (rapidly adapting) and 'Merkel's disc' (slowly adapting).

Proprioception (limb position sense), which refers to the position and movement of the limbs (kinesthesia), is determined by mechanoreceptors located in skin, joint capsules and muscle spindles. The CNS integrates information received from these receptors, while keeping track of previous motor responses that initiated limb movement – a process known as *efferent copy* or *corollary discharge* (reviewed by Matthews, 1982).

Cutaneous nociceptors

Cutaneous receptors that respond to relatively high magnitude or potentially tissue-damaging stimuli are termed *nociceptors*. They can respond to all forms of energy that pose a risk to the organism (e.g. heat, cold, chemical and mechanical stimuli). Unlike other somatosensory receptors, nociceptors are free nerve endings and are, therefore, unprotected from chemicals secreted into, or applied onto, the skin. The evolutionary strategy employed to cope with such a complex barrage of inputs has determined that some nociceptors are dedicated to respond to one stimuli (i.e. thermoception or mechanoception) and others to a range of stimuli modalities (hence termed polymodal). Further complexity lies in the observation that excitation of nociceptors does not always result in the sensation of pain – having an affective component which can alter depending on mood.

A number of different techniques have been employed in order to study the properties of nociceptors. The most convincing are microneurographical recordings of receptive fields of single afferent fibres in conscious human subjects, allowing correlation of afferent discharge and perception of pain (Wall and McMahon, 1985). Early studies used only mechanical and thermal stimuli to probe the properties of nociceptors, hence the common nomenclature of CMH and AMH for C- and A-fibre mechano-heat-sensitive nociceptors. This is a perilous differentiation, as more recent evidence suggests that most nociceptors responding to heat and mechanical stimuli will also respond to chemical stimuli.

C-fibre mechano-heat-sensitive nociceptors

These fibres are considered polymodal, as they respond to mechanical, heat, cold and chemical stimuli. Their monotonic increase in activity evokes a burning pain sensation at the thermal threshold in humans (41–49°C). CMH responses are affected by stimuli history and are subject to fatigue and sensitization modulation (see later and chapter 5 on hyperalgesia).

A-fibre mechano-heat-sensitive nociceptors

Activation of these receptors is interpreted as sharp, prickling or aching pain. Owing to their relatively rapid conduction velocities (5–36 m/s), they are responsible for *first pain*. Two subclasses of AMHs exist: types I and II.

- Type I fibres respond to high magnitude heat, mechanical and chemical stimuli and are termed polymodal AMHs. They are found in both hairy and glabrous skin.
- Type II nociceptors are found exclusively in hairy skin. They are mechanically insensitive and respond to thermal stimulation in much the same way as CMHs (early peak and slowly adapting response) and are ideally suited to signal the first pain response.

Deep tissue nociceptors

Our vast understanding of cutaneous nociceptors has lead to increased interest in understanding the complex activity of nociceptors in deep tissues. Activity of nociceptors not only depends on the origin and nature of the stimuli, but also in what tissue the receptor is located. Knowledge of how activity from nociceptors causes pain arising from deep tissues, such as muscle, joints, bone and viscera remains incomplete. Unlike cutaneous pain, deep pain is diffuse and difficult to localize, with no discernable fast (first pain) and slow (second pain) components. In many cases deep tissue pain is associated with autonomic reflexes (e.g. sweating, hypertension and tachypnoea). Nociceptors in joint capsules lack myelin sheaths. They are a mixed group of fibres, some of which have a low threshold and are excited by innocuous stimuli, while others have a high threshold and are activated by noxious pressure exceeding the normal articular range. Units that do not respond to mechanical stimuli have been termed *silent nociceptors*.

Silent nociceptors are also present within the viscera. Silent visceral afferents fail to respond to innocuous or noxious stimuli, but become responsive under inflammatory conditions. Visceral afferents are mostly polymodal C- and Aδ-fibres. In contrast to the joint, these afferent fibres have no terminal morphological specializations and are consequently sensitized to chemical mediators of inflammation and injury.

Peripheral mechanisms of injury-induced or inflammatory pain

Nociceptor activation is dynamically modulated by the magnitude of stimuli. Therefore, it is not surprising that supra-threshold or tissue-damaging stimuli alter subsequent nociceptor responses. Overt tissue damage, or inflammation, causes the sensation of pain. The most common symptom of on-going or chronic pain states is tenderness of the affected area. This tenderness, or lowered threshold for stimulation-induced pain is termed *hyperalgesia*. Hyperalgesia associated with somatic or visceral tissue injury can be assessed experimentally by observing how the response characteristics of a given fibre alter after a manipulation causing hyperalgesia. Hyperalgesia, or lowered-threshold to thermal and mechanical stimuli, occurs at the site of trauma (*primary hyperalgesia*). Uninjured tissue around this area also becomes sensitized, but to mechanical stimuli only (secondary hyperalgesia or allodynia). Divergent mechanisms mediate these phenomena. Simple cutaneous assessments have revealed the location of the neural mechanism that mediates both primary and secondary hyperalgesia. The experimental protocol is demonstrated in Figure 2.3. These experiments have illustrated that primary hyperalgesia has a major peripheral component, while the mechanism that mediates secondary hyperalgesia resides within the CNS (see Chapter 5).

Peripheral *sensitization* mediates primary hyperalgesia to thermal stimuli. Campbell and Meyer illustrated that CMHs become sensitized to burn injuries in hairy skin, but fail to do so in glabrous skin, where AMHs become sensitized for heat hyperalgesia. However, primary hyperalgesia to mechanical stimuli does not result from sensitization of either CMHs or AMHs – thresholds to mechanical stimuli (using graded von Frey filaments) being unchanged by heat or mechanical injury. Mechanical primary hyperalgesia arises as a result of receptive field expansion. Both CMHs and AMHs modestly sprout into adjacent receptive fields resulting in a greater number of afferent units being activated after mechanical stimuli (with spatial summation causing increased pain).

Sensitization of nociceptors: inflammation

Tissue injury results in complex sequelae procured in part by the recruitment of inflammatory mediators. The inflammatory reaction rapidly proceeds in order to remove and repair damaged tissue after injury. Pain develops in order to protect the organism from further damage. The affected area typically becomes:

- Red (*rubor*).
- Hot (*calor*): as a result of increased blood flow.

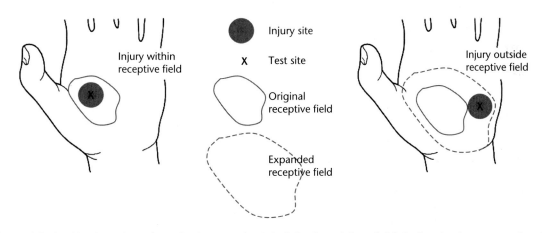

Figure 2.3 *Sensitization: primary hyperalgesia.* Hyperalgesia is defined as a leftward shift in the stimulus response function that relates magnitude of pain to stimulus intensity. This is illustrated in humans who report a lower pain threshold following burn injury. The experimental protocol commonly engaged to identify the mechanism of primary and secondary hyperalgesia is illustrated above. Firstly the response characteristics of a single fibre are established (usually response to mechanical stimulation to allow for mapping of the receptive field), subsequently the skin undergoes a manipulation (injury) that causes hyperalgesia; the test site is then re-assessed for alterations in response characteristics. Sensitization at the site of injury (i.e. of damaged tissue) is termed primary hyperalgesia, whereas sensitization outside the injury site is termed secondary hyperalgesia. If the above protocols are engaged (i.e. both test site and injury site coincide) then nociceptors are observed to have an increased response to the test stimulus, therefore primary hyperalgesia must have a significant peripheral component. However if the test stimulus and injury site do not coincide, then nociceptors fail to become sensitized; therefore the mechanism for secondary hyperalgesia must reside in the CNS.

- Swollen (*tumor*): due to vascular permeability.
- Functionally compromised (*function lasea*).
- Painful (*dolor*): as a result of activation and sensitization of primary afferent nerve fibres.

Sensitization occurs due to the release of chemical inflammatory mediators from damaged cells. A number of mediators directly activate nociceptors, while non-nociceptive afferents remain unaffected. Others act on local microvasculature causing the release of further chemical mediators from mast cells and basophils, which then attract additional leucocytes to the site of inflammation. Each of these mediators will be considered individually.

Chemical sensitivity of nociceptors

The action of injury-induced or inflammatory chemical mediators is attributed to the presence of their cognate receptors on primary afferent terminals. Figure 2.4 illustrates the location of these receptors and the possible origin of their respective ligands.

Factors that mediate the sensitivity of nociceptors, while predominantly originating from non-neuronal-damaged cells, can also emanate from the afferent terminal itself. This phenomenon is termed an *efferent nociceptor function* or *neurogenic inflammation* (for review see Black, 2002). Neurogenic inflammation is typified by two cutaneous reflexes:

- Vasodilatation (observed as a penumbral flare at the injury site).
- Plasma extravasation (observed as a wheal around the injury site).

Both of these processes are mediated by the release of neuropeptides (e.g. SP and CGRP) from primary afferent terminals (review see Richardson and Vasko, 2002).

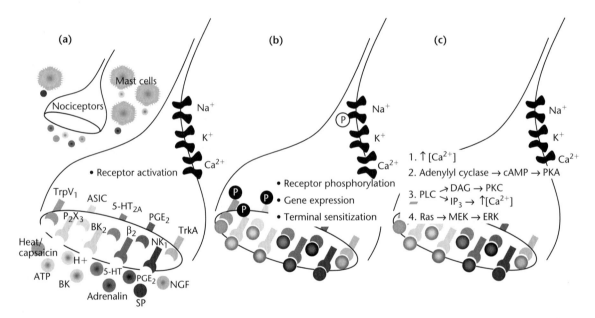

Figure 2.4 *Summary of nociceptor activation and sensitization.* Tissue damage or inflammatory insults intensify our pain experience by increasing the sensitivity of nociceptors to both thermal and mechanical stimuli. This figure summaries the mechanisms whereby the peripheral apparatus of the nociceptive pathway (the primary afferent), exacerbates this sensation. (a) Chemical mediators including ATP, BK, 5-HT, epinephrine, PGE_2, NGF and SP are released from axon terminals, damaged skin, inflammatory cells and the microvasculature surrounding the injury site. The injury site is typically very acidic owing to the increased concentration of protons in the immediate area. (b) Each of these chemical mediators bind to their high-affinity cognate receptor, present on nociceptive afferent terminals. The nociceptor-specific receptor for the irritant capsaicin, TRPV1 is also present on terminals and transduces noxious thermal stimuli. Receptor activation results in terminal sensitization or plasticity, either immediately via a post-translational mechanism (e.g. receptor phosphorylation TRPV1, P_2X_3 or ion channel phosphorylation PGE_2 or BK-mediated Na^+ phosphorylation) or over a prolonged time course which requires gene expression (NGF). (c) The pathways activated by these ligands include elevating intracellular $[Ca^{2+}]$ ([1] ASIC, P_2X_3, TRPV1), activating G-protein-coupled receptors ([2 and 3] PGE_2, BK, β_2) and subsequently elevating cAMP then PKA or elevating intracellular Ca^{2+} via PLC or the Ras-MEK–ERK/MAP-kinase pathway ([4] NGF). These pathways converge to alter the excitability of the nociceptor, ultimately lowering its threshold for activation and resulting in an increased pain sensation.

Vasodilatation is a reflex mediated by either poly-modal C- or Aδ-fibres. While flare is a more complex and incompletely understood reflex, it is considered to originate from *antidromic* activation of adjacent chemosensitive fibres after nociceptor firing. These chemosensitive fibres then release chemical mediators to act on surrounding nociceptors.

More recently, a number of nociceptor-specific receptors have been identified which have yielded great insight into modulation of nociceptors following trauma. These include:

- *Transient receptor potential vanilloid (TRPV1)* (Montell *et al.*, 2002) (formerly known as vanilloid receptor (VR1), which also mediates the action of the nociceptor-specific irritant capsaicin and the transduction of noxious heat stimuli.
- *Cold menthol receptor 1 (CMR1)*, activated by thermal stimuli in the cold range. Also a member of the TRP family of ion channels, demonstrating that TRP channels are the principal sensors of thermal stimuli in the mammalian peripheral nervous system.

Proton gated, or acid-sensing ion channels (ASICs), have been identified on nociceptors. These receptors respond to low pH (a characteristic of inflamed tissue) and have more recently been implicated in modulation of mechanosensation (Price *et al.*, 2001). Furthermore, the recent identification and cloning of two nociceptor-specific Na^+ channels, $Na_V 1.8$; formerly, SNS/PN3 (Goldin *et al.*, 2000) and $Na_V 1.9$; formerly, NaN/SNS2 (Goldin *et al.*, 2000) illustrate the immense potential for nociceptor modification. The emerging understanding of the neurobiology of nociceptor-specific ion channels is paving the way for more streamlined approaches to designing pharmacological therapies that targets nociceptor hyper-excitablility.

Direct activation of nociceptors

Building on the observation that nociceptor terminals express receptors to chemical mediators, there is convincing *in vivo* electrophysiological and psychophysical data from conscious human subjects that confirms the ability of inflammatory- or injury-induced factors to activate nociceptive afferents directly. Bradykinin (BK), a well-known *algogen* has been shown to be present at high concentration in areas of tissue damage or inflammation. The BK receptors B_1 and B_2 are known to be expressed by nociceptive afferents, and on receptor activation lead to sensitization (by increasing a Na^+ ion conductance via a protein kinase C (PKC)-dependent mechanism). Inflammation-induced mast cell degranulation causes the release of platelet

activating factor (PAF), which stimulates the release of serotonin (5-hydroxytryptamine, 5-HT) from circulating platelets. Serotonin has been shown to cause pain, extravasation of plasma proteins and hyperalgesia in rats and humans. Several 5-HT receptor subtypes have been identified on sensory neurones. However, the $5\text{-}HT_{2A}$ receptor has been shown to be localized specifically to nociceptors (Okamoto *et al.*, 2002) and is, therefore, thought to mediate the peripheral effect of serotonin during inflammation.

The excitatory amino acid glutamate is present at the site of peripheral inflammation. Sensory neurones express a full complement of glutamate receptors that are subject to modulation. Glutamate has also been shown to be released by afferent fibres, an effect exacerbated by inflammation. This highlights the possibility of autoregulation, that is a feedback mechanism where nociceptor excitability is enhanced by its own activity. Prostaglandins are cyclo-oxygenase (COX) produced metabolites of arachidonic acid (AA), released from activated membrane phospholipids during trauma or inflammation. They are considered to be archetypal sensitizing agents. Their administration fails to result in overt pain, but does decrease nociceptive thresholds and cause tenderness. Convincing evidence for a direct action on nociceptors comes from *in vitro* electrophysiological recordings of dissociated sensory neurones. Cells with nociceptor properties become hyperexcitable in the presence of prostaglandin E_2 (PGE_2) and PGI_2, and *in vivo* data illustrates direct afferent sensitization.

AA is also metabolized by lipoxygenases to leucotrienes after mechanical and thermal injury. Leucotriene B_4 (LTB_4) has been shown to indirectly cause hyperalgesia dependent on the presence of polymorphonuclear leucocytes (PMNs), but independent of the action of COX on AA. However, $8(R)$, $15(S)$-dihydroxyeicosatetraenoic acid (diHETE, 15-lipoxygenase product of arachidonic acid) has been shown to have a direct effect of afferent terminals to cause hyperalgesia (Levine *et al.*, 1986).

NGF expression rapidly increases after inflammatory lesions. It has been implicated in mediating long-term alterations in receptor properties during chronic inflammatory conditions. Local and systemic injection of NGF induces rapid onset of thermal and mechanical hyperalgesia. The high-affinity NGF receptor TrkA is expressed by around 50% of primary afferents, suggesting that a component of NGF-mediated sensitization may arise via direct activation. Indeed acute sequestration of endogenously released NGF after experimental inflammation negates the emergence of both thermal and mechanical sensitization, while chronic sequestration greatly reduced the number of nociceptors responding to thermal stimuli. Furthermore, transgenic mice over-expressing NGF in their epidermis display hyperalgesic behaviour in the absence of inflammation, confirming the potent role of NGF in mediating peripheral sensitization.

Indirect activation of nociceptors

Chemical mediators can also modulate nociceptor activity indirectly by sensitizing the response evoked by other stimuli. For instance, many non-neuronal cells (mast cells, keratinocytes and circulating eosinophils) express TrkA and therefore retain the ability to respond to injury-induced NGF. NGF has been shown to cause mast cell proliferation, degranulation and release of histamine and 5-HT. Inhibiting mast cell degranulation reduces experimental hyperalgesia and partially nullifies NGF-induced thermal and mechanical hyperalgesia. Similarly, the leucotriene LTB_4 indirectly causes hyperalgesia in both rodents and humans, by attracting neutrophils to the site of injury. The infiltrating neutrophils then release diHETE, which directly sensitizes the terminals.

Modulation of nociceptor response may also occur via the activity of the sympathetic nervous system during inflammatory states. Under normal conditions nociceptors do not respond to sympathetic stimulation. However, inflammation directly sensitizes nociceptors to catecholamines. Post-ganglionic sympathetic fibres are a source of BK-induced PG production – PGs being released from sympathetic terminals and inducing mechanical hyperalgesia. Direct intradermal injection of adrenergic agonists results in hyperalgesia. This process depends on α-adenoreceptor activation of post-ganglionic fibres producing and releasing PGs.

Sensitization of nociceptors: nerve injury

Stretch, compression or transection (axotomy) of a peripheral nerve initiates a complex reaction that alters the neurochemistry of the damaged axons. Pain associated with this type of trauma is termed neuropathic pain. Axotomy triggers an alteration of gene expression within the damaged fibres. This disruption of homoeostasis shifts the phenotype of the damaged pathways from one of the transduction and transmission of sensory information, to one that must accomplish survival and regeneration. One of the more nefarious consequences of nerve injury is the generation of spontaneous activity and hyper-excitability (sensitization) of the damaged axons. If these fibres are

nociceptors, then the result is spontaneous (and in many cases) intractable pain. Many of the reactive changes associated with nerve injury are consequent upon central sensitization (see Chapter 5). Nevertheless, several peripheral mechanisms are worth considering.

Nociceptors demonstrate a dynamic expression of receptors and ion channels. Characteristic of mechanical damage to nociceptors is the alteration in the expression and distribution of Na^+ channels. Voltage-gated Na^+ channels are important in regulating neuronal excitability, and initiating and propagating action potentials. On the basis of sensitivity to tetrodotoxin (TTX) and kinetic properties, Na^+ currents in DRG neurones can be classed as:

- Fast TTX-sensitive (TTX-S, Types I–III).
- Slow TTX-resistant (TTX-R, $Na_V1.8$ and $Na_V1.9$), with a high-activation threshold.
- Persistent TTX-R, with much lower-activation thresholds (Waxman, 1999).

Axotomy results in the downregulation of both $Na_V1.8$ and $Na_V1.9$ and an upregulation of type III TTX-S channel, $Na_V1.3$. $Na_V1.3$ reprimes post-activation much faster than either $Na_V1.8$ or $Na_V1.9$. Hence, owing to its post-injury abundance, the excitability of the damaged axon is increased by lowering its overall threshold for activation.

Anatomical reorganization is also common after peripheral nerve injury, with sprouting of large diameter A-fibres into lamina II of the spinal cord (an area that physiologically receives exclusively C-fibre nociceptor input). This purportedly aberrant localization of A-fibres may explain the touch evoked allodynia associated with nerve injury. Further maladaptive reorganization has been observed in the DRG. Post-ganglionic sympathetic fibres have been localized in baskets around sensory neurones, including nociceptors. The sensitivity of DRG neurones to catecholamines after axotomy may result from these spurious sprouts modulating sensory function.

Modulation targets

To take advantage of data regarding the modulation and altered function of nociceptors following nerve injury or inflammation, we need to understand the molecular actions that transduce these events. Unlike other sensory receptors, nociceptors are required to respond to a vast array of environmental stimuli, ranging from mechanical depression to chemical exposure. In order to comprehensively handle these challenges, nociceptors require a diverse repertoire of signalling devices (see Figure 2.4). An understanding of these devices will lead to new targets for analgesia and perhaps refine current treatments.

Among the frontline therapies for inflammatory pain are the eponymous non-steroidal anti-inflammatory drugs (NSAIDs) that inhibit the enzyme COX. COX catalyses the hydrolysis of AA to prostanoids, which contribute to peripheral sensitization by increasing cAMP levels within nociceptors. This appears to be consequent upon phosphorylation of a nociceptor-specific TTX-R Na^+ channel (possibly $Na_V 1.8$ or $Na_V 1.9$) via a cAMP- and PKA-dependent mechanism. This alteration results in a lower membrane depolarization being required to recruit an action potential, thus sensitizing an individual to pain. NSAIDs, by inhibiting this process, may provide analgesia. Similarly, other inflammatory components (e.g. BK, NGF) can modulate another nociceptor-specific cation channel, TRPV1, via PKC or phospholipase C (PLC) γ.

Unravelling the myriad of enigmatic signalling pathways activated during transient or on-going pain states will provide further targets for novel therapies. The identification of nociceptor-specific channels, such as TTX-R Na^+ channels ($Na_V 1.8$ or $Na_V 1.9$), P_2X_3, P_2X_4 and TRPV1 has already provided intriguing targets whose exploitation may ultimately result in valuable new treatments.

Key points

- Nociceptors respond to a vast array of environmental stimuli (e.g. pressure, heat, cold, chemicals).
- Nociceptors may be classified according to:
  - *Size*: Aδ- (small, myelinated) and c-fibres (small, unmyelinated).
  - *Neurochemistry*: peptidergic and non-peptidergic.
  - *Response to growth factors*: NGF and GDNF dependent.
- Nociceptors become sensitized by inflammatory components and following axotomy.
- Activation of nociceptors may be:
  - Direct (e.g. BK, 5-HT, H^+, NGF).
  - Indirect (e.g. sympathetic stimulation, BK, NGF).
- Therapeutic targets include:
  - Reduction in inflammation (e.g. NSAIDs).

- Ion channels (e.g. P_2X_3, P_2X_4, $Na_V 1.8$, $Na_V 1.9$, CMR1, TRPV1).
- Signalling pathways (e.g. PKC, PLC, PKA).

References

Black, P.H. (2002). Stress and the inflammatory response: a review of neurogenic inflammation. *Brain Behav. Immun.*, **16**: 622–653.

Cowan, W.M. (2001). Viktor Hamburger and Rita Levi-Montalcini: the path to the discovery of nerve growth factor. *Annu. Rev. Neurosci.*, **24**: 551–600.

Goldin, A.L., Barchi, R.L., Caldwell, J.H., Hofmann, F., Howe, J.R., Hunter, J.C., *et al.* (2000). Nomenclature of voltage-gated sodium channels. *Neuron*, **28**: 365–368.

Koltzenburg, M. (1999). The changing sensitivity in the life of the nociceptor. *Pain*, **Suppl. 6**: S93–S102.

Levine, J.D., Lam, D., Taiwo, Y.O., Donatoni, P., Goetzl, E.J. (1986). Hyperalgesic properties of 15-lipoxygenase products of arachidonic acid. *Proc. Natl. Acad. Sci.*, **83**: 5331–5334.

Matthews, P.B. (1982). Where does Sherrington's 'muscular sense' originate? Muscles, joints, corollary discharges? *Annu. Rev. Neurosci.*, **5**: 189–218.

Montell, C., Birnbaumer, L., Flockerzi, V., Bindels, R.J., Bruford, E.A., Caterina, M.J., *et al.* (2002). A unified nomenclature for the superfamily of TRP cation channels. *Mol. Cell*, **9**: 229–231.

Okamoto, K., Imbe, H., Morikawa, Y., Itoh, M., Sekimoto, M., Nemoto, K., *et al.* (2002). 5-HT2A receptor subtype in the peripheral branch of sensory fibers is involved in the potentiation of inflammatory pain in rats. *Pain*, **99**: 133–143.

Price, M.P., McIlwrath, S.L., Xie, J., Cheng, C., Qiao, J., Tarr, D.E., *et al.* (2001). The DRASIC cation channel contributes to the detection of cutaneous touch and acid stimuli in mice. *Neuron*, **32**: 1071–1083.

Richardson, J.D. & Vasko, M.R. (2002). Cellular mechanisms of neurogenic inflammation. *J. Pharmacol. Exp. Ther.*, **302**: 839–845.

Wall, P.D. & McMahon, S.B. (1985). Microneuronography and its relation to perceived sensation. A critical review. *Pain*, **21**: 209–229.

Waxman, S.G. (1999). The molecular pathophysiology of pain: abnormal expression of sodium channel genes and its contributions to hyperexcitability of primary sensory neurons. *Pain*, **Suppl. 6**: S133–S140.

CENTRAL MECHANISMS

3

D. Bennett

The essential message of this chapter is that pain is a perception subject to all the vagaries and trickery of our conscious mind. There is no simple relationship between a given noxious stimulus and the perception of pain. This was first highlighted by Melzack and Wall who reported that traumatic injuries sustained during athletic competitions or combat, were often initially described as being relatively painless. Psychological factors, such as arousal, attention and expectation can influence central nervous system (CNS) circuits involved in pain modulation.

Pain transmission depends on the balance of inhibitory and facilitatory influences acting on the neural circuits of the somatosensory system. Integration of these influences occurs at multiple levels of the CNS including the spinal cord, brain stem and multiple cortical regions. This chapter will elucidate some of these complex influences on central pain transmission. Derangements in these systems are often critical in the generation and maintenance of chronic pain. Some of the oldest (e.g. opioids) as well as the newest (e.g. gamma amino butyric acid (GABA) pentin) analgesics access these control mechanisms.

Modulation of pain processing at the level of the spinal cord

The dorsal horn (DH) of the spinal cord is an important area for integration of multiple inputs, including primary (1°) sensory neurones and local interneurone networks, as well as descending control from supraspinal centres.

Pain can be modulated depending upon the balance of activity between nociceptive and other afferent inputs

In the 1960s neurophysiological studies provided evidence that the ascending output from the DH of the spinal cord following somatosensory stimulation depended on the pattern of activity in different classes of 1° sensory neurones. Melzack and Wall proposed the 'gate control' theory of pain (Figure 3.1). It suggested

that activity in low-threshold, myelinated 1° afferents would decrease the response of DH projection neurones to nociceptive input (from unmyelinated afferents). Although there has been controversy over the exact neural substrates involved, the 'gate control' theory revolutionized thinking regarding pain mechanisms. Pain is not the inevitable consequence of activation of a specific pain pathway beginning at the C-fibre and ending at the cerebral cortex. Its perception is a result of the complex processing of patterns of activity within the somatosensory system. For example, this theory has led to some novel clinical therapies aimed at activating low-threshold myelinated afferents: transcutaneous electrical nerve stimulation (see chapter 36) and dorsal column stimulation.

Central sensitization

Repetitive stimulation of nociceptors leads to increased excitability of projection neurones within the DH,

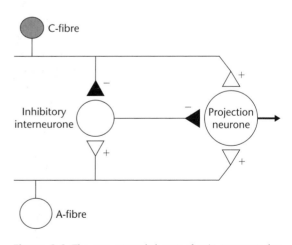

Figure 3.1 The gate control theory of pain proposes that activity in low-threshold myelinated afferents can reduce the response of DH projection neurones to C-fibre nociceptor input. An inhibitory interneurone is spontaneously active and normally inhibits the DH projection neurone reducing the intensity of pain. This interneurone is activated by myelinated (A-fibre) low-threshold afferents (responding to innocuous pressure) and inhibited by unmyelinated (C-fibre) afferents.

resulting in amplification in the processing of nociceptive information. This process is termed central sensitization (see Chapter 5). Experiments in both animals and humans have shown that central sensitization makes an important contribution to post-injury hypersensitivity in conditions, such as inflammation and nerve injury. A number of different neurotransmitters released by nociceptive afferents have been implicated in this process. The neuropeptide substance P (SP) (acting on the neurokinin-1 (NK-1) receptor) and glutamate (acting on the N-methyl-D-aspartate (NMDA) receptor) appear to be crucial. Local anaesthetic blockade of C-fibres pre-operatively, in an attempt to prevent the development of central sensitization, is the principle behind pre-emptive analgesia.

Inhibitory mechanisms within the DH of the spinal cord

Transmission in the somatosensory system can be suppressed within the DH as a result of segmental and descending inhibitory controls. This inhibition can occur (Figure 3.2):

- At the pre-synaptic level on the 1° afferent terminal.
- Post-synaptically on the DH neurone.

Inhibitory neurotransmitter systems within the DH include GABA, glycine, serotonin (5-hydroxytryptamine (5-HT)), adenosine, endogenous cannabinoids and the endogenous opioid peptides.

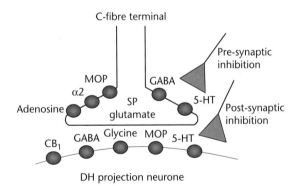

Figure 3.2 Nociceptive transmission within the DH of the spinal cord is modulated by many inhibitory compounds. GABA, glycine, noradrenaline, 5-HT , adenosine, cannabinoids and the opioid peptides act via their specific receptors on both pre- and post-synaptic inhibitory synapses. This results in reduced neurotransmitter release (SP and glutamate) by C-fibre nociceptive afferents and reduced post-synaptic depolarization. The DH response to a given 1° afferent input (and consequently pain sensibility) is therefore reduced.

The opioid system in particular plays a crucial role in regulating pain transmission. It comprises three receptor types (mu opioid receptor (MOP), delta opioid receptor (DOP) and kappa opioid receptor (KOP)) and their cognate ligands, which are encoded by the endogenous opioid genes: pro-opiomelanocortin, proenkephalin and prodynorphin. The superficial DH has a high density of these endogenous opioid peptides in the form of enkephalin and dynorphin containing interneurones. Opioid receptors are expressed both on the terminals of 1° afferent neurones and on the dendrites of post-synaptic neurones. Endogenous opioids inhibit the transmission of nociceptive information by reducing neurotransmitter release from the terminals of nociceptive afferents and causing hyperpolarization of DH neurones, hence reducing their excitability. The importance of this system was recently elegantly demonstrated by studying a gene termed DREAM, a transcription factor that represses the expression of dynorphin. Mice lacking this gene demonstrated:

- Increased expression of dynorphin within the DH of the spinal cord.
- Markedly reduced responses to acute noxious stimuli.
- Reduced pain behaviour in models of chronic neuropathic and inflammatory pain.

Inhibition at the segmental level of the spinal cord and diffuse noxious inhibitory control

The perception of pain in one part of the body can be reduced by application of a noxious stimulus to another body region. The idea that 'pain inhibits pain' has been used as the rationale behind therapeutic strategies employing counter irritation. A neurophysiological basis for this is provided by diffuse noxious inhibitory control (DNIC). The response of DH neurones to a noxious stimulus is reduced if another noxious stimulus is applied outside their receptive field. This operates as a widespread and non-somatotopic system. The inhibitory effect increases as the strength of the noxious counter-stimulus increases. The pathways involved in DNIC are not limited to the spinal cord, but also have a supra-spinal component.

Supra-spinal modulation of pain

There is a well-described descending pathway acting primarily on the DH of the spinal cord, which can inhibit the central transmission of noxious information. Initial evidence for such a pain-modulating pathway was provided by the phenomenon of stimulation produced analgesia. Electrical stimulation of the grey matter that surrounds the third ventricle cerebral aqueduct (peri-aqueductal grey (PAG)) and fourth ventricle can induce profound analgesia. This has been demonstrated in human patients; electrodes placed for therapeutic purposes in this region reduce the severity of pain, whereas tactile and thermal sensibility is unchanged. A simplified diagram of the descending pain modulating network is shown in Figure 3.3. The PAG integrates information from multiple higher centres, including the amygdala, hypothalamus and frontal lobe. It also receives ascending nociceptive input from the DH. The PAG controls the processing of nociceptive information in the DH via a projection to the rostro ventromedial medulla (RVM) and dorsolateral pontine tegmentum (DLPT).

The endogenous opioid peptides and their receptors are heavily expressed within this pathway. The actions of opioids are not restricted to the DH of the spinal cord. Opioid agonists can also stimulate the

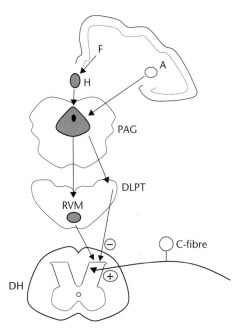

Figure 3.3 Diagram illustrating a major descending pain-modulating pathway. Regions of the frontal lobe (F), hypothalamus (H) and amygdala (A) project to the PAG in the midbrain. The PAG controls the transmission of nociceptive information in the rostroventral medulla (RVM), DH via relays in the RVM and dorsolateral pontine tegmentum (DLPT). +: nociceptive activation; −: inhibitory (anti-nociceptive) activity.

PAG and RVM resulting in activation of descending pain-modulating pathways. Other neurotransmitter systems are also involved. 5-HT and norepinephrine are transmitters found in the projection neurones from the brain stem (RVM and pons) to DH. Direct application of 5-HT or norepinephrine to the spinal cord results in analgesia, while destruction of these neurones blocks the action of systemically administered morphine. Recent studies have focussed on the role of endogenous cannabinoids, for example anandamide. These acylglycerides can inhibit the transmission of noxious information at the level of the DH via their action on cannabinoid receptor type 1 (CB_1), expressed on DH neurones. They also have anti-nociceptive actions at the level of the PAG and RVM. Some of their actions are mediated via the opioid system (e.g. via the release of dynorphin), while others are opioid independent.

With the application of an environmental stressor the normal behavioural response to pain may in fact be maladaptive. Stress results in a reduced sensitivity to pain, the duration of which depends on the timing and nature of the stimulus used. Stress induced analgesia is partially mediated by the pain inhibitory system described above. Rudimentary evidence for this comes from the fact that opioid antagonists, such as naloxone, can block stress induced analgesia. It is simplistic to think that a complex phenomenon, such as stress will only act mechanistically at the level of the spinal cord. It is also likely to have important implications for pain processing at much higher levels.

In the absence of a nociceptive stimulus, higher centre activity (induced by learning and also funnelled through the PAG) may facilitate pain, as evidenced by:

- Activity in DH nociceptive neurones.
- Activity in higher centres, demonstrated by positron emission tomography (PET) scanning.
- Subjective reports of experimentally induced pain.

Higher cognitive processing and 'the pain matrix'

The development of the techniques of functional imaging as applied to the human brain has provided fantastic insights into higher cognitive functions, including the perception of pain. One of the most striking findings from such studies is the multitude of brain regions activated following the application of a painful stimulus. These regions – 'the pain matrix' – include the thalamus, the 1° and secondary (2°) somatosensory cortex, the insular cortex, the anterior cingulate cortex and motor regions, such as the pre-motor cortex and cerebellum. Pain is not a unitary phenomenon. Affective components, such as perceived unpleasantness are distinct from the simple sensory dimension of pain (which includes location and intensity of a noxious stimulus). Using psychophysical experiments it has been demonstrated that different neural substrates appear to encode these different facets of the experience of pain. Activity in the 1° and 2° somatosensory cortex encodes the sensory component of pain, while activities in the insular and anterior cingulate cortex process its affective component. The fact that regions thought to be involved in the generation of skilled planned movement (such as pre-motor cortex and cerebellum) are activated by a painful stimulus was initially greeted with some surprise. This makes more sense however, when one considers that sensory processing does not occur in isolation, but actually in the context of an appropriate motor response.

Thunberg's thermal grill illusion provides some insight into the complexity of the central processing of pain. Temperatures of 20°C and 40°C are perceived as innocuous cool and warm, respectively. However, if they are applied simultaneously in the form of a grid, a painful burning sensation is experienced. This is thought to be secondary to an unmasking phenomenon, revealing the central inhibition of pain by thermosensory integration. Interestingly the thermal grill illusion produces activation of the anterior cingulate cortex whereas its component warm and cool stimuli do not. It has been proposed that disruption of thermosensory and pain integration can lead to the central pain syndrome, which may follow a thalamic stroke.

Gender and pain perception

Epidemiological studies suggest that the burden of pain may be greater and more varied in women. The basis of such a difference may involve genetic, hormonal and psychological differences. There are some tentative reports that there may be differences in the central processing of pain between the sexes in terms of the pattern of activity produced by a noxious stimulus. This finding however needs further confirmation. Importantly there may well be gender differences in the response to analgesic drugs, involving both pharmacodynamic and pharmacokinetic factors.

The influences of attention and emotion on pain

Many of the pain modulating mechanisms so far discussed can be accessed not only by pharmacological means, but also by contextual and/or cognitive manipulation. Pain perception can be altered by variables, such as:

- Attentional state.
- Emotional context.
- Attitude.
- Experience.

The best-studied psychological variable modifying the pain experience is attentional state. Pain is perceived as less intense when people are distracted from a noxious stimulus. A cognitively demanding task (e.g. mental arithmetic) can be used as such a distraction. Interestingly, a more cognitively demanding task produces a greater reduction in perceived pain intensity. Most levels of the CNS are thought to be involved in the attentional modulation of pain. Activation in the PAG is significantly increased during a condition in which subjects are distracted from pain. The level of PAG activity is predictive of the reduction in pain intensity produced by distraction. Attention has also been shown to modulate nociceptive responses in both sensory and limbic cortical areas.

Clinical studies demonstrate that emotional states affect the pain associated with chronic disease. Mood appears to selectively alter the affective response to pain. The anterior cingulate cortex is thought to be an important site for the modulation of pain by mood. The cognitive manipulation of pain should be remembered as a therapeutic avenue in chronic pain states.

Key points

- There is evidence for 'top-down' control, with the brain controlling its own input from lower centres.
- The endogenous opioid peptides form part of an intrinsic descending pathway inhibiting the transmission of nociceptive information.
- There are multiple cortical regions involved in the central processing of pain. The anterior cingulate and insular cortices encode its affective component. The 1° and 2° somatosensory cortices are responsible for sensory discrimination.
- Both attentional state and emotional context can have an important influence on pain perception.
- The complex central processing of sensory information means that there is no simple relationship between a given noxious stimulus and the perception of pain.

Further reading

Casey, K.L. (2000). Concepts of pain mechanisms: the contribution of functional imaging of the human brain. *Prog. Brain. Res.*, **129**: 277–287.

Cheng, H.M., Pitcher, G.M., Laviolette, S.R., *et al.* (2002). DREAM is a critical transcriptional repressor for pain modulation. *Cell*, **108**: 31–43.

Fields, H.L. & Basbaum, A.I. (1999). Central nervous system mechanisms of pain modulation. In: Wall, P.D. & Melzack, R. (eds) *Textbook of Pain*, 4th edition. Churchill Livingstone Edinburgh.

Villemure, C. & Bushnell, M.C. (2002). Cognitive modulation of pain: how do attention and emotion influence pain processing? *Pain*, **95**: 195–199.

Figures provided by Dr Sian Jaggar to illustrate relevant neuro anatomy.

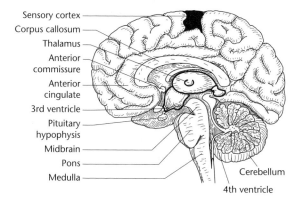

Figure 3.4 Sagital section view of the brain and brainstem.

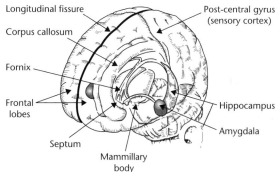

Figure 3.5 3D view of the mid-brain demonstrating the important features of the limbic system involved in the perception of pain.

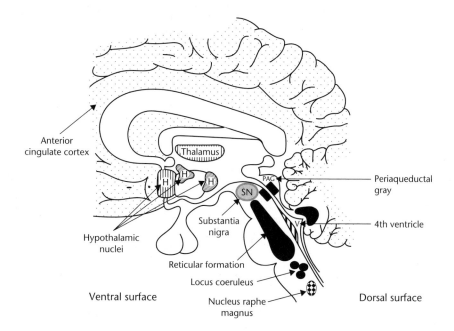

Figure 3.6 Cartoon representing the mid-brain and brainstem, localising major nuclei involved in pain pathways.

J. Riley, M. Maze & K. Welsh

Pharmacogenomics

A thorough understanding of the correlation between an individual patient's genetic make-up (genotype) and their response to drug treatment should allow for the development of:

- Patient-specific treatments.
- Population-specific treatments.
- Avoidance of adverse effects of drugs.
- Reduced inefficiency of drugs.
- Targeted drug design.

The human genome has now been documented. It is made up of 23 pairs of chromosomes. Each chromosome contains several thousand genes. Each *gene* is made up of *exons* that are interrupted by *introns*. Exons are made up of *codons* that code for a specific amino acid.

Definitions 1

Gene: An ordered sequence of nucleotides located in a particular position (locus) on a particular chromosome, which encodes a specific functional product (the gene product, i.e. a protein or RNA molecule).
Exon: A protein-coding DNA sequence of a gene.
Intron: A DNA base sequence that can be transcribed into RNA but are cut out of the message before it is translated into protein. However, introns may contain sequences involved in regulating gene expression.
Codon: Crick (1963) proposed this term now recognised to be a triplet of nitrogenous bases in DNA or RNA that specifies a single amino acid.

The word *polymorphism* comes from the Greek *poly* (several) and *morphe* (form). Thus, a polymorphism is something that can take several forms. A DNA polymorphism exists when individuals differ in their DNA sequence at a certain point in the genome. A normal form and a mutated one may represent such a difference. The mutated form can be a mutation in a single base (the commonly occurring *single nucleotide polymorphism*, i.e. SNP or 'snip'), or in a short stretch of DNA. In most regions of the genome a polymorphism is of no clinical significance since only 3% of DNA consists of coding sequences. However, when a mutation occurs inside a coding sequence it is more likely to cause disease or account for variability in the metabolism or response to drugs.

SNPs can account for diversity in *genotypes*, and can be mapped to account for diversity in *phenotypes*. Particular patterns of sequential SNPs (or alleles) found on a single chromosome are known as the haplotype. The haplotype can be inherited over time. Haplotyping (for SNPs) can be accomplished by the use of microarrays, mass spectrometry and sequencing.

Definitions 2

Genotype: An exact description of an individual's genetic constitution, with respect to a single trait or a larger set of traits (both dominant and recessive).
Phenotype: The observable properties of an individual as they have developed under the combined influences of the individual's genotype and the effects of environmental factors.

Variations in drug responses are well recognised. For example, the analgesic ladder, proposed by the World Health Organisation (WHO), recommends morphine as the primary analgesic in the treatment of moderate to severe cancer pain and codeine in the treatment of mild to moderate pain. However, inter-patient variability in the clinical response to morphine has been well documented. Clinical data shows that 10–30% of patient's do not respond to morphine, achieving poor analgesic response or intolerable side effects. Moreover, codeine is ineffective in 6–7% of Caucasians. While oral morphine remains the opioid of choice for moderate to severe cancer pain, a number of alternative opioids are now available. The decision to use an alternative strong opioid is currently based primarily on clinical observations rather than scientific rationale because the underlying neurophysiological mechanisms are unclear. The pharmacogenomics hypothesis is that a patient's response to a drug may depend on or more factors that can vary according to the alleles that an individual carries.

Pharmacogenomics of analgesic drugs

One of the aims of pharmacogenomics is to identify the genetic basis for the variability of drug efficacy and side effects within a population. The hope is, that in the future, prescribing can be tailored to individual genotype, thus maximising therapeutic effectiveness.

When investigating how genes affect the response to analgesic drugs one must consider various possibilities, including differences in genes for:

- Drug transporting proteins.
- Subunits of a receptor with effects on pain modulation (e.g. inhibitory processes).
- Drug metabolism (e.g. altered enzymatic metabolism of drug precursors or active metabolites).

Drug transporting proteins

Specific transporter proteins actively transport some drugs. Polymorphisms in genes encoding these proteins have been described, but the clinical implications of these findings are still uncertain.

Receptor targets

Opioid receptors are widely expressed:

- In the periphery (both neuronally associated, but also on various circulating immune cells).
- At a spinal level in the dorsal horn.
- In multiple regions within the brain.

MOP, KOP and DOP receptors

Over the last 20 years three opioid receptors, now termed μ opioid (MOP), κ opioid (KOP) and δ opioid (DOP), have been identified and the genes encoding them cloned. Agonist induced activation of the MOP receptor results in inhibition of neuronal transmission of painful stimuli.

Polymorphisms in many genes encoding opioid receptors are relevant to:

- Responses to endogenous opioids (and therefore possibly in pain perception).
- Treatment causing widespread variation in sensitivity to many drugs e.g. heroin (diamorphine) acts on the DOP receptor and altered drug effect may be linked to polymorphism.
- Unwanted effects (e.g. altered receptor expression which may be associated with addiction).

We now know that morphine and other commonly used opioid analgesics act at the same target, the MOP receptor. Morphine is not analgesic in the absence of MOP receptor. Variation in MOP receptor gene expression determines the analgesic potency of morphine, since through this mechanism individuals can vary in:

- Levels of MOP receptor gene expression.
- Response to painful stimuli.
- Response to opioid drugs.

One of the best candidates for contributing to these differences is variation at the MOP gene locus. This makes the MOP receptor gene a candidate gene for susceptibility or resistance to pain through endogenous or exogenous opioids. Partial KOP and DOP agonists (e.g. buprenorphine and pentazocine) can also function poorly if MOP is not present.

Humans also differ from one another in density of MOP expression. Binding studies in postmortem brain samples and *in vivo* positron–emission tomography radioligand analyses both suggest large ranges of individual human differences in MOP density. The MOP receptor is a G-protein-coupled receptor (Figure 4.1). The extracellular N-terminus of the MOP receptor has five putative *N*-glycosylation sites. The extracellular portion is important in determining the binding of different ligands, where different opioids have decreased binding affinities on mutated receptors lacking the N-terminal domain (e.g. the affinity of morphine, β-endorphin and enkephalin in binding to mutated versus wild-type MOP receptor decreases 3–8-fold, compared with methadone and fentanyl which decreases 20–60-fold).

A SNP in the human MOP receptor gene at position 118 (a putative *N*-glycosylation site) results in a receptor variant which binds β-endorphin approximately three times more tightly than at the most common allelic form of the receptor in laboratory DNA tests from human volunteers. This makes the endogenous opioid β-endorphin nearly three times more potent in people with the mutation than those without. However, this nucleotide substitution does not increase the binding and the receptor activation of morphine, methadone or fentanyl.

Drug metabolism

Different opioids are metabolised via different enzyme pathways, examples of which include:

- Cytochrome P450 2D6: codeine, oxycodone, dihydrocodeine and hydrocodone.
- Cytochrome P450 3A4: fentanyl and methadone.
- Uridine diphosphate glucuronosyltransferase (UGT) system: oral morphine, hydromorphone and buprenorphine.

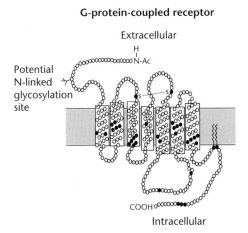

G-protein-coupled receptor

Extracellular

Potential
N-linked
glycosylation
site

COOH

Intracellular

MOP receptor
Chromosome 6 – 80 and 120 bp

Exon 1
N-terminal extracellular domain,
first TMR

Exon 2
First cytoplasmic loop to fourth TMR

Exon 3
Second extracellular loop to
carboxyterminal intracellular domain

Exon 4
Carboxyterminus

Figure 4.1 The MOP receptor demonstrating the four exon regions of this transmembrane receptor (TMR).

Cytochrome P450

Enzyme families belonging to the cytochrome P450 (CYP) system account for phase I metabolism. Nearly 70% of drugs in use today are metabolised by these enzymes.

The considerable sequence variations in the CYP genes result in a variety of functionally different phenotypes. Thus individuals may be classified as 'poor metabolisers' (PM), 'normal metabolisers', 'fast metabolisers' or 'ultrafast/extensive metabolisers' (EM). CYP2D6, CYP3A4/5/6 and CYP2C9 gene polymorphisms and gene duplication account for the most frequent variations in phase I metabolism of drugs.

CYP2D6
Codeine

More than 20 years ago, it was noted that following codeine intake, the morphine levels (responsible for analgesia) were remarkably low in some individuals. It was suggested that this could be due to a genetic polymorphism determining the *O*-demethylation of codeine. In two small parallel, randomised, double blind, crossover trials, it was found that 75 mg codeine orally increased pain thresholds (to cutaneous high energy laser light stimulation) significantly in EM but not in PM. PM are present in 6–7% of a Caucasian population due to homozygosity for non-functional CYP2D6 mutant alleles. These CYP2D6 deficient people are unable to convert codeine to morphine (Figure 4.2). Ultrafast metabolisers have been identified in several Swedish families, caused by gene amplification of CYP2D6. These individuals

are known to be particularly sensitive to codeine analgesia.

Oxycodone

Oxycodone is an opioid analgesic that closely resembles morphine. Oxymorphone, the active metabolite of oxycodone, is formed in a reaction catalyzed by CYP2D6, which is under polymorphic genetic control. The role of oxymorphone in the analgesic effect of oxycodone is not yet clear.

Alfentanil

Alfentanil is an analogue of the synthetic opioid fentanyl and is characterised by a short duration of action. A genetic defect in the inhibition of debrisoquine hydroxylation of alfentanil in human liver microsomes has been suggested to be an important determinant of the elimination of alfentanil (but the hypothesis remains under dispute).

CYP3A4
Methadone

This synthetic drug is one of the most widely used drugs for opiate dependency treatment and is a useful analgesic. It is extensively metabolised by CYP3A4 in human liver microsomes. Inter-individual variation in liver content of this enzyme is responsible for the 20-fold variability of methadone metabolism. In a study of opiate-dependent patients receiving methadone maintenance treatment, the CYP2D6 genetic status of a patient has been shown to influence methadone steady-state blood concentrations. Thus individualisation of methadone doses is clinically relevant.

Morphine metabolism

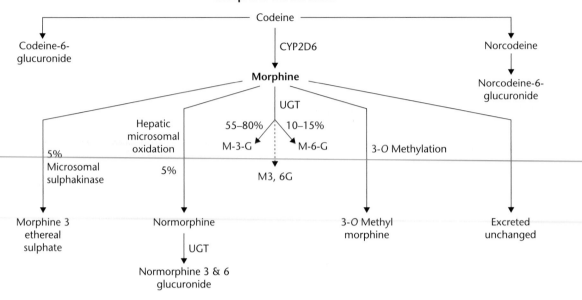

Figure 4.2 Pathways of morphine metabolism.

CYP2C9
Non-steroidal anti-inflammatory drugs
Polymorphism in the CYP2C9 gene can affect cyclo-oxygenase (COX) 1 and 2 inhibitors:

- CYP2C9 is the major enzyme for celecoxib hydroxylation *in vitro* and the CYP2C9*3 allelic variant may be associated with markedly slower metabolism.
- The pharmacokinetic variations observed for both racemic and S-ibuprofen depend on a CYP2C9 polymorphism.

UGT system

UGTs are responsible for glucuronidation of morphine, buprenorphine and some non-steroidal anti-inflammatory drugs (NSAIDs). More than 18 UGT enzymes have been described in humans. Oral morphine is primarily metabolised in the liver, through the UGT system to morphine-6-glucuronide (M6G) and morphine-3-glucuronide (M3G) (Figure 4.2). Genetic polymorphisms have been identified for the UGT family of enzymes. However, polymorphisms in the gene coding for the UGT2B7 enzyme (which catalyses the formation of M6G and M3G from the parent drug morphine) have not been shown to alter the glucuronidation ratio of M3G–M6G with mean values 5.3–6.4. In addition, a number of studies have demonstrated wide variability in morphine and metabolite plasma concentrations, despite equivalent

analgesia. An investigation of morphine responsiveness in chronic non-malignant pain did not find a significant difference in metabolite ratios between morphine responders and non-responders. Pharmacokinetic factors alone are therefore unlikely to explain the clinical observation of varied sensitivity to morphine.

Analgesics tailor made to individuals

Prescription of analgesic drugs today is based on the use of the drug in varying doses to obtain certain effects. As our knowledge of pharmacogenomics increases, drugs will be prescribed to subgroups of the population with similar matched genotypes. This advance may be possible by pre-treatment genetic testing of patients in order to choose the most suitable analgesic for the individual patient. Thus more precise tailoring of drugs to the individual patient may reduce the side-effect profiles and increase the desired analgesic effect.

Gene therapy

Gene therapies for pain conditions through peripheral opioid mechanisms are being investigated in chronic arthritic rats. When a herpes simplex virus (HSV) is used to enhance the synthesis of enkephalin in the dorsal root ganglion, not only is pain behaviour reduced, but also healing of the arthritis occurs. The use of HSV type-1 vectors to enhance endogenous neuropeptides may be a future therapeutic tool.

Key points

- Understanding the correlation between an individual patient's genetic make-up (genotype) and their response to drug treatment may in the future allow for specific targeting of treatments.
- Responses to endogenous opioids are dependent on genetic factors. This is likely to influence susceptibility to pain.
- Individual responses to analgesic drugs vary. This may be related to variation in expression of:
  – Receptors.
  – Enzymes that activate drugs.
  – Enzymes responsible for terminating drug activity.

Further reading

Eap, C.B., Broly, F., Mino, A., *et al.* (2001). Cytochrome P450 2D6 genotype and methadone steady state concentrations. *J. Clin. Psychopharmacol.*, **21**: 229–234.

de Wilt, S.N., Kearns, G.L., Leeder, J.S. & van den Anker, J.N. (1999). Glucuronidation in humans. Pharmacogenetic and developmental aspects. *Clin. Pharmacokinet.*, **36**: 439–452.

Fragerlunnd, T.H. & Braaten, O. (2001). No pain relief from codeine? An introduction to pharmacogenomics. *Acta Anaesthesiol. Scand.*, **45**: 140–149.

Lavrijsen, K.L.M., van Houdt, J.M.G., van Dyck, D.M.J., *et al.* (1998). Is the metabolism of alfentanil subject to debrisoquine polymorphism? *Anesthesiology*, **69**: 535–540.

Roses, A.D. (2000). Pharmacogenetics and the practice of medicine. *Nature*, **405**: 857–865.

Ulh, G.R., Soar, I. & Wang, Z. (1999). The mu opiate receptor as a candidate gene for pain: polymorphisms, variations in expression, nociception, and opiate responses. *Proc. Natl. Acad. Sci.*, **96**: 7752–7755.

PERIPHERAL AND CENTRAL SENSITIZATION 5

K. Carpenter & A. Dickenson

In the presence of an ongoing stimulus, most of the special senses adapt to reduce our perception of the stimulus. For example, olfactory receptors adapt to persistent odours, Pacinian corpuscles adapt completely to constant pressure, and visual receptors (rods and cones) adapt in bright light conditions. In contrast, no real adaptation is shown by nociceptors and, in fact, the opposite happens. In the presence of a repeated noxious stimulus, such as occurs during tissue injury, the perceived intensity of the painful stimulus is much enhanced – a phenomenon referred to as *hyperalgesia* – and this spreads to surrounding undamaged areas. In addition, normally non-noxious stimuli can be perceived as painful – *allodynia*. These phenomena are of obvious evolutionary importance, forcing rest of the damaged area until it is healed. But today we want to control such pain, for example to improve post-operative recovery, and to do so we must understand the underlying processes. Importantly, these basic mechanisms also underlie hard-to-treat pain conditions that outlive tissue damage or that occur without apparent cause, for example cancer pain and neuropathic pain.

Two processes contribute to hyperalgesia and allodynia: *peripheral sensitization* of nociceptors, where events around the damaged site combine to allow a lower intensity stimulus to evoke an action potential in the fibre, and *central sensitization*, where changes occur in the spinal processing of primary (1°) afferent inputs, continuing hyperalgesia and enlarging the area of hyperalgesia and allodynia.

Peripheral sensitization

Many inflammatory mediators are released by tissue injury. These can directly activate and sensitize nociceptor terminals to subsequent thermal, mechanical and chemical stimuli. They may also stimulate antidromic release of transmitters from collateral branches of sensory nerves (neurogenic inflammation). Peripheral inflammation is discussed in more detail in Chapters 2 and 6 so, to avoid repetition,

the release, effects and interactions of inflammatory mediators are summarized in Table 5.1. This chapter discusses the events and interactions that go on in the nociceptor terminal to produce the sum effects of peripheral inflammation, rather than focusing on single transmitters. In particular, some intracellular second messengers (e.g. cyclic adenosine monophosphate (cAMP) and protein kinase Cε (PKCε) and molecular sensors (e.g. the capsaicin vanilloid receptor 1 (VR1) (also known as TRPV1) and the sensory-nerve-specific sodium channel (SNS) (also PN3)) are emerging as important molecules in integrating signals and generating peripheral sensitization.

Peripheral consequences of nociceptor activation

Normally, for a stimulus to be perceived as painful it must be strong enough to generate action potentials in nociceptors. As well as the action potential being propagated to the central terminals of the sensory fibre, electrical activity will also spread back down to the peripheral terminals of collateral branches, where the membrane depolarization will open voltage-dependent Ca^{2+} channels. Ca^{2+} influx can then trigger release of transmitters in the area surrounding the original injury, spreading the inflammatory processes and activating surrounding nociceptors. In addition, the second messengers generated by the many mediators involved can interact to enhance the sensitivity of each nociceptor terminal in the inflamed area.

Important second messengers

Cellular cAMP, PKA and PKC are probable secondary mediators of nociceptor sensitization. Such intracellular signalling cascades seem to converge on 'effector' channels like VR1 and SNS. Cellular cAMP and PKA activity have been shown to be essential for maintaining peripheral hyperalgesia. Of the five PKC isoforms present in sensory nerves, it appears that PKCε mediates nociceptor sensitization. Guanylyl cyclase activation and cGMP formation appears to play an opposite role to cAMP, reducing nociceptor sensitivity.

Table 5.1 Mediators of peripheral sensitization and how they act

Mediator	Receptor(s)/ion channel(s)	Effectors/ions	Effects and interactions
BK	B_2	PLC, PKC (especially PKCε)	Nociceptor activation PLA_2 activation (and PGE_2 release) Sensitizes nociceptors to: heat, IL-2, prostanoids, 5-HT and histamine Effects require intact sympathetic post-ganglionic neurones and nerve growth factor NGF
5-HT	$5-HT_{1-4}$		Nociceptor activation
Histamine	H_1	PLC, PKC/DAG	Nociceptor activation
PGE_2	EP_{1-4}	cAMP, PKA, IP_3/DAG	Release of IL-2, histamine and 5-HT Potentiates conductance through SNS Enhances currents through VR1 May mediate many effects of BK
Protons	ASIC1–3, VR1	Na^+/K^+	Nociceptor activation Sensitizes VR1, reducing temperature threshold to body temperature
Adenosine	A_2	cAMP	Nociceptor activation and hyperalgesia (Note: A_1 receptor is inhibitory and may be antinociceptive)
ATP	P_2X_3	Na^+/K^+	Nociceptor activation May convey subnoxious information (warm currents and bladder stretch)
Glutamate	AMPA, kainate, NMDA	Na^+/Ca^{2+}	Thermal hyperalgesia, mechanical allodynia

PGE_2: Prostaglandin E2; IP_3: Inositol triphosphate; DAG: diacyl glycerol; COX: cyclo-oxygenase; LOX: Lipoxygenase.

The capsaicin vanilloid receptor VR1

The VR1 ion channel can be activated by heat, capsaicin and hydrogen ions (e.g. pH $<$ 5.5) allowing the influx of cations (Na^+) and action potential generation. Thus, capsaicin, heat and low pH all produce pain in human volunteers.

Smaller reductions in pH, such as those that occur during inflammation (e.g. to pH 6.4) enhance VR1 responses to capsaicin and to heat. Under these moderately acidic conditions, the temperature threshold for VR1 activation is reduced so much that the channel may be activated at the raised cellular temperatures that occur at sites of inflammation.

As well as integrating extracellular stimuli, VR1 also integrates intracellular signals. Heat-activated currents through VR1 are enhanced by PKC, rises in intracellular calcium ($[Ca^{2+}]_i$) are required for both capsaicin- and proton-induced heat sensitization in rat nociceptors, and PKA activation (by Ca^{2+}- and PGE_2-stimulated cAMP formation) can increase capsaicin-evoked currents (Figure 5.1(a)). Elevated $[Ca^{2+}]_i$ can lead to substance P (SP) and calcitonin gene related peptide (CGRP) release, but can also feed back to desensitize VR1. A direct interaction has also been suggested between intracellular adenosine triphosphate (ATP) and the VR1.

The importance of VR1 in peripheral sensitization was demonstrated in VR1-null mice (which do not express the VR1 receptor). Recordings from C-fibres show that they lack the normal well-characterized capsaicin-, acid- and noxious-heat-gated currents. Thus, they lack normal behavioural responses to capsaicin injection and have limited development of thermal hyperalgesia after peripheral inflammation. However, the mice have normal responses to acute noxious mechanical and thermal stimuli, indicating that other, as yet unidentified, heat-gated channels must exist (Caterina et al., 2000; Davis et al., 2000).

Acid-sensing ion channels

Protons not only activate and sensitize VR1, they also activate a range of acid-sensing ion channels (ASICs), some of which are only expressed by sensory nerves. Whether these simple channels are modulated by events during inflammation is not yet clear.

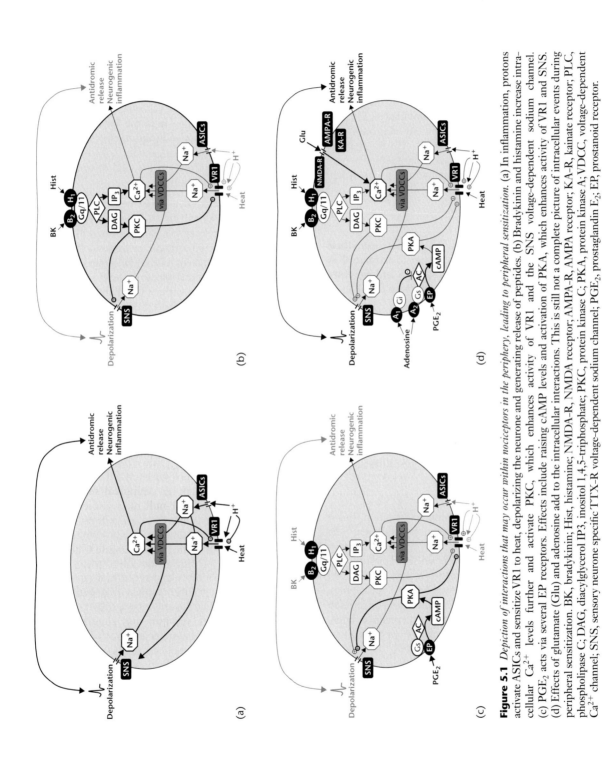

Figure 5.1 *Depiction of interactions that may occur within nociceptors in the periphery, leading to peripheral sensitization.* (a) In inflammation, protons activate ASICs and sensitize VR1 to heat, depolarizing the neurone and generating release of peptides. (b) Bradykinin and histamine increase intracellular Ca^{2+} levels further and activate PKC, which enhances activity of VR1 and the SNS voltage–dependent sodium channel. (c) PGE_2 acts via several EP receptors. Effects include raising cAMP levels and activation of PKA, which enhances activity of VR1 and SNS. (d) Effects of glutamate (Glu) and adenosine add to the intracellular interactions. This is still not a complete picture of intracellular events during peripheral sensitization. BK, bradykinin; Hist, histamine; NMDA-R, NMDA receptor; AMPA-R, AMPA receptor; KA-R, kainate receptor; PLC, phospholipase C; DAG, diacylglycerol IP3, inositol 1,4,5–triphosphate; PKC, protein kinase C; PKA, protein kinase A; VDCC, voltage–dependent Ca^{2+} channel; SNS, sensory neurone specific TTX–R voltage–dependent sodium channel; PGE_2, prostaglandin E_2; EP, prostanoid receptor.

A sensory neurone specific, tetrodotoxin-resistant sodium channel

Voltage-gated sodium channels are found in excitable tissues throughout the body and most are blocked by the application of tetrodotoxin (TTX). At least three TTX-resistant (TTX-R) sodium channels are expressed in sensory neurones, and these channels in nociceptors may be important sites for the integration of sensitizing stimuli. PGE_2 modulates TTX-R sodium currents in primary afferent neurones and antisense neutralization of the SNS channel reversibly blocks PGE_2-induced inflammatory hyperalgesia. PKA and PKC also interact to modulate TTX-R currents in nociceptors.

Inflammatory mediators

Bradykinin, histamine and PGE_2 act via their different G-protein-coupled receptors to activate PKA and PKC. This sensitizes VR1 and SNS and increases $[Ca^{2+}]_i$ levels (see Figure 5.1(b) and (c) for details).

Adenosine, ATP and purine channels

ATP is released by damaged tissues and causes pain in human volunteers both by direct activation of its own receptors and by the generation of adenosine. Adenosine A_2 receptors couple to G_s, generating cAMP. Thus adenosine can both activate and sensitize nociceptors (Figure 5.1(d)). Eight ATP receptors have been identified so far. Of these the purine ion channel P_2X_3 seems of importance in nociceptive pathways and appears to be sensitized by warm temperatures.

Peripheral glutamate

Glutamate is important in central sensitization, but it may also contribute to peripheral hyperalgesia. The three ion channel receptors for glutamate (alpha-amino-3-hydroxy-5-methyl-4-isoxazolepropionic acid (AMPA), kainate and N-methyl-D-aspartate (NMDA) receptors) have been detected on nociceptors. Glutamate can activate C-fibres and can also be released from peripheral afferent terminals. Intracellular interactions also seem to occur, as effects of peripheral glutamate application can be potentiated by SP.

Central sensitization

The end result of peripheral sensitization is to generate more activity in primary afferent nociceptors. When this information arrives at the dorsal horn (DH) of the spinal cord, mechanisms are in place to detect increased afferent activity. This peripheral activity is either further augmented before signals proceed to higher brain centres, or inhibited with reduction in the perception of pain. This ability to enhance or modulate incoming activity is possible because of the complex pharmacology of the DH of the spinal cord. Many different transmitters are stored and released by afferent and spinal cord neurones, with several descending inhibitory and excitatory pathways modulating activity. This rich chemistry also provides us with many potential pharmacological targets for manipulation. It is the balance between activity in the excitatory and inhibitory systems of the DH that determines the 'amount' of information entering ascending tracts to the higher centres and the subsequent perception of pain.

Spinal hyper-excitability describes the increased excitability of DH neurones after persistent noxious stimulation. A more excitable DH neurone will respond to weaker inputs from afferent neurones – those that are not normally sufficient to drive an action potential – expanding the peripheral receptive field and increasing the peripheral area within which stimulation will evoke a response. Thus, more DH cells will respond to a given stimulus, increasing the spinal nociceptive drive. The end result of this is central sensitization (secondary (2°) hyperalgesia), which can be observed behaviourally in many tests. One example is the reduced latency of response to noxious heat in the hotplate test (described as thermal hyperalgesia). Electrophysiological correlates include:

- The observation that after inflammation, non-noxious stimuli can release SP in the spinal cord.
- The phenomenon of wind-up, where repeated stimulation causes responses of DH neurones to increase, even though the strength of the stimulus remains the same.

Analogous to the situation in the periphery, interactions between different transmitters determine the state of excitability of the system. Eliminating any one single transmitter molecule or receptor may well have little effect on nociception unless that entity has a dominant role. So far, the only prime substrate identified is the NMDA receptor for glutamate. This glutamate-gated ion channel is a powerful switch and coincidence detector, which requires a specific combination of events for its activation. Once these conditions are met, intracellular interactions between the various cascades that are instigated continue the process of central sensitization.

Events combine to activate the NMDA receptor

Both low-threshold and high-threshold sensory afferent fibres contain and release glutamate. AMPA

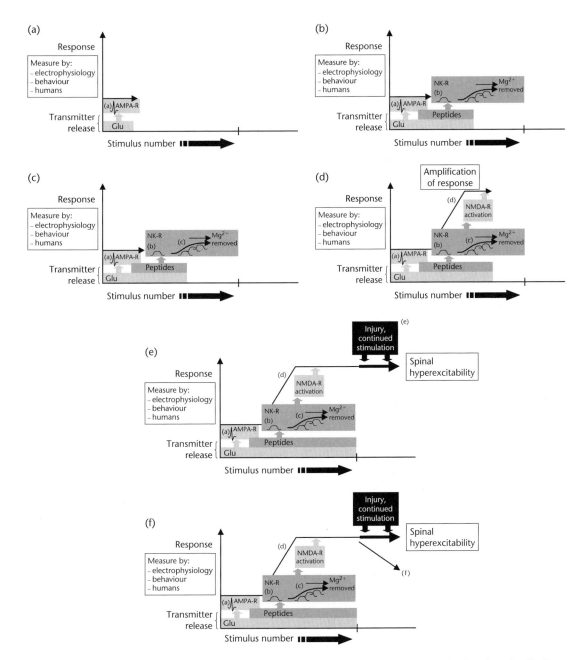

Figure 5.2 *Illustration of the involvement of the NMDA receptor in neuronal hyper-excitability.* (a) The first few stimuli release glutamate (Glu), which acts via the AMPA receptor (AMPA-R) to produce a rapid excitatory post-synaptic potential (epsp), action potential propagation, and faithful representation of the stimulus. (b) After repeated stimulation, peptides are released, and act via G-protein-coupled receptors (e.g. the tachykinin receptors, NK-R), to give rise to longer-lasting epsps. (c) These summate to give a sustained membrane depolarization, relieving the Mg^{2+} block from the pore of the NMDA receptor channel. (d) Released Glu can now activate the NMDA receptor, and the ensuing Ca^{2+} influx leads to a state of hyper-excitatability in the post-synaptic neurone, greatly increasing its response to subsequent stimuli. (e) If the stimulus continues (e.g. injury), the elevated level of response will be maintained, and spinal hyper-excitability will follow. (f) If the stimulus stops, or if the NMDA receptor is blocked, the neurone returns to resting state and responses return to normal. Repeated stimulation (at sufficient intensity to activate C-fibres) leads to an elevated level of response that can be measured in electrophysiology and behavioural experiments in animals, and psychophysical experiments in humans. This phenomenon is referred to as wind-up, and illustrates the importance of NMDA receptor activation in starting the processes of central sensitization. The sequence of events during a train of stimuli is explained in these four figures. AMPA-R, AMPA receptor; Glu, glutamate; NK-R, neurokinin receptor; NMDA-R, NMDA receptor; Hist, histamine.

receptors for glutamate are Na^+ selective ion channels, which, when glutamate binds, produce short-lived (~2 ms) post-synaptic depolarizations. In response to a noxious stimulus glutamate is released, AMPA receptors are activated and action potentials are generated in second order and projection neurones, transmitting the stimulus to higher centres. This is a fast and faithful transmission of the nociceptive information (Figure 5.2(a)).

The NMDA receptor differs from the AMPA receptor in that, when activated it passes a large Ca^{2+} influx, in contrast with the AMPA and other glutamate receptors. Consequences of unchecked elevated Ca^{2+} could be severe, so the channel is tightly regulated. It is blocked by Mg^{2+} ions at physiological membrane potentials, the block only being released during sustained membrane depolarization. So, during the situation described above when the AMPA receptor is active, although the released glutamate will still be binding to the NMDA receptor, the channel cannot open to pass Ca^{2+} ions.

In the presence of a more persistent noxious stimulus, peptides are released along with glutamate from afferent fibre terminals. This delay in peptide release occurs partly because peptides are located in terminals of high-threshold C-fibre afferents, but also because neuropeptide vesicles are stored at some distance from release sites, ensuring that peptides may not be released from the afferent fibre terminal except in conditions of high frequency stimulation and significant Ca^{2+} entry.

The tachykinins and CGRP are the predominant excitatory peptide transmitters in the DH. There are three tachykinin peptides – SP, neurokinin A (NKA) and neurokinin B (NKB) – which prefer the tachykinin receptors NK_1, NK_2 and NK_3 respectively (although a large degree of cross-affinity exists). SP and the NK_1 receptor have been studied in more detail than the others. Most spinal cord neurones that respond to SP are in lamina I and express NK_1 receptors. These SP-responsive neurones are not absolutely required for normal responses to acute noxious stimuli, but they are needed for the generation of spinal hyper-excitability and manifestation of behavioural inflammatory hyperalgesia. Many behavioural and electrophysiological pharmacological studies using NK_1 receptor antagonists have revealed a role for SP in generating spinal hyper-excitability. However, despite this convincing pre-clinical evidence that SP and its receptors form an important part of the nociceptive pathway, NK_1 receptor antagonists have been disappointing in human trials for analgesia in a variety of clinical pain states.

The substantial heterogeneity among mammalian tachykinin receptors has been blamed for this.

Importantly, the membrane depolarizations caused by tachykinin receptor activation are slower to rise than AMPA currents and are longer lasting (Figure 5.2(b)). With repeated stimuli, the peptide post-synaptic potentials begin to summate and the membrane is depolarized sufficiently to remove the Mg^{2+} block from the NMDA receptor (Figure 5.2(c)). The released glutamate can now activate the channel, allowing a large Ca^{2+} influx (Figure 5.2).

Subsequent intracellular interactions

It is probably not an overstatement to say that the mechanisms discussed below all depend absolutely on NMDA receptor activation for their initiation and in turn, full development of NMDA receptor-mediated hyper-excitability depends on each of these mechanisms. The key element is increased $[Ca^{2+}]_i$, which is only generated in sufficient amounts from influx through the NMDA receptor channel.

Effects on the NMDA receptor

Ca^{2+} influx through NMDA receptors feeds back to increase channel open probability. This is thought to be mediated through PKC phosphorylation of sites in the C-terminus of the NMDA receptor NR1 subunit. Whereas PKCε appears to be the major isoform responsible for sensitization of nociceptors in the periphery, evidence indicates a specific role for PKCγ in spinal neurones, particularly in neuropathic pain (Malmberg et al., 1997b). However, PKC may also mediate Ca^{2+}-dependent inactivation of the NMDA receptor. Tyrosine kinases also enhance NMDA receptor function, mediating the effects of several transmitters and maybe also PKC itself.

PKA, activated by increased intracellular cAMP, may also enhance NMDA receptor function. It is certainly an important molecule in inflammatory hyperalgesia, as a neuronal-specific modulatory subunit of PKA (R1β) is required for the development of inflammatory, but not neuropathic pain (Malmberg et al., 1997a) (in contrast to the situation described above for PKCγ). It is an intriguing possibility that in different injury states distinct subsets of afferent neurones may drive the development of DH hyper-excitability by distinct intracellular pathways.

Brain-derived neurotrophic factor (BDNF) can be released from afferent neurones, and acts via its tyrosine kinase B (TrkB) receptor to activate an Src kinase that further enhances NMDA receptor function (Figure 5.3).

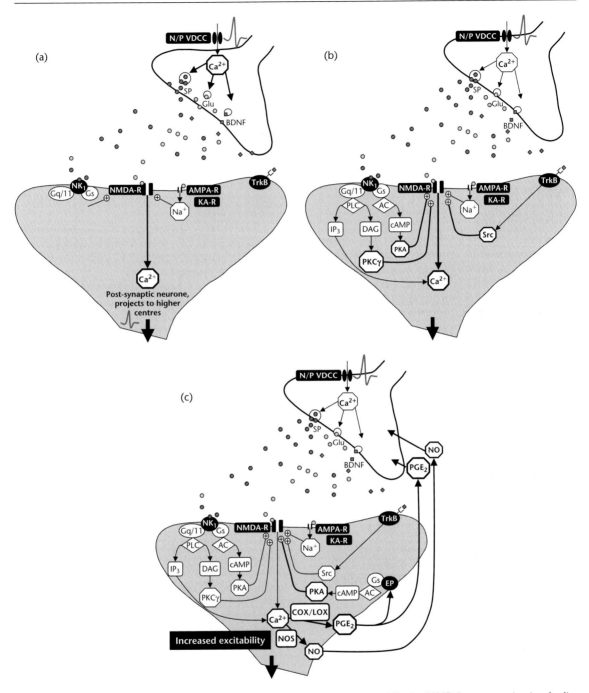

Figure 5.3 *Depiction of several interactions that may occur in dorsal horn neurones following NMDA receptor activation, leading to neuronal hyper-excitability.* (a) Action potential arrives at pre-synaptic terminal and via activation of N/P-type voltage-dependent Ca^{2+} channels (VDCCs) generates release of transmitters (SP, glutamate and BDNF). Receptor effects combine to depolarize the membrane, generate action potentials and activate the NMDA receptor (see Figure 5.2), allowing Ca^{2+} influx. (b) Activation of NK receptors generates PKA and PKCγ, and TrkB receptors activate Src kinase, all of which augment NMDA-R function. (c) Activation of NK receptors generates PKA and PKCg, and TrkB receptors activate Src kinase, all of which augment NMDA-R function. For clarity, interactions with inhibitory systems are not shown. N/P VDCC, N- and P-type voltage-dependent Ca^{2+} channel; Src, pp60c-src, a well-characterized protein tyrosine kinase; COX/LOX, cyclooxygenase/lipoxygenase.

Phospholipase pathway products

Elevated $[Ca^{2+}]_i$ activates PLA_2 and leads to formation of COX and LOX products. Many noxious events and injury have been shown to generate PGE_2, and application of NMDA receptor antagonists, NK_1 receptor antagonists and morphine can all attenuate this release. These connections again demonstrate the importance of interactions between several systems rather that the absolute importance of any one system. PGE_2 may also function as a retrograde messenger in the spinal cord, with release from the post-synaptic neurone signalling changes back to the pre-synaptic terminal (Figure 5.3).

Nitric oxide

Nitric oxide synthase (NOS) is expressed by spinal cord neurones and its activation is Ca^{2+} dependent. There is much evidence that nitric oxide (NO) plays a role in nociceptive transmission, particularly after inflammation or noxious stimulation sufficient to activate the NMDA receptor (with sufficient increase in $[Ca^{2+}]_i$). NO activates guanylyl cyclase and generates cGMP, but subsequent cellular mechanisms underlying its effects are not completely understood. Some suggested interactions are illustrated in Figure 5.3.

Receptor pathways

Tachykinins activate several intracellular pathways such as:

* cAMP-mediated PKA activation.
* IP_3/DAG-mediated calcium entry and subsequent activation of Ca^{2+}-dependent kinases (PKCγ).
* Activation of NOS and NO release.
* Activation of the arachidonic acid pathway and release of PGE_2.

PKCγ and PKA (particularly the R1β modulatory subunit) are required for the development of neuropathic and inflammatory pain, respectively (Malmberg et al., 1997a, b). Released PGE_2 can then act via EP_4 receptors on both the post-synaptic and the pre-synaptic neurone to elevate cAMP and activate PKA.

Metabotropic glutamate receptors (G-protein-coupled) add more diversity. Of the eight receptors identified so far, two are excitatory (activating IP_3/DAG) and six are inhibitory (inhibiting adenylyl cyclase and reducing cAMP formation) (Figure 5.3).

Key points

* Inflammatory mediators act via their receptors to initiate intracellular signalling cascades of key second messengers – Ca^{2+}, cAMP, PKA (R1β isoform), PKCε.

* These messengers interact and converge on key effector channels – VR1 and SNS (Figure 5.1).
* The resulting increased activity in nociceptors leads to increased afferent drive in the DH of the spinal cord.
* Glutamate and peptides are released from afferent terminals and the peptide post-synaptic potentials summate to deloparize the post-synaptic membrane. This allows NMDA receptor activation such that significant Ca^{2+} influx occurs (Figure 5.2).
* Second messengers (e.g. PKCγ and PKA) interact to enhance NMDA receptor function, with among other effects Ca^{2+} activating NO and PGE_2 (Figure 5.3).
* These changes increase the excitability of the DH neurone (spinal hyper-excitability), allowing:
  – DH neurones to respond to weaker inputs from afferent neurones.
  – Expansion of the peripheral receptive field.
  – Increase in the spinal nociceptive drive.

In this way, weak peripheral inputs that impinge upon a hyper-excitable spinal cord can produce high levels of perceived pain.

Further reading

Caterina, M.J., Leffler, A., Malmberg, A.B., et al. (2000). Impaired nociception and pain sensation in mice lacking the capsaicin receptor. Science, 288: 306–313.

Davis, J.B., Gray, J., Gunthorpe, M.J., et al. (2000). Vanilloid receptor 1 is essential for inflammatory thermal hyperalgesia. Nature, 405: 183–187.

Dickenson, A.H. (1995). Spinal cord pharmacology of pain. Br. J. Anaesth., 75: 193–200.

Hunt, S. & Mantyh, P. (2001). The molecular dynamics of pain control. Nature Rev., 2: 83–91[AQ2].

Malmberg, A.B., Brandon, E.P., Idzerda, R.L., Liu, H., McKnight, G.S. & Basbaum, A.I. (1997a). Diminished inflammation and nociceptive pain with preservation of neuropathic pain in mice with a targeted mutation of the type I regulatory subunit of cAMP dependent protein kinase. J. Neurosci., 17: 7462–7470.

Malmberg, A.B., Chen, C., Tonegawa, S. & Basbaum, A.I. (1997b). Preserved acute pain and reduced neuropathic pain in mice lacking PKC-γ. Science, 278: 279–283.

6

INFLAMMATION AND PAIN

W.P. Farquhar-Smith & B.J. Kerr

Inflammation and pain

Tissue injury, irritation or infection can induce inflammation. The classical observations of redness (rubor), heat (calor) and swelling (tumour), are invariably accompanied by pain (dolor). Each reaction contributes to the prevention of further insult and the resolution of damaged tissue. Post-operative pain exhibits the classical features of inflammatory pain. In some disease states, such as arthritis, the inflammation persists and causes chronic inflammatory pain. Inflammation and inflammatory pain are mediated by a plethora of diverse substances released by tissue damage itself and the subsequent cascade of inflammatory processes. Some inflammatory mediators directly activate and sensitize primary (1°) afferent nerve fibres (C and Aδ). Others stimulate the release of further mediators from immune cells, attracted by yet other chemicals in the inflammatory 'soup', which is a term used to refer collectively to all the pro-inflammatory mediators. Immune cells are recruited to the site of injury and act as a potent source of growth factors and cytokines. These are important in the generation and maintenance of hyperalgesia. This system exhibits enormous potential for interaction and escalation between each of the contributing processes. The polymorphonuclear leucocyte, of which the neutrophil is most plentiful, appears to be the principle immune cell involved in the generation of inflammatory pain.

Different components of the inflammatory 'soup' can activate or sensitize 1° afferent neurones, or induce the influx of immune cells at the inflamed site that release further pro-inflammatory mediators. Sensitization of 1° afferent neurones leads to a decreased threshold of pain activation and an increased response to a noxious stimulus. Electrophysiologically, in the 1° afferent nociceptor, this is evident not only by a lowered threshold for nociceptor activation, but also by increased spontaneous activity and an increased frequency of firing. These changes are manifest clinically as an increased response to a noxious stimulus: hypersensitivity. The resultant increase in afferent input to the spinal cord leads to the development and maintenance of secondary

(2°) (or central) sensitization, which may lead to chronic pain, even after the resolution of inflammation.

The list of inflammatory mediators is long and research continues to add many more. This chapter will discuss only the fundamental elements of inflammation and the key mediators that play a pivotal role in the generation of inflammatory pain. In addition to the myriad pro-inflammatory mediators, intrinsic inhibitory systems exist to mitigate the cascade of inflammation that is potentially damaging if left unchecked. Exploitation of these systems provides a therapeutic avenue in the treatment of inflammatory pain. The inflammatory response is also thought to contribute to the generation of other pathological pain states, such as neuropathic pain (reviewed in Chapter 7 & 20).

Inflammatory mediators produced locally

Protons

Tissue damage releases a number of substances directly from cells. Protons are produced in inflamed tissue and, in common with serotonin (5-hydroxytryptamine (5-HT)), can act directly on 1° afferent neurones. This probably occurs by increasing ion permeability, a process that shares characteristics with the noxious stimulation of nociceptors by capsaicin. Exposure of C- and Aδ-fibres to pH of 6 or less can activate acid-sensing ion channels (ASICs). A lowered pH of the inflammatory milieu also enhances the direct effects of other mediators. Moreover, local generation of heat acts upon heat activated ion channels (which share many characteristics of the vanilloid receptor the transient receptor potential vanilloid receptor 1 (TRPV1) formerly known as VR1 at which capsaicin acts) and may contribute to hyperalgesia.

Kinins

Kinins are peptides cleaved from circulating proteins that are activated at the site of injury. The archetypal kinin, bradykinin (BK), is produced by action of high molecular weight kininogen on kallikrein and is found in raised concentrations in inflamed tissue. BK both activates and sensitizes nociceptors. These actions of BK are mediated by G-protein-coupled BK B_1 and B_2 receptors that activate protein kinase C (PKC). As with many of the key inflammatory mediators, BK is synergistic with other algogenic substances (including prostaglandins (PGs) and nerve growth factor (NGF)) and can stimulate the release of other pro-inflammatory cytokines.

Adenosine triphosphate

Adenosine triphosphate (ATP) is released locally by inflammation and like many other mediators, can reproduce pain when injected locally. ATP acts upon P_2X receptors (of which the purine channel P_2X_3 is selectively expressed by non-peptidergic 1° afferent nociceptors) and contributes to hyperalgesia and pain.

NGF

NGF is released locally from a number of cells (including fibroblasts) and performs a central role in the inflammation cascade. Its increased concentration in inflamed tissue (in human inflammatory pain states and animal models) is associated with hyperalgesia. Via its receptor tyrosine kinase A (TrkA), NGF can directly sensitize the NGF-dependent subset of nociceptors, in addition to potentiating the actions of other sensitizing agents (e.g. BK). NGF signalling has also been

found to enhance responsiveness to heat and capsaicin, via interactions with TRPV1. Moreover, NGF degranulates mast cells, releasing more mediators (including NGF) and amplifying the inflammatory signal.

The release of chemoattractants provokes the influx of neutrophils, that release further sensitizing lipoxygenase (LOX) enzyme products, thought to maintain inflammatory hyperalgesia. This hyperalgesia is attenuated by sequestration or neutralization of NGF. Furthermore, in animal models, prior degranulation of mast cells inhibits the increase in NGF and hyperalgesia. Moreover, exogenous administration of NGF itself provokes hyperalgesia associated with local neutrophil influx. Some of the interactions of NGF on other pro-inflammatory systems are displayed in Figure 6.1.

Inflammatory mediators released and produced from immune cells

Products of COX and LOX metabolism

Prostanoids are produced by the enzymatic activity of cyclo-oxygenase (COX) and LOX on arachidonic acid (AA) and perform a number of pro-inflammatory tasks. The anti-inflammatory action of corticosteroids is in part related to the prevention of AA release, by inhibition of phospholipase A_2 (PLA_2). In inflammation, a number of PGs are produced. Prostaglandin E_2 (PGE_2) is produced predominantly by the COX-2 isoform and can directly activate and sensitize nociceptors via the PGE_2 EP receptors. Prostaglandins also enhance the effects of BK and augment neuropeptide release (including substance P (SP) and calcitonin gene-related peptide (CGRP)). Non-steroidal anti-inflammatory drugs (NSAIDs) act by inhibition of COX and reduce the production of these sensitizing PGs. Contemporary evidence suggests that PGs may be important in the development of inflammation-induced 2° hypersensitivity in the central nervous system (CNS), implicating a novel central role for NSAIDs in the CNS. Indeed, immune-like cells in the CNS, such as microglia, appear to release similar pro-hyperalgesic substances in the spinal cord much like peripheral immune cells.

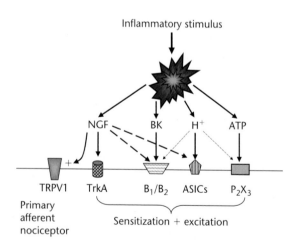

Figure 6.1 Interactions of elements of inflammation. NGF, BK, protons (H^+) and ATP all act on their respective receptors to excite and/or sensitize the 1° afferent nociceptors. However, as with many elements of the inflammatory soup, NGF interacts with other receptor systems to enhance their effect. NGF also increases activation of the transient receptor potential vanilloid (TRPV1) receptor, previously known as VR1.

Leucotriene B_4 and LOX

Certain products of LOX activity from immune cells (e.g. leucotriene B_4 (LTB_4) which is a product of the 5-LOX pathway) sensitize nociceptors by increasing cyclic adenosine monophosphate (cAMP). Activation of adenylate cyclase by LTB_4 results in the production of cAMP, which may then stimulate downstream kinases including PKA. Indeed, an increase in cAMP

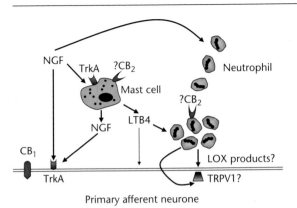

Primary afferent neurone

Figure 6.2 The role of NGF in neutrophil accumulation and pain. By its action on TrkA, NGF not only sensitizes 1° afferent neurones directly, but also causes mast cell degranulation. Among many pro-inflammatory substances, LTB_4 and more NGF are released. LTB_4 is considered a major influence on neutrophil accumulation. Release of products of LOX metabolism are thought to provoke pain, by action on the transient receptor potential vanilloid (TRPV1) (VR1) receptor. The anti-hyperalgesic action of cannabinoids could be mediated by CB_1 receptors on 1° afferent neurones or by modulating neuroimmune interactions via CB_2 receptors on immune cells.

is thought to be the basis of sensitization of 1° afferent nociceptors of many aetiologies. LTB_4 is also a powerful chemoattractant to immune cells, recruiting them into the inflammatory mêlée and stimulating more LTB_4 release and the release of other metabolites of the LOX pathways (such as the sensitizing substance 8(R),15(S)-dihydroxyeicosatetraenoic acid).

Particular LOX metabolites produced by neutrophils have been postulated to act on TRPV1 receptors and may be responsible for the link between neutrophils and inflammatory hyperalgesia. Animal studies have shown that inflammation-induced neutrophil accumulation is associated with an increase in LTB_4. Both neutrophil accumulation and LTB_4 are reduced in mast cell deficient animals. Thus the NGF–mast cell–LTB_4–neutrophil axis is of paramount importance. Some of the key processes involved in neutrophil accumulation and pain are shown in Figure 6.2.

Cytokines

Histamine and 5-HT are well-known products of mast cell degranulation, yet many cytokines with disparate and varied functions are also released. Of these, interleukin-1β (IL-1β) and tumour necrosis factor α (TNFα) exert powerful pro-inflammatory effects that result in hyperalgesia. Indeed, exogenous administration of both these substances can evoke inflammatory hyperalgesia. Furthermore, they are capable of synergistic

interaction with NGF. Each of these substances can increase the levels of the other two, further amplifying inflammation. IL-1β also mediates neutrophil chemotaxis. Similarly, administration of the IL-1 endogenous antagonist (IL-1ra) attenuates NGF levels and inhibits the resultant inflammatory hyperalgesia, highlighting the importance of these substances. These and many more cytokines (up to IL-18 have been described!) are released by other immune cells (including macrophages), further demonstrating the complexity and the potential augmentation of the inflammatory signal.

Neurogenic inflammation

Part of the inflammatory process is mediated by neuropeptides released from sensory nerve endings. Neurogenic inflammation is responsible for the 'flare' reaction following a scratch injury, mediated by neuropeptides released from sensory nerve endings. NGF increases neuropeptide content of sensory nerves and local inflammation-induced release. Neurokinins (e.g. SP and neurokinin A (NKA)) and CGRP act via specific receptors causing vasodilation and plasma extravasation. These changes facilitate the entry of recruited immune cells to the affected area and promote the development of oedema. Although these substances can directly depolarize sensory neurones, the action of neuropeptides is probably more important in the facilitation of central sensitization.

Endogenous anti-inflammatory systems

Anti-inflammatory cytokines

Given that NGF, IL-1β and TNFα (and many others) potentiate and enhance each other's actions, intuitively an intrinsic inhibitory system would appear necessary to temper potentially damaging pro-inflammatory processes. One line of defence is afforded by release of naturally anti-inflammatory cytokines. These include IL-10 and IL-1ra. Evidence for such anti-inflammatory effects includes:

- IL-1ra (an endogenous IL-1 antagonist) reduces IL-1β-induced rise in NGF concentration and hyperalgesia.
- Inflammation increases macrophage-derived IL-10, and IL-10 exhibits anti-inflammatory actions including inhibition of neutrophil influx.
- Treatment with IL-10 attenuates local release of IL-1β, TNFα and NGF in animal models of inflammation.

Peripheral endogenous opioids

Endogenous opioids also act to moderate excessive inflammation. Although opioid receptors are expressed predominantly in the CNS they are also found in the periphery. Such peripheral receptors (both mu opioid (MOP) and kappa opioid (KOP) receptors have been implicated) are upregulated in inflammatory states and thus increase the efficacy of endogenous agonists. Exogenous administration of MOP agonists display naloxone-reversed anti-inflammatory and analgesic activity when injected into sites of painful inflammation. Immune cells (principally neutrophils) conscripted to the inflamed tissue not only produce pro-inflammatory substances, but also release endogenous opioids in biologically significant amounts. Interestingly, peripheral opioid analgesia displays a relative lack of tolerance under inflammatory conditions.

Endogenous cannabinoids

More recently the endogenous cannabinoid system has been elucidated. This comprises of G-protein-coupled cannabinoid receptors (CB_1 and CB_2) and a number of endogenous cannabinoids (including anandamide (AEA), 2-arachidonylglycerol and palmitoylethanolamide (PEA)). These receptors mediate some of the therapeutic and recreational aspects of cannabis.

The predominantly neuronal CB_1 receptors are expressed in brain, spinal cord and peripheral 1° afferent neurones. Levels of PEA are raised in inflamed tissue, and activation-dependent neuronal production of AEA may inhibit neuronal excitability by activation of CB_1 receptors.

The CB_2 receptor is almost exclusively expressed peripherally, on immune cells, but is also present on CNS glia. CB_2 receptor activation has been shown to prevent mast cell degranulation in animal models (representing a potent upstream site for anti-hyperalgesia), potentially attenuating the amplificatory release of NGF and other mediators. Endogenous PEA has been postulated to modulate mast cell degranulation *in vivo*, in a process coined 'autocoid local inflammation antagonism'. Exogenous administration of PEA attenuates inflammation-induced neutrophil accumulation. In addition, neutrophils may also release anti-inflammatory cannabinoids (Figure 6.2).

Eicosanoid endocannabinoids (including AEA) share a similar biochemistry to leucotrienes; both can be metabolized by LOX. Exogenous administration of certain cannabinoids not only mitigates release of cytokines (including TNFα and IL-6) but may also increase levels of the anti-inflammatory IL-10.

Potential drug therapies

Knowledge of the mechanisms and substances involved in inflammation and inflammatory processes indicates potential analgesic strategies. Anti-inflammatory analgesics could be developed on the basis of:

- Reduction of pro-inflammatory processes.
- Accentuation of inhibition of inflammation.

Already widely used, NSAIDs are analgesic and anti-inflammatory by reduction of PGs. Since inhibition of the constitutive COX-1 (as opposed to the inducible COX-2) is thought to be responsible for side effects, recent additions to the NSAID armamentarium are more COX-2 selective.

Inhibition of 5-LOX is anti-hyperalgesic in certain animal models of inflammatory pain, but problems of toxicity have meant these compounds have yet to be used in clinical trials. Toxicity problems have also hampered the development of BK antagonists. Nevertheless, many other targets have been identified that may have promise. For example, manipulation of ASICs has been postulated as a therapeutic and selective mechanism for pain relief.

Exogenous administration of anti-inflammatory compounds, or manipulation of metabolism to enhance levels of inhibitory endogenous compounds, also offer novel analgesic approaches. Upregulation of peripheral opioid receptors has been exploited by local administration of opioids after arthroscopy and topical application of opioids may offer a novel analgesic strategy. Exploitation of peripheral cannabinoid-induced neuroimmune modulation of inflammation offers analgesic potential without central psychoactive side effects.

Key points

- Tissue damage induces inflammation, causing release of numerous inflammatory mediators that activate and sensitize 1° afferent nociceptors. Many pro-inflammatory substances promote the release of and accentuate the actions of other inflammatory mediators.
- Resultant electrophysiological changes lead to inflammatory hyperalgesia. The augmented afferent barrage to the spinal cord from this peripheral (1°) sensitization drives central (2°) sensitization.
- Degranulation of mast cells releases not only inflammatory mediators that act directly and indirectly on 1° afferent nociceptors, but also powerful chemotactic substances to promote influx of neutrophils and macrophages. These recruited immune

cells also release pro-inflammatory and hyperalgesic molecules.

- The role of NGF is pivotal since it:
  - Is released by inflammation.
  - Can sensitize 1° afferent neurones.
  - Acts synergistically with other sensitizing substances.
  - Precipitates mast cell degranulation.
  - Potentially amplifies inflammation by release of further mediators including NGF.
- Several endogenous systems exist to assuage the potentially damaging augmentation of inflammatory processes. These include release of anti-inflammatory cytokines and the endogenous cannabinoid and opioid systems.
- Pharmacological manipulation of inflammatory mechanisms may provide analgesic opportunities.

Further reading

Boddeke, E.W. (2001). Involvement of chemokines in pain. *Eur. J. Pharmacol.*, **429**: 115–119.

Burnstock, G. (2000). P2X receptors in sensory neurones. *Br. J. Anaesth.*, **84**: 476–488.

DeLeo, J.A. & Yezierski, R.P. (2001). The role of neuroinflammation and neuroimmune activation in persistent pain. *Pain*, **90**: 1–6.

Rice, A.S.C., Farquhar-Smith, W.P., Bridges, D., Brooks, J.W. (2003). Cannabinoids and pain. In: Dostrovsky, J.O., Carr, D.B. & Koltzenburg, M. (eds) *Proceedings of the 10th World Congress on Pain*, Vol. 24. Progress in Pain Research and Management, IASP Press, Seattle; Chapter 37, pp. 437–468.

Stein, C., Machelska, H., Binder, W., *et al.* (2001). Peripheral opioid analgesia. *Curr. Opin. Pharmacol.*, **1**: 62–65.

7

NERVE DAMAGE AND ITS RELATIONSHIP TO NEUROPATHIC PAIN

N.B. Finnerup & T.S. Jensen

Introduction

The nociceptive system was previously thought of as a hard-wired system, mediating information about tissue damage to the brain in a fixed and static manner. However, injury to the peripheral or central nervous system (CNS) triggers a cascade of changes, which alter the structure and function of the nervous system. The result is a high degree of plasticity in those systems that mediate information about tissue damage, with neuronal modifications occurring at several levels of the neuraxis from the peripheral receptor to the cortex. These changes after nerve damage may result in peripheral or central neuropathic pain.

Neuropathic pain is characterized by pain in an area with sensory loss corresponding to the damaged nerve or central lesion. The qualities may be burning, smarting, shooting, aching, and pricking. The pain may be accompanied by dysesthesia (unpleasant abnormal sensations), allodynia (the elicitation of pain in the affected area by non-noxious stimulation with light touch or innocuous cold or warmth), and hyperalgesia (increased pain response to a normal noxious stimulus). Other features frequently seen in neuropathic pain are wind-up-like pain (abnormal temporal summation of pain), aftersensations (pain continuing after stimulation has ceased), and referred pain (pain felt in a place apart from the stimulated area). We will discuss the mechanisms that can be relevant for neuropathic pain after nerve damage as seen in animals and in humans.

Peripheral nerve damage

Sensitization of primary afferent nociceptors

Experimental

Pain is normally elicited by activating receptors of unmyelinated (C) and thinly myelinated (Aδ) primary afferents. Under normal conditions, C- and Aδ-nociceptors are silent. They respond only when stimulated, and respond in a more vigorous manner to stimuli that are potentially noxious. Abnormal nociceptor sensitization, in the absence of acute tissue injury, inflammation, or abnormal spontaneous afferent activity, has been demonstrated in models of peripheral nerve injury. After lesioning peripheral nerve fibres they exhibit:

- Spontaneous activity.
- Increased sensitivity to various chemical, thermal, and mechanical stimuli.

Abnormal activity not only occurs at the peripheral terminal, but also along the peripheral nerve (ectopic activity) and in the dorsal root ganglion (DRG) cells. This indicates that the CNS receives an abnormal input from at least three sources:

- Sensitized nociceptors.
- Ectopic foci along the nerve.
- Spontaneously active neurones within the DRG.

This ectopic activity following nerve injury is accompanied by increased expression of ion channels (particularly sodium channels) and receptors. The accumulation of sodium channels and receptors at sites of ectopic impulse generation may be one of the mechanisms responsible for lowering action potential threshold and for spontaneous activity in damaged primary afferents.

Patients

Microneurographic recordings from transected nerves in human amputees with phantom limb pain show spontaneous afferent activity. Likewise, recordings from patients with mechanical or heat hyperalgesia exhibit sensitized C-nociceptors innervating the painful region. Thus, sensitized nociceptors may not only be a source for spontaneous pain, but also a site from which evoked pains may arise.

Indirect evidence for C-fibre sensitization has also been obtained from patients with postherpetic neuralgia (PHN) where topical application of the C-fibre excitant capsaicin can increase pain. Topical application of the local anaesthetic lidocaine, which blocks ectopic impulse transmission in primary afferent nociceptors, produces pain relief.

Inflammation of the peripheral nerve trunk

Experimental

Nervi nervorum are small nerves that innervate the connective tissue sheaths of peripheral nerves. These nerves may be another source of pain in diseases of peripheral nerves, particularly when there is an inflammatory element. Inflammation within a nerve facilitates access of new substances that can alter nerve function. For example, following experimental injury to nerves and DRG by nerve transection activation of macrophages associated with endoneurial blood vessels has been demonstrated. Tumour necrosis factor (TNF)-α, produced by activated macrophages, has the ability to induce ectopic activity in primary afferent nociceptors and thereby contributes to both spontaneous and evoked types of pain.

Patients

While there is firm evidence that nerve lesions represent an important source of neuropathic pain, the evidence that inflammation plays such a role is much weaker. However, acute herpes zoster is accompanied by intense inflammation along the affected peripheral nerve that typically resolves in several weeks. A small subgroup of patients with PHN has inflammatory infiltrates throughout the affected peripheral nerve, DRG and dorsal root. In patients with acute demyelinating polyradiculopathy, deep proximal aching pain, in addition to paroxysmal types of pains, is a characteristic phenomenon. Although the evidence is lacking, it is possible that inflammation of proximal parts of nerve sheaths by activity in nervi nervorum contributes to such deep proximal pain. It is interesting to note that in patients with polyneuropathy the deep aching pain is most prevalent. It remains to be seen whether this pain is in part explained by an abnormal activity in small primary afferents from nervi nervorum.

Sympathetic activity and damaged peripheral nerves

Experimental

Under normal conditions, nociceptors do not respond to sympathetic stimulation or catecholamines. However, after experimental nerve injury, cutaneous afferent fibres develop noradrenergic sensitivity and neurones express functional adrenoceptors. After a peripheral nerve injury, coupling between sympathetic and sensory nerves occurs at three different sites:

1 The peripheral skin, corresponding to the receptive end of nociceptive afferents projecting into the nerve territory of a lesioned nerve.

2 The axotomized nerve end or its neuroma.

3 DRG containing cell bodies that have been lesioned.

Stimulation of sympathetic efferents in contact with neuromata can excite afferent nociceptors. When peripheral nerves have been lesioned, it is possible (by electrical stimulation of the sympathetic trunk at physiological stimulus frequencies) to activate C-fibres via α_1-adrenergic mechanisms. In addition to this peripheral interaction, the coupling of sympathetic and afferent neurones may also take place within the DRG. After nerve lesioning, sympathetic vasoconstrictor fibres innervating blood vessels within the DRG start sprouting and form basket-like terminals around large primary afferent cell bodies. In addition, when stimulating sympathetic neurones, it is possible to activate primary afferents by an α_2-adrenergic-mediated mechanism.

Patients

Evidence indicates that persistent pain in some patients is maintained by sympathetic neuron activity:

- Locally administered catecholamines (in the vicinity of injured nerves) induce or exacerbate pain, which is abolished in some patients by sympatholytic therapy.
- In amputees, injection of noradrenaline/norepinephrine around a stump neuroma produces intense pain.
- In PHN, intra-cutaneous adrenaline and phenylephrine increase spontaneous pain and allodynia in the affected limb.
- In post-traumatic neuralgias, intra-cutaneous application of norepinephrine into a symptomatic area rekindles spontaneous pain and dynamic mechanical hyperalgesia that had been relieved by sympathetic blockade.

These findings suggest that noradrenergic activity contributes to sensitization of human nociceptors after partial nerve lesion. There are also reports that sympathetic blocks (intravenous (i.v.) phentolamine or topical clonidine) transiently relieve neuropathic pain.

Central sensitization: increased peripheral input

Central sensitization is a plastic change of cellular excitability in second or higher order transmission neurones. While usually described after tissue damage, such sensitization can also occur after nerve injury.

Experimental

Animal work indicates that the central sensitization following complete or partial nerve injury is due to pathological activity in sensitized C-nociceptors, which in turn sensitizes dorsal horn (DH) neurones. Central sensitization involves a series of molecular events including:

- Presynaptic release of substance P and glutamate.
- Activation of ligand gated ion channels and voltage-dependent calcium ions (Ca^{2+}) channels.
- Activation of metabotropic *N*-methyl-D-aspartate (NMDA) receptors and neurokinin-1 (NK1) receptors in postsynaptic cell membranes, causing release of intracellular Ca^{2+}. This in turn results in a release of protein kinase C (PKC).
- Release of PKC in response to Ca^{2+}. This is important because it phosphorylates several receptors (including the NMDA receptor) resulting in a lowering of sensitivity to glutamate. The biochemical events after nerve injury become more profound in later stages, where excitotoxic cell death may contribute to a persistent stage of hyperexcitability.

The neuronal manifestations of such sensitization are multiple and include at least the following:

- Increase of neuronal activity to noxious stimuli.
- Expansion of neuronal receptive field size.
- Spread of spinal hyperexcitability to other segments and higher structures, such as thalamus and cortex.

Patients

Central sensitization is clinically manifested by various forms of hyperalgesia including: mechanical, thermal, and chemical hyperalgesia.

At least three types of mechanical hyperalgesia have been described: dynamic allodynia, static hyperalgesia, and punctate hyperalgesia (Table 7.1). The central sensitization elicited from the periphery is thought to be the cause of the dynamic mechanical allodynia, produced by light tactile stimuli. Once central sensitization is established (with allodynia mediated by Aβ-input), it can be maintained by input from C-fibres. Further

stimulating these nociceptors (e.g. by heating) increases not only ongoing pain, but also the touch-evoked pain. Selective block of Aβ-fibres eliminates the touch-evoked pain, while the ongoing pain is maintained. Furthermore, central sensitization also allows Aδ-afferents to gain access to 2° pain signalling neurones. This is suggested to be the cause of punctate mechanical allodynia and perhaps also cold allodynia.

Thermal hyperalgesia is of two kinds:

- Heat hyperalgesia is exceedingly rare in neuropathic pain.
- Cold hyperalgesia is common. There are several postulated mechanisms involved:
  - Disinhibition caused by lesioning of cool sensory pathways, thus reducing inhibition of cold-evoked pain.
  - Loss of Aδ-fibres with a relative sparing of C-fibres.
  - Central sensitization.

Central sensitization: decreased peripheral input

Experimental

Some studies suggest that lost C-fibre input, as a consequence of degeneration or de-afferentation, leads to a reduction of synaptic contacts in the outer laminae of the DH. Consequently, Aβ-mechanoreceptive afferents, which normally terminate in deeper laminae (III and IV), grow into lamina II and directly contact the de-afferented cells. While these findings would explain the touch-evoked allodynia in patients with reduced or lost C-fibre input, more recent experimental findings have questioned this explanation.

Patients

Although the experimental evidence for a de-afferentation hyperexcitability is unclear, clinical observations

Table 7.1 Assessment and mechanisms of different types of hyperalgesia after nerve damage

Types	Stimulus	Mechanism
Mechanical		
Dynamic allodynia	Light tactile stimuli (e.g. brush)	Central sensitization; due to increased or decreased C-fibre input
Static hyperalgesia	Gentle mechanical pressure	Peripheral sensitization
Punctate hyperalgesia	Punctate stimuli (e.g. von Frey hair)	Central sensitization due to Aδ-fibre input
Thermal		
Heat hyperalgesia	Heat stimuli (e.g. warm metal roller)	Peripheral sensitization
Cold hyperalgesia	Cold stimuli (e.g. cold metal roller/acetone)	Central sensitization or disinhibition
Chemical	Topical capsaicin, histamine, menthol	Peripheral sensitization

show that such hyperexcitability does occur. Pathological studies have utilized:

1 Direct axonal markers (e.g. anti-protein gene product (PGP) 9.5 antibodies) to demonstrate dendritic loss.
2 Functional activity markers (e.g. vascular responses to histamine iontophoresis) and quantitative sensory testing).

These demonstrate that there is a subgroup of neuropathic pain patients with pain and loss of cutaneous C-fibres and co-existing allodynia. In such patients degeneration of central terminals of unmyelinated primary afferents induces a synaptic re-organization within the DH, leading to aberrant direct connections between Aβ-mechanoreceptive fibres and DH neurones that have lost their normal nociceptor input.

Central nerve damage

Neuronal hyperexcitability

Experimental

Glutamate and other excitatory amino acids are briefly released in response to a CNS lesion. This may contribute to sensitization of central neurones, similar to that seen in response to excess afferent input, consequent upon peripheral nerve damage. Moreover, de-afferentation of higher order neurones may contribute to changes in neuronal hyperexcitability.

- Gamma amino butyric acid (GABA) is a widely distributed inhibitory neurotransmitter in the CNS and plays an important role in the control of pain transmitting pathways.
- GABAergic inhibitory neurones have a high susceptibility to hypoxia and inhibitory fibres descending from medulla oblongata, pons, and the midbrain (including serotonergic, noradrenergic, and enkephalinergic) may also be damaged.
- Loss of tonic inhibition generated by these systems contributes to the increased responsiveness and enlargement of receptive fields of neurones in pain pathways.

Patients

The importance of neuronal spontaneous and evoked hyperactivity for central pain has been confirmed in human studies. At cord level, spinal cord injury (SCI) patients with central pain have significantly more sensory hypersensitivity at-level than pain-free SCI patients. This suggests a role for at-level neuronal hyperexcitability in central SCI pain. High levels of spontaneous activity and evoked hyperactivity during C-fibre electrical stimulation are recorded in the dorsal root entry zone (DREZ) during DREZ microcoagulation in SCI pain patients. Ablation of this focal hyperactivity results in pain relief.

In the thalamus, abnormal neuronal hyperactivity has been recorded in patients with central pain. Low frequency potentials detected in the ventroposterolateral (VPL) thalamic nucleus are decreased during periaqueductal grey (PAG) stimulation and this is associated with pain relief.

Drug administration in patients with central nerve lesions supports the notion that NMDA-mediated excitation and decreased GABA-mediated inhibition occurs in central pain. In addition, general blockade of sodium channels (using lidocaine) relieves spontaneous and evoked pain. Blockade of ectopic discharges in the injured pain pathway may explain this effect.

Inflammation

Experimental

The anti-inflammatory cytokine interleukin-10 reduces mRNA levels of inflammatory-related genes and pain-related behaviour after SCI. As in peripheral nerve damage, neuroinflammation and neuroimmune activation (actively involved in CNS injury) are likely to play a role in persistent central pain. Human studies to support this are currently lacking.

Central re-organization

Experimental

CNS plasticity is likely involved in the development of central pain. After spinal cord lesion there is an increased deposition of calcitonin gene-related peptide (CGRP) in the deeper layer of the DH. This is interpreted as a sprouting of fine primary afferents (containing CGRP) from the superficial to the deep laminae of the DH. Antibodies to nerve growth factor (NGF) suppress this redistribution of CGRP as well as pain-related behaviours and abnormal responsiveness of wide dynamic range neurones.

Patients

Referred sensations to a de-afferented region, after stimulation in a reference zone at or above the level of a lesion, suggest a re-organization of the CNS. Functional magnetic resonance imaging (MRI) has demonstrated co-activation of non-adjacent cortical representations after contact in a reference zone of a patient with a spinal lesion. This supports a subcortical re-organization projecting to the cortex after a central injury. Central nerve lesions are also related to re-organization in the thalamus. Receptive and projected field dissociation is observed, with receptive fields located on the border zone and projected fields referred to anaesthetic body areas.

Key points

- Peripheral nerve injury may have effects both peripherally and centrally:
  - Peripheral effects:
    Abnormal nociceptor activity.
    Spontaneous neuronal activity.
    Axonal sprouting.
    Spontaneous activity in DRG.
    Increased sympathetic activity.
  - Central effects:
    Central sensitization due to increased input.
    Central sensitization due to decreased input.
    Spinal and cortical re-organization.
- Central nerve injury is associated with:
  - Abnormal activity in spinal cord and higher centres.
  - Spinal and cortical re-organization.

Further reading

Baron, R. (2000). Peripheral neuropathic pain: from mechanisms to symptoms. *Clin. J. Pain*, **16**: 12–20.

Coderre, T.J. & Katz, J. (1997). Peripheral and central hyperexcitability: differential signs and symptoms in persistent pain. *Behav. Brain Sci.*, **20**: 404–419.

Jensen, T.S., Gottrup, H., Sindrup, S.H. & Bach, F.W. (2001). The clinical picture of neuropathic pain. *Europ. J. Pharmacol.*, **429**: 1–11.

Koltzenburg, M. & Scadding, J. (2001). Neuropathic pain. *Curr. Opin. Neurol.*, **14**: 641–647.

Woolf, C.J. & Salter, M.W. (2000). Neuronal plasticity: increasing the gain in pain. *Science*, **288**: 1765–1769.

Yezierski, R.P. (2000). Pain following spinal cord injury: pathophysiology and central mechanisms. *Prog. Brain. Res.*, **129**: 429–449.

RECEPTOR MECHANISMS

E.E. Johnson & D.G. Lambert

Pain serves a vital biological defensive function, often associated with other psychological and central disturbances. It is a physiological condition, which is detected by refined receptors within the damaged body tissues. It has two components: the motivational-affective (emotional) component and the sensory-discriminative component. Nociception and pain are not necessarily analogous. Nociception is the term applied to perception of nociceptor activation by noxious stimuli, whereas pain refers to a subjective response. One pain classification describes: physiological, inflammatory (from tissue damage) and neuropathic pain (from changes in nerves) with peripheral and central nervous system (PNS and CNS, respectively) changes some of which may be permanent, altering the brain's future perspective of pain. We describe basic receptor pharmacology and then some of the more important and unusual receptors in the 'pain pathway'.

General terminology

Some of the terms used in receptor pharmacology are described below:

- *Ligand*: General term for a molecule (peptidic, chemical, ionic or synthetic), which binds at a receptor site.
- *Agonist*: Ligand that binds at, and activates, a regulatory receptor to produce a pharmacological response (can be a full or partial response).
- *Antagonist*: Ligand that binds at a receptor site but does not produce a response. Binding is generally, but not exclusively, reversible (competitive) and attenuates the effect of an agonist.
- *Inverse agonist*: Ligand that binds and activates the receptor, but produces a response opposite to that observed on activation with an agonist.
- *Affinity*: The tenacity of ligand binding to a receptor site. Statistically, it is the probability of the ligand binding to a free receptor at any given time.
- *Efficacy*: The ability of ligand to produce a response after binding to a receptor.
- *Constitutive activity*: Activity at a receptor in the absence of a ligand.

- *Selectivity*: The ability of a ligand to be selective (i.e. only binding to a precise receptor type).
- *Stereoselectivity*: The selectivity of a receptor for a particular stereoisomer of a ligand.
- *Co-localization*: Similar anatomical distribution patterns (e.g. such patterns of a ligand and its receptor).
- *Down- and upregulation*: Decrease or increase in levels of expression of cellular components. Generally controlled by feedback mechanisms.
- *Desensitization*: The diminishing effects of a ligand when given continuously or repeatedly.
- *Tolerance*: A more gradual diminishing in the effects of a ligand.
- *Metabotropic*: A receptor that is coupled to some metabolic reaction. For example, G_q-protein-coupled receptors activate the enzyme phospholipase C (PLC) and hence produce a metabolic action.
- *Ionotropic*: A receptor whose activation leads to a flow of ions.

Basic receptor function

A basic principle of pharmacology is that a drug must exert an effect on one or more of the cell's chemical constituents to produce a pharmacological response; for this, two important properties are required by receptors: (a) recognition of extracellular molecules and (b) transduction of information intracellularly.

Firstly, the ligand molecule must come into contact with a receptor for which it has selectivity, and collide in such a manner that an interaction is possible. Receptors have native-binding sites or pockets, which must be accessible to the ligand for binding to occur. Numerous mathematical models have been proposed to describe these interactions; the Law of Mass Action governs the formation of the reversible receptor–ligand complex. Receptors can exist in two states: 'resting' (R) and 'activated' (R*), and can be described by a two–state model. In the case of a therapeutic drug, the amount bound is important, since this must oe controlled within a desired range. Outside of this dosage other properties of the drug may complicate therapy.

In the unbound state, a receptor is functionally silent except when constitutive activity occurs. Appreciable activation without a ligand was first observed for β-adrenoceptors, either with mutations in the third extracellular loop or in cases of over-expression. Other examples of receptors with constitutive activity are the benzodiazepine receptors.

The ability of a receptor to couple with an intracellular effector molecule is important for continuing signal transduction. There are a large number of effectors (discussed below) found in cells. Examples of intracellular responses observed on activation of these include:

- Movement of ions (such as K^+, Ca^{2+} and Cl^-) in or out of the cell.
- Increase or decrease in the enzymatic activity.
- Protein phosphorylation.
- Altered transmitter release.
- Control of protein synthesis.

Transduction signals can be amplified within a cell (e.g. a receptor may activate more than one guanine–nucleotide-binding protein (G-protein) and also, an active G-protein α-subunit can activate more than one effector molecule). Therefore, a maximal cellular response can generally be achieved at low ligand concentrations. Some pathways have feedback mechanisms, so that they are able to regulate the synthesis and catabolism of messengers to control response as required. The overall response observed generally depends on the cell type activated and the signal-transduction components within this cell (e.g. acetylcholine receptors and β-adrenoceptors in cardiac muscle are both G-protein coupled but produce different cellular responses as they activate different classes of G-proteins).

The kinetics of the pharmacological response depends on receptor type activated and signal-transduction pathway followed. For example, ion influx is seen within milliseconds of an ion channel being activated, whereas effects through a G-protein receptor are observed after several seconds. Long-term changes, such as modulation of gene transcription and protein synthesis, take hours to show and are generally much longer lasting. Desensitization, that is loss of effect of a ligand, can occur within a cell by several possible mechanisms: loss of receptors, depletion of messengers or cell components, physiological adaptation, or increased metabolism.

Basic receptor pharmacology

Receptors can reside either at the level of the plasma membrane, intracellularly, or associated with intracellular organellar membranes. These major groups can be further subdivided as below, though the plasma membrane-bound receptors (Figure 8.1) will be the main focus of this chapter.

- Plasma membrane-bound receptors:
  - Ligand-gated ion channels.
  - Tyrosine kinase-coupled receptors.
  - G-protein-coupled receptors.
- Nuclear (steroid) receptors.
- Inositol (1,4,5) triphosphate $(Ins(1,4,5)P_3)$ and ryanodine receptors.

Plasma membrane-bound receptor classes

Ligand-gated ion channels

Ligand-gated ion channels are also termed ionotropic. Examples include nicotinic and γ-aminobutyric acid (GABA A). They are composed of multiple subunits coming together to form an ion channel. The agonist binds to the extracellular surface of one of these subunits (precise site is receptor dependent) to directly open the channel (i.e. the receptor and channel are one and the same protein). Opening allows the transfer of ions down an electrochemical gradient and can be mediated indirectly by G-proteins. Such receptors are involved in fast synaptic transmission.

Tyrosine kinase-coupled receptors

Tyrosine kinase-coupled receptors are also termed metabotropic. Examples of these include growth factors. The agonist binds to the extracellular surface causing a conformational change and two receptors dimerise. Autophosphorylation of the intracellular domain in each receptor enables the dimer to interact with -SH_2 domain containing proteins (e.g. Grb2) mediating a response within minutes.

G-protein-coupled receptors

Opioid receptors are an example of G-protein-coupled receptors. These receptors are also termed metabotropic. They span the plasma membrane seven times and utilise a G-protein transducer. A G-protein is a heterotrimeric complex consisting of three subunits (α, β and γ) and can generally be classed as inhibitory $(G_{i/o})$ or excitatory $(G_s/G_{q/11})$. On activation, a conformational change of the receptor protein occurs, leading to an interaction between receptor and G-protein.

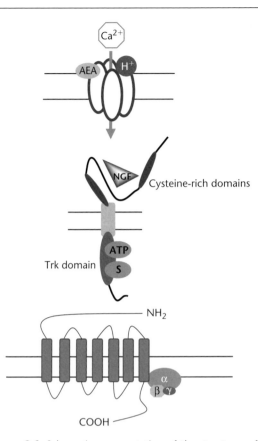

Figure 8.1 Schematic representation of the structures of the three most important plasma membrane-bound receptor types involved in pain transmission. The upper panel shows a ligand-gated ion channel (the vanilloid, receptor VR1 is given as an example showing the Ca^{2+} pore, and H^+ and anandamide (AEA-binding sites)). The middle panel shows a typical tyrosine kinase receptor (e.g. NGF which requires dimerisation for activation) with ATP and phosphorylation sites(S). The lower panel depicts a typical G-protein-coupled receptor (e.g. opioid) with seven transmembrane domains and the G-protein interaction. For abbreviation see text.

Guanosine diphosphate (GDP) is exchanged for guanosine triphosphate (GTP) on the α-subunit, promoting the cleavage of the G-protein complex to the active state ($G_{\alpha\text{-GTP}}$ and βγ). Classically $G_{\alpha\text{-GTP}}$ then activates subsequent effector molecules (discussed below) to modulate second messenger formation. A response is observed within seconds. G-proteins can also directly influence ion channels.

Intracellular effectors

A variety of effectors can couple to receptors. The cell type and effectors present generally determine the signal-transduction pathway followed on activation of a particular receptor. The first four described below are the key G-protein-coupled effectors, with the other examples relating to tyrosine kinase receptors and ion channels.

Adenylyl cyclase

On activation, adenylyl cyclase (AC) converts adenosine triphosphate (ATP) to cyclic adenosine monophosphate (cAMP), an important regulatory second messenger with many physiological roles. cAMP can then activate protein kinase A (PKA), which has a variety of cellular effects. For example, activation of β_1-adrenoreceptors in the heart stimulates PKA to increase the release of Ca^{2+} from intracellular stores by opening voltage-gated Ca^{2+} channels, and so regulates contraction of the cardiac muscle. Some G-protein-coupled receptors inhibit AC and, therefore, decrease cAMP production. In the case of opioid receptors, this can lead to decreased neuronal activity.

Guanylyl cyclase

Similar to AC, guanylyl cyclase (GC) converts GTP to cyclic guanosine monophosphate (cGMP) in response to peptides, such as atrial natriuretic peptide. cGMP (like cAMP) has many cellular effects, including activation of protein kinase G, which regulates contractile proteins and ion channels.

Phospholipase C

This is a membrane-bound enzyme family which converts phosphatidylinositol bisphosphate (PIP_2) to $Ins(1,4,5)P_3$ and diacylglycerol. These second messengers then activate intracellular Ca^{2+} ion channels and PKC, respectively. Other isoforms of PLC can be activated directly by tyrosine kinase receptors. An example of this mechanism is epinephrine acting on α_1-adrenoreceptors in vascular smooth muscle cells, which activates PLC and so causes an increase in $Ins(1,4,5)P_3$. This in turn increases intracellular Ca^{2+}, which leads to constriction of the vessel.

Phospholipase A_2

Receptor-mediated activation of phospholipase A_2 (PLA_2) is similar to the activation of PLC and produces arachidonic acid (AA) and eicosanoids, which have recently been shown to control K^+ channels in some neurones. Eicosanoids can also be released as local hormones.

Cations

G-protein coupled receptors can directly interact with ion channels within the plasma membrane. One of the major roles of Na^+ within the cell is the generation of an action potential. Opening and closing of the voltage-gated Na^+ and K^+ channels at a particular point in the membrane can result in membrane depolarisation and hence propagation of an impulse. K^+ is responsible for the hyperpolarisation phase, which hinders impulse firing until the membrane potential has returned to normal.

Some ions channels, such as the Ca^{2+}-activated K^+ ion channel, are voltage and ligand gated. Binding of Ca^{2+} to the cytoplasmic side of the channel causes the channel to open and increase K^+ efflux, again effecting membrane polarity. G-protein-coupled opioid receptors enhance an outward K^+ conductance to hyperpolarize and close voltage-sensitive calcium channels (VSCCs).

Ras

Ras is a membrane-bound proto-oncogene product, which conveys the signal from the SH_2 domain of the tyrosine kinase receptor dimer through the kinase cascade. Activation of Ras mediates a cascade of phosphorylation through various serine/threonine kinases, until the final component (mitogen-activating protein kinase) is phosphorylated. This then activates one or several transcription factors, so initiating long-term cellular responses including gene expression and cell division.

Jak

Activation of a tyrosine kinase receptor (by cytokines) causes dimerisation and association with the cytosolic tyrosine kinases or Jaks. These then target a family of transcription factors (Stats), which migrate to the nucleus and regulate gene expression.

Potentiating nociceptors

There are three main stages in the perception of pain:

- Pain sensitivity.
- Transmission of signals from periphery to dorsal horn (DH) of the spinal cord.
- Signals to and from the higher brain.

Sensory endings activated by noxious stimuli are known as nociceptors and are the first stage in pain sensitivity. Chemical inflammatory mediators (e.g. H^+, AA, 5-hydroxytryptamine (5-HT), bradykinin (BK), nerve growth factor (NGF) and nucleotides) released from primary ($1°$) sensory terminals and non-neural cells or synthesised as required, can alter sensitivity or directly excite nociceptors (Table 8.1).

Table 8.1 Mediators acting on nociceptive neurone surface receptors and neuromodulators whose release they control

	Mediator	Receptor	Neuro-modulator
Metabotropic	BK	BK2	SP
	NGF	TrkA	CGRP
Ionotropic	Capsaicin	VR1	Glutamate
	H^+	VR1/ASIC	CCK
	Heat	VR1/VRL-1	Somatostatin
	ATP	P_2X_3	
	5-HT	$5-HT_3$	

ASIC: acid-sensing ion channel; CCK: cholecystokinin; Trk: tyrosine kinase. For abbreviations see text.

Kinins

Following tissue damage, proteolytic cleavage of kininogen produces two closely related mediators: bradykinin (BK) and kallidin. BK induces its potent nociceptive actions via G-protein-coupled receptors, BK1 and BK2. Its effects are directly enhanced by the release of prostaglandins (PGs). BK receptor stimulation can activate membrane-bound PLA_2 which catabolises the production of AA from membrane esters. This can then be converted to PG by cyclo-oxygenase (COX) enzymes. The BK2 receptor is the predominant subtype found on nociceptor endings.

Prostaglandins (PGs)

PGs do not directly cause pain, but enhance the effects of other mediators, (particularly 5-HT or BK) via G_s-proteins. Interestingly, BK may cause PG release, so exerting a 'self-sensitizing' effect. Other eicosanoids and prostacyclins may be important, though evidence for these is so far limited.

Capsaicin

Capsaicin (8-methyl-N-vanillyl-6-noneamide), a lipophilic vanilloid molecule, is the active ingredient of *Capsicum* chilli peppers, responsible for the hot burning sensation. It acts specifically through a ligand-gated cation channel, on the surface of small and medium nociceptors. Vanilloid receptor type 1 (VR1) has been identified on dorsal roots of C- and Aδ-fibres (immunoreactivity co-localise its expression with that of the lectin, IB4 and P_2X_3 purinoceptors). VR1 is activated by: capsaicin, acidification and temperatures above $43°C$. Inflammatory mediators (e.g. BK and NGF) potentiate sensitivity to capsaicin and heat. This sensitization is mediated by activation of PLCγ (possibly reducing PIP_2 inhibition on the receptor). The VR1 protein of 838 amino acids is a member of the transient receptor potential (TRP) superfamily of ligand-gated ion channels, whose core transmembrane structure resembles that of a voltage-gated K^+ channel (Figure 8.1). This receptor has high permeability to Ca^{2+}, which is responsible for the many cellular effects observed with capsaicin. VR2 has also been identified and this is activated by noxious heat (threshold of 52°C). A VR-like (VRL-1) receptor has also been postulated to exist on nociceptors.

Since anandamide (AEA, see later), an endocannabinoid, is structurally related to capsaicin (with amide bonds and aliphatic side chains) it has been postulated to act at VR1. Indeed, AEA induces vasodilation via VR1, accompanied by the release of calcitonin generelated peptide (CGRP). There is also a possible link between capsaicin and glutamate release. Capsaicin can induce anti-nociception.

Nerve Growth Factor (NGF)

NGF is a known mediator of persistent pain. Polymodal C-fibre neurones can be classified depending on their need for neurotropic mediators:

- NGF-dependent nerves are also known as tyrosine kinase A (TrkA)-positive neurones, since they express the NGF tyrosine kinase receptor.
- Glial cell line-derived neurotropic factor neurones are important in neuropathic pain. They do not express TrkA, but rather P_2X_3. They are also known as c-Ret-positive neurones.

Serotonin (5-HT)

5-HT is an indolamine mediator released on nerve injury, capable of inducing hyperalgesia. It is found in brain cells, platelets, enterochromaffin and mast cells. There are many serotonergic pathways originating in the raphe nuclei; paralleling those of norepinephrine (NE). Since NGF is important for degranulation of mast cells, it is probable that 5-HT has a role in controlling NGF-mediated inflammatory hyperalgesia.

Several receptors for 5-HT have been identified: $5-HT_1$–$5-HT_7$. These are G-protein coupled, with the exception of $5-HT_3$ that is a member of the ligand-gated ion channel family. The effects of 5-HT can be either excitatory or inhibitory. $5-HT_{1A}$, localised on raphe nucleus neurones, is an autoreceptor since it modulates its own release. The major subtypes expressed in the rat DH (mainly on small fibres) are $5-HT_{2A}$ and $5-HT_3$. These subtypes are responsible for 5-HT-mediated nociception, particularly hyperalgesia. 5-HT mRNA is co-localised with that for CGRP, indicating that 5-HT neurones belong to the TrkA- and NGF-dependent group of neurones, important in modulating inflammatory pain.

Adenosine Triphosphate (ATP)

ATP is an important intracellular messenger, now also recognised as a vital extracellular signal. Following release from secretory vesicles or lysed cells, it can modulate ion channel activity. This is achieved through specific receptors, found peripherally in the skin and centrally on second-order neurones located in the DH. In the periphery, its effects can be potentiated by SP, H^+ and BK. ATP is metabolised to adenosine by surface-located enzymes, ectonucleotidases. Adenosine then acts at P1 (A_1- or A_2-types) receptors, further modulating pain transmission both peripherally and centrally (though the effects observed are usually opposing).

ATP and other adenosine nucleotides activate purinergic G-protein-coupled (P_2Y) or ionotropic (P_2X) receptor subtypes. Seven subtypes, P_2X_1–P_2X_7 have been cloned so far. Of these, at least six (P_2X_1–P_2X_6) are expressed on sensory neurones. These (with the exception of P_2X_7) can combine to form functional heteromeric receptors. Recently, trimeric complexes of identical subunits, which model a required structural core of the P_2X channel, have been proposed.

Of greatest interest is P_2X_3, as this is the primary subtype expressed in small C-fibres. During inflammation, an upregulation of P_2X receptors is observed, possibly due to the H^+ sensitivity of the receptors. These receptors are responsible for processing the majority of nociceptive information from peripheral ATP. Centrally, ATP can act pre- or post-synaptically at P_2X receptors, the two being distinct populations with an apparent different subunit composition. Spinally it is co-released with GABA. ATP can also act pre-synaptically on nociceptors to increase glutamate release.

Primary nociceptive modulators

Several neuromodulators are released from, and play important regulatory roles in, the central terminals of

Table 8.2 Summary of neurotransmitters in ascending and descending non-nociceptive and nociceptive pathways of the nervous system

Pathway	Effect of transmitter	Neurotransmitter	Localisation	
			Spinal cord	Supra-spinal
Ascending	Excitatory	Glutamate	Sensory afferent neurones to DH	Efferent neurones from cortex and cerebellum (descending)
	Inhibitory	Tachykinins	Sensory afferent neurones to DH	
		GABA	Inter-neurones and motor neurones	Cerebellum, neocortex, thalamus and hypothalamus
Descending	Excitatory	5-HT (also inhibitory)	Motor neurones	Raphe nuclei
		Acetylcholine	Synapses	Synapses in brain stem
	Inhibitory	NE		Locus coeruleus, neocortex, thalamus and cerebellum
		Opioids	Spinal cord	Thalamus and hypothalamus
		Nociceptin	Spinal cord	Thalamus and hypothalamus

the primary ascending afferents and the descending tracts from the higher brain centres (Table 8.2).

Tachykinins

SP an undecapeptide was the first neuropeptide discovered and is now recognised as one of the tachykinins, along with eledoisin, and neurokinin A (NKA) and B (NKB). These neuropeptides are formed by the proteolytic cleavage of larger precursor proteins (pre-protachykinins) in the spinal ganglia. They show sequence homology to opioid peptides. SP is expressed in approximately 50% of C-fibre afferents (predominantly polymodal C-fibres), 20% of Aδ-fibres, and not at all in Aα/Aβ-fibres. It is a co-transmitter with other peptides and glutamate in response to both nociceptive and non-nociceptive inputs. Its actions are mediated through the tachykinin receptor NK1.

All NK receptor subtypes are G-protein coupled (similar to BK1 and BK2 receptors) and act by increasing intracellular Ca^{2+}. The receptors are localised in the DH and bind to SP (NK1), NKA (NK2) and NKB (NK3).

Calcitonin Gene Related Peptide (CGRP)

CGRP is a 37 amino acid neuropeptide, distributed widely throughout the nervous system. It has an important role in inflammation and pain modulation. It is found in the majority of primary afferent nerves (in approximately 50% of polymodal C-fibre afferents, 33% of Aδ-fibres and 20% of Aα/Aβ-fibre neurones), after synthesis in the dorsal root ganglion (DRG). It is released in the periphery where it can

potentiate the excitatory effects of SP and increase intracellular Ca^{2+} release. Several subtypes of CGRP receptors have been identified, as well as a calcitonin-like receptor. These are all G-protein coupled and are localised in the nucleus accumbens, indicating a CNS role for CGRP in pain transmission.

Gamma-amino-butyric-acid (GABA)

GABA is the most widely distributed inhibitory transmitter in the vertebrate CNS. GABAergic neurones occur in abundance in the neocortex and cerebellum, though they are also found in spinal cord inter-neurones. At least three subtypes of GABA receptor have been identified on GABAergic neurones:

- GABA A is an ionotropic pentameric ligand-gated Cl^- channel. It is composed of several subunits, with α, β, δ and γ being essential for receptor function. There are several isoforms of each subunit; hence at least 13 subclasses of this receptor exist. GABA A binds GABA, muscimol, bicuculline (on α- and β-subunits) and also has binding sites for barbiturates, ethanol and benzodiazepines. These all potentiate the channel-opening action of GABA.
- GABA B is a G-protein-coupled receptor that can inhibit cAMP formation. This receptor binds GABA and the muscle relaxant, baclofen. It is generally found on nerve terminals mediating pre-synaptic neurotransmitter release.
- GABA C receptors (recently discovered) are also ligand-gated Cl^- channels, found mainly in the retina. These bind GABA, muscimol and the agonists, cis- and trans-4-aminocrotonic acid and are sensitive to picrotoxin, but not bicuculline.

GABAergic neurones involved in pain transmission are mainly concentrated in the brain. Long projections are found between the striatum and the substantia nigra and also between the hypothalamic nuclei and the forebrain. However, they are also found in the spinal cord, mediating release of peptides.

Glutamate

This is one of the most important transmitter pathways modulating nociception. It is co-located closely in the CNS with opioid systems. Glutamate, released from central terminal afferents, is the major excitatory output along:

- Ascending nociceptive pathways from the DRG and lamina I.
- From the cortex and cerebellum to other brain areas (secondary ($2°$) response neurones).

Several transmitters are co-released with glutamate (namely SP, NKA and CGRP) as a result of noxious, thermal, mechanical or electrical stimuli. Fast transmission is mediated through two major classes of receptor:

- Ionotropic receptors are directly gated ion channels, with subtypes including:
  - $(\pm)$-α-amino-3-hydroxy-5-methylisoxazole-4-propionic acid (AMPA).
  - NMDA.
  - Kainate.
- Metabotropic (mGlu) are G-protein coupled and can be divided further into three groups based on pharmacology, signal transduction and sequence homology (these will not be considered further).

AMPA receptors mediate the largest component of synaptic currents and are responsible for baseline activity, whereas NMDA activation induces windup and mediates long-term plastic changes. Kainate receptors also contribute to responses induced by noxious stimuli.

Functional NMDA receptors exist as heteromeric combinations of various subunits. This generally includes an NMDA receptor (NR) 1 subunit plus one or more of NR2A, NR2B, NR2C and NR2D (determined by subunit-dependent localisation). They have binding sites for glutamate, glycine, magnesium, zinc and phencyclidine. However, activation only occurs when the noxious input is above threshold level and pore blockade (by extracellular Mg^{2+}) is removed. Simultaneously, glutamate must bind to NMDA and an impulse must cause depolarisation of the post-synaptic membrane. Activation of NMDA receptors causes elevation of intraneural Ca^{2+}, which stimulates a series of transduction messengers (protein kinases, protein phosphatases and immediate early genes) within the post-synaptic cell. Recently it has been proposed that nitric oxide (NO) and prostanoids can also activate NMDA receptors.

Opioid peptides

Several classification systems for the three classical opioid receptor subtypes have been proposed. The more recent system uses DOP (δ or OP_1), KOP (κ or OP_2), MOP (μ or OP_3) nomenclature and is in line with recent IUPHAR (International Union of Pharmacologists) guidelines. Further opioid subtypes, such as λ, ι, ζ, σ and ε, have been postulated, though are not generally accepted. Classical opioid receptors belong to the G-protein-coupled receptor superfamily and couple to pertussis toxin-sensitive inhibitory $G_{i/o}$-proteins. Activation leads to:

- An inhibition of AC activity that decreases cellular cAMP.
- Stimulation of K^+ efflux.
- Inhibition of voltage-gated Ca^{2+} channels.

The overall effect is inhibition of transmitter release. Opioids modulate transduction in two main ways:

- Indirect action on the DH, by pre-synaptic inhibition of the release of excitatory peptides from afferent fibres.
- Direct post-synaptic actions on DH neurones.

Opioid receptor subtypes show approximately 60% sequence homology on alignment of the amino acid sequences. Further subdivision on pharmacological grounds has been suggested, but there is no structural evidence for this. Pharmacology here is still controversial. There is now evidence to demonstrate the existence of homo- and heterodimers and several splice variants of each subtype.

Localisation of these receptor proteins is subtype dependent, with MOP having the widest distribution in the CNS – correlating well with its major role in pain regulation. Central and peripheral binding sites have been identified for the other subtypes (DOP and KOP), again consistent with their roles in: water balance, food intake, pain perception and neuroendocrine modulation. While there is some overlap in subtype distribution – distribution for MOP and DOP generally appears complementary – their precise anatomical localisation differs markedly. KOP immunoreactive neurones are sometimes co-localised with immunostaining for CGRP, NO synthase, vasoactive intestinal peptide and choline acetyltransferase.

Endogenous opioids, such as endorphins, enkephalins and dynorphin, are derived mainly from three

Table 8.3 Selectivity of opioid peptides for classical opioid receptor subtypes. Nociceptin does not bind to MOP/DOP/KOP. Peptide sequences are presented in standard single letter amino acid code and those in bold show sequence homology to nociceptin (FGGFTGARKSARKLANQ)

Precursor	Ligand	Peptide sequence	MOP	DOP	KOP
?	Endomorphin-1	YPWF-NH$_2$	+++	−	−
?	Endomorphin-2	YPFF-NH$_2$	+++	−	−
Pro-opiomelanocortin	β-endorphin	**YGGF**MTSE**KS**QTPLVTLFKNAIIKNAYKKGE	+++	+++	++
Pro-enkephalin	Leu-enkephalin	**YGGF**L	+	+++	−
		YGGFMRF			
		YGGFMRGL			
	Met-enkephalin	**YGGF**M	++	+++	−
Pro-dynorphin	Dynorphin A	**YGGF**LRRIRPKLKWD**NQ**	++	+	+++
	Dynorphin B	**YGGF**LRRQFKVVT			
	α-neoendorphin	**YGGF**LRKYPK			
	β-neoendorphin	**YGGF**LRKYP			

+: denotes affinity; − : denotes no binding affinity.
A: alanine; D: aspartic acid; E: glutamic acid; F: phenylalanine; G: glycine; I: isoleucine; K: lysine; L: leucine; M: methionine; N: asparagine; P: proline; Q: glutamate; R: arginine; S: serine; T: threonine; V: valine; W: tryptophan; Y: tyrosine.

pre-cursors in mammals: pro-opiomelanocortin, pro-dynorphin and pro-enkephalin (Table 8.3), though a fourth (pro-endomorphin) is proposed but remains to be identified.

Enkephalins, key neurotransmitters of the opioid family, are present in cell bodies, fibres and nerve endings in many areas of the CNS. These bind to the MOP opioid receptor subtype and are thought to be of major importance in pain modulation through descending efferent pathways. Neutral endopeptidase (NEP) is a zinc metalloendopeptidase which catabolises the degradation of many neuropeptides, such as SP, BK and enkephalin. Its importance has been investigated using knock-out studies. When NEP is inhibited pharmacologically, increased concentrations of enkephalin result in anti-nociception. In contrast, in knock-out mice (lacking the gene for NEP), hyperalgesia was observed in the hot plate, tail withdrawal and writhing tests. This indicates NEP-knock-out results in BK-induced hyperalgesia, in place of enkephalin-mediated analgesia.

Pro-enkephalin encodes Leu and Met enkephalin. The pro-dynorphin gene codes for several bioactive peptides, including dynorphin A and B. These show considerable structural and sequence homology with nociceptin (N/OFQ), produced from the precursor, pro-nociceptin. Dynorphin A does not bind significantly to nociceptin receptors (NOPs) and N/OFQ does not bind to KOP.

The classical response to opioid agonists is analgesia. However, a variety of other physiological and pathological effects have been reported, indicating the complex central role of the opioid system. These non-pain effects must be appreciated when developing analgesics acting at opioid receptor subtypes. Analgesic effects are mediated through all receptor subtypes, particularly MOP (DOP and KOP are also responsible for addiction and dysphoria). Interactions between the MOP and DOP systems are possibly necessary to elicit some responses, though KOP receptors generally act independently.

There is evidence that opioid peptides modulate the release of other excitatory and inhibitory mediators in the pain pathway. One example is the action of dynorphin A at KOP receptors. This suppresses the release of SP associated with nociceptive transmission, so diminishing the perceived intensity of noxious stimuli.

Nociceptin (N/OFQ)

N/OFQ was isolated after the discovery of its opioid-like receptor, NOP (previously known as ORL-1 or OP$_4$). This 17-amino acid neuropeptide is derived from post-translational processing of its precursor, proN/OFQ (pN/OFQ). There are several basic cleavage sites upstream and downstream of N/OFQ, indicating that pN/OFQ may code for further biologically active peptides, such as nocistatin.

NOP is also a G-protein-coupled receptor that couples with pertussis toxin-sensitive $G_{i/o}$-proteins. It is found pre-synaptically on sympathetic, parasympathetic and sensory nerves, where it can modulate release of neuropeptides. Functional NOP also occurs post-synaptically on spinal nerves. Spinally N/OFQ mediates similar cellular effects to opioids. However, supraspinally hyperalgesia/anti-opioid actions are observed. The distribution of pronociceptin and its transcripts in the CNS differs to that for opioid precursors and peptides (though is qualitatively similar to the anatomical localisation of NOP). This difference in localisation could explain the opposite effects of opioids and N/OFQ on pain thresholds, despite activation of similar signal-transduction mechanisms.

Norepinephrine (NE)

The catecholamine NE (the principle neurotransmitter of the adrenergic pathways, of which epinephrine and dopamine are further examples) is synthesised in nerve terminals from the dietary amino acid, phenylalanine. This is converted to tyrosine and then to DOPA by tyrosine hydroxylase, in the rate-limiting step of an anabolic pathway. The enzyme requires iron, oxygen and a cofactor. Accumulation of NE or dopamine in the cytoplasm can inhibit the cofactor and so control DOPA synthesis. DOPA is used to synthesise dopamine, which enters the vesicles of the nerve terminals where it becomes NE. In the adrenal medulla and several nerve terminals, NE can also be converted to epinephrine by methylation. NE is stored in vesicles until an action potential increases Ca^{2+} in the nerve terminal, causing vesicles to fuse with the pre-synaptic membrane, releasing NE into the synaptic cleft. NE then travels across the cleft to activate receptors on the post-synaptic membrane.

The adrenoceptors are members of the G-protein-coupled receptor superfamily and there are several subtypes with differing affinities for catecholamines: α_1, α_2, β_1 and β_2. The α_1- and β-receptors predominantly occur post-synaptically, whereas α_2-receptors are found pre-synaptically in the nervous system.

α_2-adrenoceptors are further examples of inhibitory autoreceptors. They inhibit the release of NE (and other transmitters such as 5-HT and glutamate) via actions at $G_{i/o}$ (inhibition of Ca^{2+} channels, enhancement of K^+ conductance and reduced cAMP formation). Thus, activation of these receptors (e.g. with clonidine) may reduce nociceptive afferent firing (pre-synaptically) leading to an analgesic response. Evidence for different

isoforms of α_1 and α_2 exists, though the significance of these findings is unclear. β-receptors couple to G_s-proteins, which are stimulatory. Activation thus stimulates AC and increases cAMP. Termination of the action of catecholamines is achieved by uptake of the transmitter into the nerve terminal via uptake 1. Uptake 2 in non-neuronal sites is also involved. NE is metabolised by monoamine oxidase (MAO), found mainly in glial and neuronal cells in two isoforms, MAO-A and MAO-B. Catechol-O-methyltransferase is also involved in catecholamine metabolism.

Cannabinoids

Δ^9-tetrahydrocannabinol (Δ^9-THC) is the major psychoactive constituent isolated from *Cannabis sativa*. It interacts with a small family of $G_{i/o}$-coupled receptors. Like opioid, NOP and α_2-adrenoceptors, activation results in:

- Inhibition of AC.
- Closure of voltage-gated Ca^{2+} channels.
- Stimulation of K^+ efflux.

Two G-protein-coupled receptor subtypes have been identified. Cannabinoid receptor type 1 (CB_1) is located on neurones and CB_2 on immune cells (a third subtype, CB_{1a}, has also been suggested).

CB_1 receptors show a high level of expression (pre- and post-synaptically) in many areas of the brain and spinal cord. Low expression in the brain stem may explain the lack of respiratory depression associated with cannabinoids. Cannabinoid receptors are also located in the skin, where they can produce anti-nociceptive effects via modulation of SP, NO and particularly CGRP secretion. CB_1 mRNA expression correlates well with distribution of large diameter A-fibres (24% of which co-express SP and CGRP). Mechanisms for the anti-nociceptive effects of cannabinoids are described at all levels of pain modulation in the brain and spinal cord (Walker *et al.*, 1999). Endogenous ligands for CB_1 receptors, including AEA have been identified. Administration to animals via a range of routes produces an anti-nociceptive response. Moreover, this lipid also activates VR1 receptors (see above).

The anti-inflammatory roles of cannabinoids may be induced through CB_2. Activation prevents degranulation of mast cells and secretion of pro-inflammatory mediators.

Table 8.4 summarises a range of ligands (research and clinical) for some of the receptor systems described earlier. It is far from comprehensive. Note that for several of the well-characterised receptor systems, no selective clinical ligands are available.

Table 8.4 Summary of research tools and clinical drugs for the main receptor classes involved pain transmission

Receptor	Mechanism	Endogenous ligand	Research agonist	Research antagonist	Clinical drug
Glutamate					
NMDA	Ligand-gated ion channel	Glutamate	NMDA	DL-AP5 CP-101606 Ifenprodil Ro 25-6981 (NR2B)	Ketamine[a] CPP[a] Amantidine[a] Dextromethorphan[a]
				APV (+)-HA966 2,3 benzo-diazepines	Phenylcyclidine Nitrous oxide
AMPA			AMPA		
Kainate		Kainate			
I mGlu	G-protein coupled	Glutamate	CPCCOEE MPEP S-DHPG AIDA		
II mGlu					
III mGlu				Ethylglutamic acid MSOP	
Tachykinin					
NK1	G-protein coupled	SP		CP 96345 CI-1021 CP-99,994 Spantide	
NK2		NKA			
NK3		NKB			
CGRP					
CGRP1	G-protein coupled	CGRP		CGRP8-37	
Kinin					
BK1	G-protein coupled	Bradykinin		[desArg,^{9}Leu^8]-BK	
BK2				[desArg,^{9}Leu^8]-Lys^{0}BK	
GABA					
GABA A	Ligand-gated Cl$^-$ channel Benzodiazepines	GABA	Muscimol Isoguvine	Bicuculline Songorine	Barbiturates Ethanol
GABA B	G-protein coupled		Baclofen	CGP 35348 SCH 50911	
GABA C	Ligand-gated Cl$^-$ channel				
5-HT					
5-HT$_2$	G-protein coupled	5-HT	DOI	Methysergide Ketanserine Sarpogrelate HCl Tropisetron	
5-HT$_3$	Ligand-gated ion channel				

Receptor	Mechanism	Endogenous ligand	Research agonist	Research antagonist	Clinical drug
ATP					
P_2X	G-protein coupled	ATP>ADP>AMP	α,β-meATP	Suramin[b] PPADS[b] TNP-ATP IP_5I NF023	
P_2Y	Ligand-gated ion channel		2MeSADP		
NE					
α_1	G-protein coupled	NE	NS-49 methoxamine	L-765,314	
α_2			MPV-2426 Mivazerol MED	Yohimbine OPC-28326	
β_1			T-0509	LK 204-545 Vaninolol	
β_2			TA-2005 trimetoquinol	ICI 118 551	
Opioid					
MOP	G_i-protein coupled	β-Endorphin Endomorphin-1 Endomorphin-2	DAMGO PL017 Dezocine	CTOP Cyprodime Naloxone[b] β-funaltrexamine Quadazocine	Morphine Fentanyl Diamorphine (heroin) Hydromorphone Codeine Sufentanil Oxymorphone Dextropropoxyphene Methadone Pethidine
DOP		Leu-enkephalin Met-enkephalin	DPDPE DSLET DADLE	Naltrindole ICI174864	Etorphine (vetrinary medicine)
KOP		Dynorphin	U50488H CI-977 U69593	Nor-BNI	Etorphine Pentazocine Ketocyclazine Buprenorphine Nalbuphine
Nociceptin					
NOP	G_i-protein coupled	N/OFQ	N/OFQ (1–13)NH_2 Ro 64-6198 *rac*-5a ZP120 CTD [Arg[14],Lys[15]] N/OFQ	[Nphe[1]] JTC-801 J-113397	
Cannabinoid					
CB_1	G_i-protein coupled	AEA	Noladin ether HU210 AEA[b]	SR141716A LY320135 AM281	Δ^9-THC Cannabidiol

Continued

Table 8.4 *Continued*

Receptor	Mechanism	Endogenous ligand	Research agonist	Research antagonist	Clinical drug
			2-AG[b] O-1057[b] Levonantradol[b] Nabilone[b] CP55,940[b] WIN55212-2[b] Δ^9-THC	Virodhamine	
CB$_2$		PEA	JWH-015 JWH-051 HU-308 DMH-Δ^8-THC- 11-oic acid GW405833	SR144528	

Vanilloid
VR1
	Ligand-gated ion channel (TRP superfamily)	Capsaicin	Olvanil
			Gingerols
			2-iodo-
			  resiniferatoxin
				Capsazepine
				Ruthenium red
				5-iodo-
				  resiniferatoxin
				KJM429
				JYL1421
					Resiniferatoxin (in trials)

2-AG: 2-arachidonylglycerol; AIDA: (*RS*)-1-aminoindan-1,5-dicarboxylic acid; APV: (2-amino-5-phosphonovalerate; CI-1021: 1-(1*H*-indol-3-ylmethyl)-1-methyl-2-oxo-2-[(1-phenylethyl)amino]ethyl]-2-benzofuranylmethyl ester; CP-99,994: (2S,3S)-3-(2-methoxybenzylamino)-2-phenylpiperidine; CPCCOEt: 7-(Hydroxyimino)cyclopropa[*b*]chromen-1α-carboxylate ethyl ester; CTD: Ac-RYYRWK-NH$_2$; DAMGO: Tyr-D-Ala-Gly-MePhe-Gly(ol)-enkephalin; DL-AP5: DL-2-amino-5-phosphonovaleric acid; DMH:-Δ^8-THC-11-oic acid, 1'-1'-dimethylheptyl-Δ^8-THC-11-oic acid; DOI: (+/−)-2,5-dimethoxy-4-iodoamphetamine; DPDPE: [D-Pen^2,D-Pen^5]-enkephalin; GW405833: 1-(2,3-dichlorobenzoyl)-5-methoxy-2-methyl-(2-(morpholin-4-yl)ethyl)-1*H*-indole; IP$_5$I: diinosine pentaphosphate; JYL1421: [*N*-(4-*tert*-butylbenzyl)-*N*′-[3-fluoro-4-(methylsulfonylamino)benzyl]thiourea; KJM429: [*N*-(4-*tert*-butylbenzyl)-*N*′-[4-(methylsulfonylamino)benzyl]thiourea; α,β-meATP: α,β-methylene-ATP; MED: Medetomidine; 2MeSADP: 2-methylthioadenosine 5′-diphosphate; MPEP: 2-methyl-6-(phenylethynyl)pyridine; Nor-BNI: Nor-binaltorphimine; [Nphe^1]: [Nphe^1]N/OFQ(1–13)NH$_2$; PEA: palmitoylethanolamide; *rac*-5a: hexahydropyrrolo[3,4-*c*]pyr-role; PPADS: pyridoxalphosphate-6-azophenyl-2′,4′-disulfonic acid; S-DHPG: (*S*)-3,5-dihydroxyphenylglycine; SR141716A: *N*-(piperidin-1-yl)-5-(4-chlophenyl)-1-(2,4-dichlorophenyl)-4-methyl-1*H*-pyrazole-3-carboxamide; SR142948A: 2-{[5-(2,6-dimethoxyphenyl)-1-(4-(*N*-(3-dimethylaminopropyl)-*N*-methylcarbamoyl)-2-isopropyl-phenyl)-1*H*-pyra-zole-3-carbonyl]amino}adamantine-2-carboxylic acid; SR48692: 2-{[1-(-7-chloroquinolin-4-yl)-5-(2,6-dimethoxyphenyl)-1*H*-pyrazole-3-carbonyl]amino}adamantine-2-carboxylic acid; Suramin: (8-(3-benzamido-4-methylbenzamido)-naphthalene-1,3,5-trisulfonic acid; TNP-ATP: 2′,3′-*O*-(2,4,6-trinitrophenyl)-ATP; Virodhamine: *O*-arachidonoyl ethanolamine; ZP120: Ac-RYYRWKKKKKKK-NH$_2$.
[a] Antagonist.
[b] Non-selective.

Key points

- Receptors (involved in pain transmission) are classified into G-protein-coupled receptors (e.g. opioid), ligand-gated ion channels (e.g. GABA A) and tyrosine kinase-linked receptors (e.g. NGF).
- Based on *in vivo* and *in vitro* studies with laboratory animals and recombinant cell lines, a plethora of receptor systems modulate nociceptive afferent inflow, spinal transmission and descending inhibitory control.
- Primary excitatory and inhibitory receptors are those for glutamate and GABA, respectively.

- Clinically, receptor modulation of nociceptive transmission is currently centred on the use of opioids and α_2 adrenergic agonists.

Further reading

Boehm, S. & Kubista, H. (2002). Fine tuning of sympathetic transmitter release via ionotropic and metabotropic presynaptic receptors. *Pharmacol. Rev.*, **54**: 43–99.

Caterina, M.J. & Julius, D. (2001). The vanilloid receptor: a molecular gateway to the pain pathway. *Annu. Rev. Neurosci.*, **24**: 487–517.

Chizh, B.A. & Illes, P. (2001). P2X receptors and nociception. *Pharmacol. Rev.*, **53**: 553–568.

Dhawan, B.N., Cesselin, F., Raghubir, R., Reisine, T., Bradley, P.B., Portoghese, P.S. & Hamon, M. (1996). International Union of Pharmacology. XII. Classification of opioid receptors. *Pharmacol. Rev.*, **48**: 567–592.

Furst, S. (1999). Transmitters involved in antinociception in the spinal cord. *Brain Res. Bull.*, **48**: 129–141.

Mogil, J.S. & Pasternak, G.W. (2001). The molecular and behavioural pharmacology of the orphanin FQ/nociceptin peptide and receptor family. *Pharmacol. Rev.*, **53**: 381–415.

Walker, J.M., Hohmann, A.G., Martin, W.J., Strangman, N.M., Huang, S.M. & Tsou, K. (1999). The neurobiology of cannabinoid analgesia. *Life Sci.*, **65**: 665–673.

PAIN ASSESSMENT

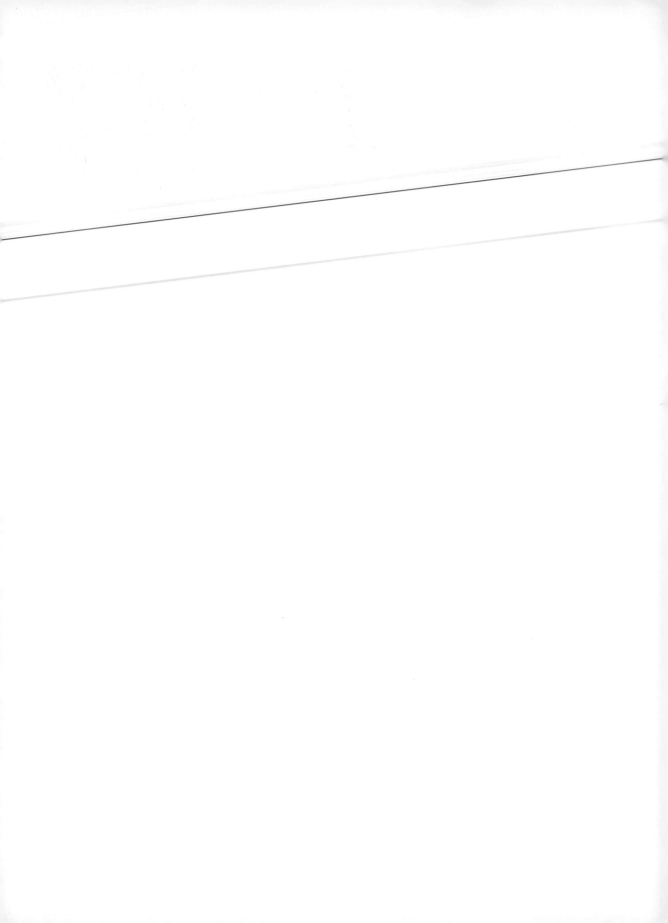

PAIN MEASUREMENT

MEASUREMENT OF PAIN IN ANIMALS

9

B.J. Kerr, P. Farquhar-Smith & P.H. Patterson

Introduction

At the turn of the last century, Sir Charles Sherrington established many of the fundamental concepts regarding how mammals respond to noxious stimuli. He proposed that specialized cells, which he termed nociceptors (from the Greek *nocere*, meaning 'to harm'), serve to alert the animal to situations where real or potential tissue damage may occur. Pain or 'nociception' as Sherrington referred to it, is a sensory experience that triggers a type of 'alarm system' in the animal. This sensory 'alarm system' can then initiate the appropriate motor output programmes that will remove the animal away from the threat. In higher vertebrates, and especially humans, the sensation of pain can often involve far more complex processes than a simple, stimulus–response reflex arc. In this case, higher cognitive functions, such as attentional state, emotion and memory are also considered critical factors in the perception of pain.

This complexity requires that many lines of scientific investigation be pursued. Reductionist approaches alone will be insufficient if advances in the development of new therapeutic strategies for pain are to be made. A mechanistic approach demands that careful study of complex animal systems at the behavioural level be carried out. Thus we will summarize:

- Fundamental principles.
- Common behavioural assays.
- Basic concepts of experimental design (referring to rodents unless otherwise stated).

Basic parameters

While it is true that the use of a behavioural model in pain research can lend a greater degree of complexity to the study, it still remains the case that these experimental 'models' are carried out in organisms that cannot verbally report their perception of sensation. In the laboratory, the examination of nociception involves the observation and estimation of reactions and reflexes to various experimental stimuli. The majority of these assays involve the brief delivery of a stimulus of sufficient intensity to activate nociceptive sensory fibres. The outcome measure or dependent variable is the presence or absence of a characteristic flexion reflex or withdrawal response. In some cases, the latency for the onset of the withdrawal response may be measured. Certain paradigms may also measure the duration of this response (i.e. when a flexion reflex is produced and the animal keeps the stimulated paw elevated for several seconds before returning to a weight bearing posture). It should be noted, however, that the presence of a flexion reflex does not necessarily imply that the stimulus was nociceptive. In certain circumstances, flexion responses may be initiated by non-painful stimulation of large diameter (non-nociceptive) mechanoreceptors that are more directly related to locomotor function than to nociceptive withdrawal. However, nociceptive withdrawal responses are more robust and can be easily distinguished from non-nociceptive, locomotor reflexes if the chosen stimulus parameters are in the range to activate nociceptive C-fibre afferents. These assays can assess an animal's sensitivity to acute noxious stimuli.

In most cases, the stimulus is presented over several trials and the mean latency to respond, or the general responsiveness (i.e. the number of responses over the trials), is recorded. A nociceptive threshold can then be established for a given animal or group of animals (often referred to as the baseline sensitivity). Experimental manipulation (i.e. pharmacological treatment) that shifts this baseline mean in subsequent trials can then be regarded as affecting the animal's nociceptive sensitivity. For example, a manipulation that shifts the response threshold or response latency above the established baseline can be regarded as antinociceptive, while a decrease in the mean is often indicative of enhanced nociceptive sensitivity or hyperalgesia.

In addition to these common stimulus–response assays, other models study more complex nociceptive behaviours. Such activity includes defensive guarding or persistent elevation of a paw, licking or vigorous shaking of the paw that is outside the animal's normal grooming pattern. These types of assays are often performed with little or no experimental intervention. That is, the experimenter is not delivering the stimulus continuously, for example, where the stimulus is a chemical algogen (see the formalin test in the next section). Moreover, in certain nerve injury paradigms (used to model neuropathic pain) spontaneous nociceptive behaviours are often measured and quantified by frequency or duration.

Models

Acute sensitivity to thermal stimuli

The standard four paradigms to measure sensitivity to noxious thermal stimuli (most commonly heat) include:

- Hot plate test (HP).
- Plantar test (PT) sometimes referred to as the 'Hargreaves test'.
- Tail flick test (TF).
- Tail immersion test (TI).

These qualitatively similar assays, deliver a thermal stimulus ($\geqslant 49°C$) to:

- A discreet region of the hind paw or tail (e.g. PT, TF).
- A broad surface area of tissue (either by direct placement of the animal on a heated surface (HP) or by immersing the animal's tail in a heated volume of water (TI).

In all four assays, the latency for a nociceptive withdrawal response is measured (i.e. tail movement, a rapid flexion of the hindlimb, a jump or licking of the stimulated area). During measurements a cutoff duration of stimulus application should always be established to prevent tissue damage (which may itself alter responsiveness) from occurring with repeated testing.

Acute sensitivity to mechanical stimuli

Several paradigms have also been designed to measure sensitivity to noxious mechanical stimuli. Again these may deliver the stimulus to a discrete or broad area of tissue.

Assays, including those using von Frey hair monofilaments, assess the animal's sensitivity to punctuate mechanical stimuli. These monofilaments are calibrated to deliver a prescribed amount of force (in grams) to the stimulated region (such as the dorsal or ventral aspect of the hindpaw skin). Again, the presence or absence of a nociceptive flexion reflex in response to the stimulus is measured. Different scoring methods have been devised, depending on the

type of model or experimental manipulation used. For the most part, the determination of a 'threshold force' to elicit nociceptive withdrawal is calculated. Hairs are applied in ascending order of bending force, with each hair being applied several times in succession. The presentation of hairs of different bending force is generally separated by several minutes. The von Frey hair that elicits a nociceptive response in greater than 60% of the trials (i.e. three responses out of five applications) is considered to be threshold. However, in some instances the experiment may be designed to record the frequency of responses to a single filament. This type of paradigm is usually carried out when determining the development of mechanical allodynia (nociceptive responsiveness to a previously innocuous stimulus) in models of neuropathic pain. In this case, the von Frey hair chosen is one that elicits few or no behaviours prior to the experimental manipulation. Following the manipulation (i.e. induction of cutaneous inflammation or an injury to a peripheral nerve) the animal may display a heightened sensitivity or allodynia by responding to this stimulus.

In contrast, assays such as the tail clip test or the Randall–Silleto test characterize an animal's threshold to a mechanical stimulus. Pressure is delivered over a larger area of tissue – analogous to the hot plate or tail immersion assays. Instruments deliver a calibrated amount of pressure and the force or weight that evokes a withdrawal response or vocalization is then recorded.

Persistent/tonic nociception

The basic feature of models of persistent or tonic nociception is that they involve a single injection of a neuroactive compound that will stimulate nociceptive fibres for a prolonged period. One of the most commonly used paradigms, the formalin test, was developed in the late 1970s by Dubuisson and Dennis. In this model, a small volume (50–100 µl) of a dilute solution of formaldehyde in saline is injected subcutaneously into the ventral or dorsal hindpaw. Concentrations are in the range of 0.5–5%. This results in a characteristic, bi-phasic behavioural response (see Figure 9.1). The first phase is brief (5–10 min) and very robust responses are observed: licking, biting or vigorous shaking of the injected paw. A quiescent interphase is then observed, lasting 5–10 min with the animal resuming normal locomotion and weight bearing on the injected paw. It is followed by a prolonged 'second phase' of nociceptive behaviours characterized by much milder responses, such as flinching, excessive guarding or lifting of the

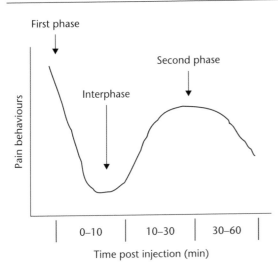

First phase

Second phase

Interphase

Pain behaviours

| 0–10 | 10–30 | 30–60 |

Time post injection (min)

Figure 9.1 Characteristic formalin response.

injected paw. A multitude of different strategies are used for the scoring and quantification of formalin-evoked behaviours.

Other models of persistent or tonic nociception have been developed to investigate visceral pain (e.g. the writhing test). In this commonly used model, a dilute solution of acetic acid is injected intraperitoneally. Within a few minutes characteristic upper abdominal wall contractions are observed and the number of these contractions over a set time period, usually 5 min, is noted. However, it is currently unclear what clinical scenario such a stimulus models, or how the activity relates to human behaviour patterns.

Inflammatory models

The common mediators used to model inflammatory injuries are carageenan and complete Freund's adjuvant (CFA) which effectively model the classical observations of rubor (redness), calor (heat), and swelling (tumour) seen after tissue injury. After subcutaneous injection in the dorsal or ventral surface of the paw both substances reliably induce cutaneous inflammation, which is accompanied by oedema, swelling and erythema of the tissue. Nociceptive sensitivity is then assessed using behavioural paradigms described above (e.g. HP). Hypersensitivity to both thermal and mechanical stimuli is generally observed within minutes to hours after the injection. This can last from days to weeks, depending on the concentration and site of injection. In general, the use of carageenan produces a much milder syndrome. Normal sensitivity may return approximately 24 h after injection if relatively low concentrations of carageenan (i.e. a 2% solution) are used.

Injection of inflammatory mediators into hollow viscera, such as the urinary bladder and gut has also been used to model visceral inflammatory pain. For example, intravesicular turpentine induces many characteristics of visceral hyperalgesia including visceral hyper-reflexia and referred somatic pain.

Nerve injury–neuropathic pain models

A significant amount of pain research has focused on chronic pain of neuropathic origin. Several animal models of neuropathic pain have been developed to reflect the aberrant sensitivity to thermal and mechanical stimuli known to occur in humans with neuropathic pain. Each of these neuropathic models evokes a unique set of physiological and anatomical changes at the level of the nerve, the dorsal root ganglia and the spinal cord. However, they have all been found to produce robust and reliable changes in nociceptive behaviours in response to both thermal and mechanical stimulation.

Chronic constriction injury

Chronic constriction injury (CCI) serves as a model of partial nerve injury. The sciatic nerve is exposed at mid-thigh level and the nerve is constricted with four loose, chromic catgut ligatures, separated by approximately 1 mm. The ligatures do not completely sever axons but induce a constriction of the nerve in which subsets of fibres die off gradually. Concern about the variability of ligature placement and the degree of constriction produced by this procedure led to further models:

- *Partial sciatic nerve injury or Seltzer model*: In this model the sciatic nerve is exposed and a single ligature is used to tie off and completely ligate approximately one half to one-third of the diameter of the nerve.
- *Spinal nerve ligation or 'Chung' model*: This model involves a complete ligation of a spinal nerve in close proximity to the dorsal root ganglion (DRG). Although much more invasive, its use has become widespread due to the diminished variability in the injury produced. In its original conception, this involved the exposure and tight ligation of both the L5 and L6 but a modified version where only the L5 spinal nerve is tightly ligated is preferred.

Inflammatory injury (neuritis model)

Since human neuropathic pain only rarely involves complete transection of nerve fibres, a neuropathic model has been developed where the injury arises from a focal inflammatory reaction around the nerve induced by:

- Carageenan.
- CFA.
- Extract of yeast cell walls.
- Zymosan.

These stimuli model the role of inflammatory and immune cells in the development of chronic nociceptive hypersensitivity after peripheral nerve injury in the absence of overt axon transection.

Limitations of behavioural assays

These behavioural models have been rigorously characterized for their validity and reproducibility and are in common use today. They are however limited because the measurement of pain is often an approximation. Measurement involves a high degree of subjectivity between:

- The responsiveness of different animals.
- Observers quantification of these behaviours.

Thus, the subjectivity of these types of observations can produce a high degree of experimental bias. These common pitfalls can be remedied by designing experiments with the proper controls:

- Experimenter blindness (i.e. the observer is unaware of any treatment the animal has received).
- Use of proper negative control or sham groups.
- Using a single observer throughout the course of an experiment.

Key points

Behavioural methods of measuring pain in animals involve observing activities and comparing them to normal. Thus, locomotor activity may be altered (e.g. licking, biting):

- Spontaneous responses to stimuli, which may be:
  - Inflammatory (e.g. sub-cutaneous formalin).
  - Neuropathic (e.g. nerve ligation).
  - Visceral (e.g. intra-luminal chemicals).

- Induced responses to stimuli observed in a number of domains:
  - Thermal (applied to discrete or broad tissue areas).
  - Mechanical (applied to discrete or broad tissue areas).

Further reading

Overviews on nociceptive testing in animals

Dubner, R. & Ren, K.E. (1999). Assessing transient and persistent pain in animals. In: Wall, P.D. & Melzack, R. *Textbook of Pain*, 4th edition. Churchill Livingstone, Edinburgh; pp. 359–369.

Le Bars, D., Gozariu, M. & Cadden, S.W. (2001). Animal modes of nociception. *Pharmacol. Rev.*, 53: 597–652.

The formalin test and scoring strategies

Debuisson, D. & Dennis, S.G. (1977). The formalin test: a quantitative study of the analgesic effects of morphine, meperidine, and brain stimulation in cats. *Pain*, 4: 161–174.

Watson, G.S., Sufka, K.J. & Coderre, T.J. (1997). Optimal scoring strategies and weights for the formalin test in rats. *Pain*, 70: 53–58.

The use of the plantar test for thermal nociceptive testing

Hargreaves, K., Dubner, R., Brown, F., Flores, C. & Joris, J. (1988). A new and sensitive method for measuring thermal nociception in cutaneous hyperalgesia. *Pain*, 32: 77–88.

Models of neuropathic pain

Bennett, G.J. & Xie, Y.K. (1988). A peripheral mononeuropathy in rat that produces disorders of pain sensation like those seen in man. *Pain*, 33: 87–107.

Chacur, M., Milligan, E.D., Gazda, L.S., Armstrong, C., Wang, H., Tracey, K.J., Maier, S.F. & Watkins, L.R. (2001). A new model of sciatic inflammatory neuritis (SIN): induction of unilateral and bilateral mechanical allodynia following acute unilateral peri-sciatic immune activation in rats. *Pain*, 94: 231–244.

Eliav, E., Herzberg, U., Ruda, M.A. & Bennett, G.J. (1999). Neuropathic pain from an experimental neuritis of the rat sciatic nerve. *Pain*, 83: 169–182.

Kin, S.H. & Chung, J.M. (1992). An experimental model for peripheral neuropathy produced by segmental spinal nerve ligation in the rat. *Pain*, 50: 355–363.

Seltzer, Z., Dubner, R. & Shir, Y. (1990). A novel behavioural model of neuropathic pain disorders produced in rats by partial sciatic nerve injury. *Pain*, 43: 205–218.

10

R.B. Fillingim

Pain measurement is a critical issue, because it serves as the primary basis for determining pain-related diagnoses and treatment efficacy. However, pain is by definition an internal and personal phenomenon; therefore, clinicians and scientists must infer a patient's pain experience entirely from indirect measures. This chapter will discuss the multiple methods of pain assessment that are available, including consideration of the circumstances under which each method may be most useful. Before reviewing specific methods, a brief overview of important issues in pain measurement will be provided.

Issues in pain measurement

Pain assessment must accommodate the complexity and multidimensionality of the pain experience. For example, the International Association for the Study of Pain's definition of pain states 'pain is an unpleasant sensory and emotional experience....' Optimal pain assessment should include measurement of both the sensory and emotional dimensions of pain. Unfortunately, the most commonly used pain scales represent one-dimensional measures of pain severity (e.g. a single 0–10 pain rating), which fail to separate affective and sensory components. In addition, pain involves not only a perceptual experience, but also behavioural, physiological and psychological responses (e.g. see Table 10.1). Therefore, the assessment of pain must extend beyond the perceptual experience to incorporate responses from these different domains.

Self-report methods for assessing pain

In clinical settings, the most common method for assessing pain severity is an 11-point (i.e. from 0 to 10) numerical rating scale (NRS). Advantages of this method are convenience for the assessor, ease of use for the patient and relative sensitivity to treatment-related changes in pain. One criticism has been that NRSs do not actually provide ratio-level scaling of pain. Therefore, if a patient's pain is reduced from 8 to 4 after treatment, it cannot be inferred that she or he has experienced a 50% reduction in pain. From a statistical point of view this can be problematic; however, from a clinical standpoint, a reduction of such magnitude would be welcomed (whether or not it represents a true 50% decrease).

Another common method of pain assessment is verbal rating scales (VRS) in which patients choose a word that most accurately reflects their pain level (e.g. no pain, mild, moderate, severe). While numbers are often assigned to each descriptor, VRS are actually categorical and not ordinal or ratio scales (unless numerical weights for the descriptors have been empirically determined and validated).

Visual analogue scales (VAS), which involve presenting patients with a line of predetermined length anchored

Table 10.1 Multiple components of the pain response			
Perceptual	**Behavioural**	**Physiological**	**Psychological**
Pain intensity	Withdrawal	Autonomic activation	Emotional responses (e.g. anger, fear, depression)
Pain unpleasantness	Avoidance	Neuroendocrine (e.g. cortisol)	Cognitive responses (e.g. coping, appraisal)
Pain localization	Facial expression	Increased muscle activity	Cognitive performance (e.g. reaction time, memory)
Pain quality	Posture/gait		

at each end with descriptors (e.g. 'no pain' and 'most intense pain imaginable') are frequently used to assess pain. Patients place a mark bisecting the line to provide an estimate of their pain level. The length of the line leading up to the mark is recorded. VAS have excellent statistical properties, including ratio-level scaling. However, they require more time to administer and score, and some individuals have difficulty in understanding the concept. Both mechanical and

electronic VAS are available, which can enhance usability and reduce scoring errors (Figure 10.1).

In addition to these single item pain measures validated and reliable multiple item pain measures, providing more detailed assessment of pain are available. These include: the McGill pain questionnaire (MPQ), the descriptor differential scales (DDS) and the brief pain inventory (BPI).

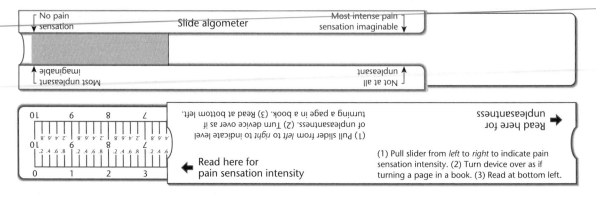

Figure 10.1 An example of a mechanical visual analogue scale (MVAS) for pain assessment. The patient views the MVAS as shown at the top and moves the sliding insert to the right. This reveals the red fill to the point that reflects his/her pain level. The clinician or investigator then turns the MVAS over (as shown at the bottom) and notes the length of the line that the patient revealed. In this example the MVAS score would be 36 mm (range is 0–100 mm). After assessing pain intensity, the same MVAS can also be used for pain unpleasantness, by rotating the MVAS 180° and instructing the patient to rate the unpleasantness of his/her pain.

Table 10.2 MPQ descriptors

1 Flickering
  Quivering
  Pulsing
  Throbbing
  Beating
  Pounding
	6 Tugging
	  Pulling
	  Wrenching
	
	7 Hot
	  Burning
	  Scalding
	  Searing
		12 Sickening
		  Suffocating
		
		13 Fearful
		  Frightful
		  Terrifying
		
		14 Punishing
			18 Tight
			  Numb
			  Drawing
			  Squeezing
			  Tearing
			
			19 Cool

2 Jumping
  Flashing
  Shooting
	8 Tingling
	  Itchy
	  Smarting
		14 Punishing
		  Grueling
		  Cruel
		  Vicious
			Cold
			  Freezing

3 Pricking
  Boring
  Drilling
  Stabbing
  Lancinating
	Stinging
	
	9 Dull
	  Sore
	  Hurting
	  Aching
	  Heavy
		Killing
		
		15 Wretched
		  Blinding
			20 Nagging
			  Nauseating
			  Agonizing
			  Dreadful
			  Torturing

4 Sharp
  Cutting
  Lacerating
	10 Tender
	  Taut
	  Rasping
		16 Annoying
		  Troublesome
		  Miserable
		  Intense
		  Unbearable	

5 Pinching
  Pressing
  Gnawing
  Cramping
  Crushing
	Splitting
	
	11 Tiring
	  Exhausting
		17 Spreading
		  Radiating
		  Penetrating
		  Piercing	

- The MPQ consists of 20 groups of single-word pain descriptors (see Table 10.2) with the words in each group increasing in rank order intensity. It yields an overall score (the pain rating index) and four subscales: sensory (sum of items 1–10), affective (sum of items 11–15), evaluative (item 16) and miscellaneous (sum of items 17–20).
- The DDS (see Table 10.3) consists of two lists of 12 words, one for pain intensity and the other for pain affect, with patients rating the extent to which each word describes their pain level. This scale has excellent statistical properties but is somewhat cumbersome.
- The BPI (see Table 10.4) asks patients to rate their worst, least, average and current pain levels using 11-point NRSs. Patients also rate the degree to which pain interferes in multiple aspects of life. A pain drawing is also included. This tool has been widely used with cancer patients. It provides information not only about pain severity, but also pain-related interference and pain location.

These scales have the disadvantage of requiring more time for administration and scoring compared to single item measures; however, they afford considerably more information. For example, the MPQ provides data regarding the quality of the pain, which can be helpful in determining diagnoses, while the BPI includes items related to the temporal characteristics and bodily location(s) of pain. Thus, the increased time required for administration of these scales offers the advantage of more detailed information regarding the nature of the patient's pain.

Quantitative sensory testing

Self-report methods are typically used in the assessment of clinical pain. However, these (and other assessment methods) can also be employed to quantify responses to pain induced via the application of controlled sensory stimuli. Quantitative sensory testing (QST) refers to the evaluation of somato-sensory responses to controlled and quantifiable physical stimuli, administered under standardized conditions. QST can be used to address a variety of questions relevant to pain:

- To examine individual difference variables (e.g. age, sex, ethnicity) and environmental factors (e.g. stress) that influence pain perception. This has relevance for both basic research and clinical pain management.
- To investigate the bio-psychosocial mechanisms involved in both normal and abnormal pain responses.
- To provide diagnostic information among patients with chronic pain and related sensory dysfunction, including mechanistically based identification of patient subgroups.
- In the assessment of clinical pain severity. For example, patients match an experimentally induced pain stimulus to their clinical pain. More sophisticated approaches, such as triangulation, may also help. Triangulation refers to a psychophysical procedure in which patients rate both their clinical pain and an experimental pain stimulus using the same measurement scale, following which they are asked to match their clinical pain to the experimental pain stimulus (see Figure 10.2). By triangulating their responses it is possible to determine whether patients are using the pain scales consistently.
- As a valuable outcome measure for documenting patients' responses to treatment. Investigators are increasingly using QST in clinical outcome studies.

Multiple sensory stimuli have been used for QST. They differ along important dimensions including temporal and spatial qualities, anatomical site stimulated,

Table 10.3 DDS for pain intensity and pain effect

DDS intensity	DDS effect
Faint	Slightly unpleasant
Moderate	Slightly annoying
Barely strong	Unpleasant
Intense	Annoying
Weak	Slightly distressing
Strong	Very unpleasant
Very mild	Distressing
Extremely intense	Very annoying
Very weak	Slightly intolerable
Slightly intense	Very distressing
Very intense	Intolerable
Mild	Very intolerable

Table 10.4 Items included on the BPI

Pain ratings (0–10)	Interference of pain in activities (0–10)
Current pain	General activity
Worst pain (last 24 h)	Mood
Least pain (last 24 h)	Walking ability
Average pain (last 24 h)	Normal work
	Relations with other people
	Sleep
	Enjoyment of life

specificity of afferent fibres stimulated and whether the evoked pain mimics clinical pain (Table 10.5). The most common forms of stimulation are thermal and mechanical, due to their ease of administration and convenience. However, stimulation method(s) should be chosen based on the scientific or clinical purpose for which the QST is being used. For example, if an investigator wishes to examine alterations in pain perception among patients with musculoskeletal pain,

then a clinically relevant stimulation method that can be applied to muscle may be ideal (e.g. ischaemic). Alternatively, to investigate mechanisms associated with neuropathic pain, an experimental stimulus that mimics those pain qualities would be preferred (e.g. intra-dermal injection of capsaicin). In many situations, using multiple stimulation methods that differ along important dimensions will be most informative.

In addition to deciding on the stimulation technique, the method of assessing pain-related responses must also be considered. A common measure used in QST is the pain threshold, defined as the minimum amount of stimulation required to produce a pain. Another measure is pain tolerance, which refers to the maximum amount of stimulation an individual is willing to experience. These measures have the advantages of being intuitively appealing and quantitative. However, they are also one dimensional and likely represent some unknown combination of behavioural and perceptual measures. The self-report methods described above can also be used to assess perceptual responses to supra-threshold painful stimuli. These methods offer the advantages of permitting assessment of multiple pain dimensions and determining responses to stimuli dispersed throughout the noxious range (e.g. stimulus–response functions). Behavioural and physiological measures can also be obtained.

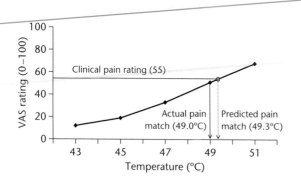

Figure 10.2 This shows a stimulus response function created by plotting a patient's ratings of thermal pain intensity across a range of temperatures. On the Y-axis, the patient's clinical pain rating is depicted (55 VAS units), from which it is *predicted* that the patient will match his/her clinical pain to a temperature of 49.3°C. The actual temperature (49°C) to which the patient matched his/her clinical pain is quite close to the predicted temperature, suggesting that this patient used the VAS scale consistently to rate both clinical and thermal pain. Triangulation provides a measure of clinical pain anchored to an experimental pain stimulus as well as an index of how consistently the patient is rating pain across modalities (i.e. clinical versus experimental).

Behavioural measures

Research in non-human animals has long relied on behavioural responses to noxious stimuli as indices of nociceptive processing. Similarly, pain can be inferred from behavioural responses in humans.

Table 10.5 Characteristics of common experimental pain stimuli

	Electrical	Thermal	Mechanical	Cold pressor	Ischaemic	Chemical
Tissue depth	Superficial or deep	Superficial	Superficial and deep	Superficial and deep	Primarily deep	Superficial or deep
Anatomical structure	Skin, muscle, viscera	Skin	Skin, muscle, viscera	Skin, muscle	Muscle	Skin, muscle
Afferent selectivity	Poor	Good	Moderate	Moderate	Moderate	Good
Temporal characteristics	Brief, repeatable	Brief or tonic, repeatable	Brief or tonic, repeatable	Tonic	Tonic	Tonic
Spatial characteristics	Small area, localized pain	Variable area, localized pain	Variable area, localized pain	Variable area, diffuse pain	Large area, diffuse pain	Variable area diffuse pain
Clinical relevance	Poor	Moderate	Moderate	Moderate	Good	Good
Quantifiable stimulus	Yes	Yes	Yes	Somewhat	Somewhat	Somewhat

Adapted from Fillingim (2002).

Technically, self-reports of pain, such as those described above, can be construed as verbal pain behaviours; however, pain behaviour typically refers to non-verbal actions. Detailed systems for coding and quantifying overt pain behaviours exhibited by patients with clinical pain have been described and validated. Commonly observed pain behaviours include guarding (e.g. limping), rubbing the painful area and facial grimacing. These behavioural measures have been correlated to patients' self-reported pain and depression. Pain behaviours increase in the presence of a solicitous spouse and are reduced by multidisciplinary pain treatment. A specific aspect of pain behaviour that has received considerable attention is the analysis of facial expressions. Methods for classifying facial expressions have been well validated in emotion research. For example, the facial action coding system provides specific criteria for judging facial expressions viewed on videotape. While this system was originally developed for the study of emotion, it has been successfully applied to experimental and clinical pain.

Heretofore, these behavioural and facial observation methods have primarily been employed in research settings, due to the time and expertise required for implementation. However, less complex systems for behavioural observation in the clinical setting have been developed, which greatly increase the practical utility of behavioural pain assessment. The major advantage of behavioural measures is their accessibility to investigators; that is, they can be directly observed and quantified. This can be particularly useful when attempting to quantify pain in patients unable to provide verbal ratings (e.g. infants, cognitively impaired patients). Moreover, both in scientific and clinical arenas, concerns are frequently expressed over the complete reliance on patients' self-reports of pain. Behavioural measures provide an additional source of data on which to base treatment decisions. Interestingly, pain behaviours and self-reported pain can provide conflicting information, presenting a dilemma for the clinician or scientist. It is important to remember that pain behaviour, while more directly observable than self-report, is not necessarily a more valid or accurate measure of patients' pain. Indeed, understanding the conditions under which self-reported pain and overt pain behaviour diverge represents an important clinical and scientific issue.

Physiological and neurological measures

Physiological measures of pain have long been sought, as clinicians and scientists desired more objective indices of pain. Autonomic responses were thought to be viable candidates, since noxious stimuli reliably elicit changes in measures including blood pressure, heart rate, electro-dermal responses and pupil dilatation. However, these responses are not specific to painful stimuli. Other emotional and physical stressors are able to evoke similar patterns of autonomic activation. Moreover, the experience of pain can be accompanied by increased responses on some autonomic indices, but blunted responses on others. Indeed, substantial individual differences are present in physiological responses to painful stimulation. A variety of muscle reflexes that appear to be related to nociceptive processing (e.g. the nociceptive flexion reflex, exteroceptive suppression of the temporalis muscle) have been described. Such reflexes have been correlated with pain reports and are sensitive to analgesic treatments. However, due to the required expertise and resources for measuring these responses, they are primarily relegated to laboratory research. In addition, they actually represent neuromuscular nociceptive responses and as such should be considered supplementary measures, rather than a substitute for assessing the perceptual experience of pain.

In recent years, functional imaging has garnered tremendous attention in pain research. In humans, techniques such as single photon emission computed tomography (SPECT), positron emission tomography (PET) and functional magnetic resonance imaging (fMRI) have been applied to quantifying cerebral activity associated with clinical and/or experimentally induced pain. These imaging methods actually detect changes in regional cerebral blood flow (rCBF), which is closely related to synaptic activity. A discussion of the advantages and disadvantages of these various imaging methods is beyond the scope of this chapter and readers are referred to Casey and Bushnell's (2000) book *Pain Imaging* for more detailed information. Imaging studies have revealed considerable, though not always consistent, information regarding pain-related cerebral responses. For example, some (but not all) clinical chronic pain conditions have been associated with decreased resting thalamic activation and many clinical pain states are characterized by increased activity in the anterior cingulate cortex. These findings in clinical populations appear to vary depending on the nature of the pain (e.g. nociceptive versus neuropathic). In experimentally induced cutaneous pain, activation in the thalamus, somatosensory cortex, anterior cingulate and insular cortices are observed. The pattern of results appears to be influenced by:

1 Temporal attributes (e.g. phasic versus tonic).
2 Location (e.g. cutaneous versus visceral).
3 Intensity of the painful stimuli.

For example, pain-related activation in multiple brain regions becomes more robust and bilateral with increased stimulus intensity, suggesting good correspondence between cerebral and perceptual responses. Brain imaging has also been used to examine endogenous pain modulation. Elegant studies, using hypnotic suggestions, have elucidated the neuroanatomical pathways involved in pain affect versus pain sensation.

Despite its successes, several limitations to these methods must be recognized. First, whether cerebral activation is 'pain related' is typically determined by measuring rCBF in areas of interest during pain stimulation and subtracting out rCBF occurring during some control stimulation (typically an innocuous stimulus from the same modality). This approach assumes that the only difference between the painful and control stimulation conditions is pain. However, this is rarely the case. For example, painful stimulation typically demands more attention and is more anxiety provoking. In addition, it may involve greater cortical effort devoted to suppressing motor responses. It may be these components of the pain condition, rather than the pain itself, that produce increased activation in some brain regions. Furthermore, increased rCBF, which reflects increased synaptic activity, could indicate either excitatory or inhibitory neural responses. In the latter case, one would expect increased activation to be related to decreased intensity of pain. Finally, these technologies remain quite expensive, require highly specialized equipment and facilities and demand considerable expertise. Therefore, their integration into routine clinical assessment is unlikely to be imminent. Nonetheless, pain imaging represents a promising approach for translational pain research and will undoubtedly expedite our understanding of the neural transmission of pain in humans.

Response bias

Response bias is another important and vexing issue in pain measurement. Response bias refers to a general phenomenon in which factors other than a patient's pain influence the values obtained from the pain response measures used. While response bias is often assumed to refer to intentional misrepresentation of pain by the patient, it actually includes a wide range of factors. For example, errors in measurement can result from patients not understanding how to use the pain scale. In addition, subtle or overt influence of the investigator or clinician on subjects' pain responses represent a form of response bias. Moreover, patients may display unwitting, but systematic inaccuracies in reporting pain based on influences, such as psychological factors, environmental contingencies or cultural variables. Obviously, response bias can substantially affect the interpretation of pain assessment results.

While it is not possible to remove all sources of response bias, several steps can be taken to reduce it:

1 Use only reliable and validated pain measures, whose psychometric properties have been demonstrated in prior research.
2 Provide specific and detailed instructions to patients regarding the use of the pain scales, for example in a practice trial ensure that the instructions are understood by explicitly stating the end points of an NRS or VAS, for example 0 represents 'no pain' and 10 represents the 'most intense pain imaginable.' These anchors are extremely important, and changing them slightly can alter the properties of the scale.
3 Use multiple measures of pain response to reveal potential response biases. For example, patients may report high levels of clinical pain on an NRS, while behavioural observation reveals minimal pain behaviour. Such discrepancies can occur for multiple reasons, but response bias is one possible explanation.
4 Incorporate QST into clinical pain assessment helping reveal response biases through methods such as triangulation. In triangulation, patients rate their clinical pain and some experimental pain stimulus using the same measurement scale, following which they are asked to match their clinical pain to the experimental pain stimulus. By triangulating their responses, it is possible to determine whether patients are using the pain scales consistently.
5 When assessing experimentally induced pain use signal detection methods, which yield two indices: discriminability and response bias. The former refers to subjects' ability to differentiate among stimuli of different intensity, while the latter refers to the tendency to describe any stimulus as painful. Thus, a direct measure that may reflect response bias is obtainable in experimental settings.

Key points

- Pain measurement serves as the foundation for determining pain-related diagnoses and documenting treatment efficacy. Therefore, valid and reliable pain measures are vital.
- Pain measurement should accommodate the multidimensional nature of pain, including assessment of both the sensory and affective qualities of pain.

- In addition to perceptual measures, assessment of behavioural and physiological pain responses can be highly valuable, especially in populations that are unable to communicate verbally.
- Recent advances in functional brain imaging have revealed important information regarding the neuroanatomical structures involved in the experience of both clinical and experimental pain. Such imaging promises to further elucidate the neural mechanisms underlying human pain responses.
- Response bias is a significant concern in pain assessment and can emanate from multiple sources. Several steps can be taken to reduce response bias, which will permit more reliable and valid pain measurement.

Further reading

Casey, K.L. & Bushnell, M.C. (eds) (2000). *Pain Imaging*. IASP Press, Seattle.

Fillingim, R.B. (2002). Sex differences in analgesic responses: evidence from experimental pain models. *Eur. J. Anaesthesiol. Suppl.*, **26**: 16–24.

Jensen, M.P., Chen, C. & Brugger, A.M. (2002). Postsurgical pain outcome assessment. *Pain*, **99**: 101–109.

Keefe, F.J. & Smith, S. (2002). The assessment of pain behavior: implications for applied psychophysiology and future research directions. *Appl. Psychophysiol. Biofeedback*, **27**: 117–127.

Price, D.D. (1994). Psychophysical measurement of normal and abnormal pain processing. In: Boivie, J., Hansson, P. & Lindblom, U. (eds) *Touch, Temperature, and Pain in Health and Disease: Mechanisms and Assessments*. IASP Press, Seattle; pp. 3–25.

Turk, D.C. & Melzack, R. (eds) (2001). *Handbook of Pain Assessment*. Guilford Press, New York.

DIAGNOSTIC STRATEGIES

11

S.I. Jaggar & A. Holdcroft

A working knowledge of pain evaluation is critical, because it serves to:

- Monitor the clinical condition over time.
- Analyse changes in response to treatment.
- Advance the principles and practice of pain management.

Moreover, The Joint Commission on Accreditation of Healthcare Organizations (JCAHO) set a standard in 2000 for all healthcare organizations. It stated that all patients have a right to appropriate assessment (and management) of pain. As with all medical interactions, such evaluation will involve history, examination and appropriate special investigations.

Issues in pain measurement

The International Association for the Study of Pain (IASP) definition of pain states that 'Pain is an unpleasant sensory and emotional experience associated with actual or potential tissue damage, or described in terms of such damage'. Full assessment therefore requires:

- Multidimensional approaches to pain evaluation.
- An awareness that it is not necessary to be able to visualize an obvious nociceptive stimulus (directly, or by means of special investigations) for spontaneous pain or a central sensitization evoked response to occur.

Both the over-worked clinician and wider society frequently overlook these central features. Medical and para-medical staff are commonly observed utilizing unidimensional (e.g. visual analogue scale (VAS) and verbal rating scale (VRS)) pain assessment tools, thus failing to address other components of pain, for example affective and cognitive responses. And how often does one hear the judgemental phrases 'a lot of the problem is in their mind' or 'this cannot be that painful' in the context of a patient (or relative) complaining of pain.

Self-report methods for assessing pain – history

Self-reporting of pain is still the most reliable indicator of pain (as opposed to nociception). This can be achieved by means of a full pain history (Chapter 12) and/or the use of specific pain assessment tools (Chapter 10). The particular method used will depend upon both the patient and the scenario. A full pain history and some of the multidimensional assessment tools (e.g. Magill Pain Questionnaire (MPQ), Descriptor Differential Scales (DDS)) are time consuming and will be inappropriate in a trauma patient in acute, severe pain – at least until a measure of analgesia has been achieved. Conversely, using a unidimensional VAS score in the context of a complex pain problem will miss important features of the syndrome. This is perhaps most likely to occur in the setting of the post-operative patient in whom neurological damage (and potential neuropathic pain) is overlooked. Choice of tool will change with time and consideration should be given to this whenever faced with an individual in pain.

There will of course be situations where the practitioner is faced with barriers to communication, complicating pain assessment. This is most common in patients: at the extremes of age (Chapters 27 and 28), who are seriously ill or intubated (Chapter 16), with emotional or cognitive difficulties, or where there is a language or cultural barrier. Pain problems in such patients are as important as in those who communicate their distress clearly. The general principles to apply when faced with such patients is to ensure (JCAHO, 2003):

- Adequate time is allowed for assessment.
- Carers, family members and translators are available to improve communication.
- Appropriate tools are available for use (e.g. MPQ has been translated and validated for at least 15 languages).
- Secondary measures (e.g. behavioural changes) are utilized only when no other alternative exists.

In general terms, pain tools may be either unidimensional, or multidimensional. They should in general have the following features:

- Easy to administer for the practitioner.
- Easily understandable by the patient.
- Be valid (does indeed measure pain).
- Highly sensitive (i.e. elicits few false negatives so that the test does not inappropriately fail to identify patients suffering pain).
- Demonstrate reliability and internal consistency:
  - Between tests (repeated testing of a patient produces consistent results).
  - Between raters (different examiners achieve the same results when applying the test to the same patient).

Unidimensional tools are highly sensitive in assessing the specific feature measured (such as pain intensity), but rarely address the other components of pain (Katz and Melzack, 1999). They have the advantage of being easy and quick to administer, in addition to being easy to score. They have been incorporated into many clinical systems (e.g. A&E evaluation, pain diaries for repeated measures, post-operative pain charts). Moreover, many (e.g. VAS, numerical rating scale (NRS)) have been widely used and validated, demonstrating internal consistency and reliability. However, each is slightly different and some patients will find different systems easier to use. It is therefore important to be familiar with a range of measures. The major features of these tools are:

- VAS – this consists of a line with an anchor at each end (Figure 11.1). The line may be horizontal or vertical, but it has been found that patients find the vertical scale easier to use and it is more sensitive than the horizontal scale.
- NRS – consists of a line with anchors at either end, but in addition numbers between the anchors (Figure 11.2). It is sometimes used in response to the request 'give me a number for your pain intensity from 1 to 10'.
- VRS – a group of ranked words is used (e.g. for pain intensity: mild, moderate and severe). This type of verbal scale is useful if a person has visual or motor impairment.

Multidimensional tools, such as MPQ (Melzack, 1975) or brief pain inventory (BPI), can be extremely sensitive at assessing all the pain components. Many have been validated across a range of languages and cultures and demonstrate high levels of consistency and reliability. However, they take some time to become familiar with, so that they can be appropriately administered. Furthermore, they may take some time to complete, score and analyse the results, limiting

their use in some circumstances. Examples of these tools are given in Chapters 10.

Examination

Currently there is no bedside examination, analogous to performing a non-invasive blood pressure recording, that can be performed to document the amount of pain a patient is suffering (as opposed to their degree of hypertension). However, full physical examination may provide clues to the causes, effects and associated features of such pain. Thus the practitioner should actively search for:

- Known causes of pain, e.g. obvious trauma (old or new), sites of infection, abnormal mass lesions, inflammatory conditions.

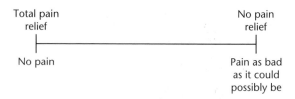

Figure 11.1 Example of a VAS for pain assessment. A 10 cm line is anchored at either end with a description of the pain level appropriate to mark at that site. No other descriptions are given. The patient is asked to mark the line at the level that best describes their pain. The assessor then measures the distance along the line. As shown in this VAS, the scale can be manipulated to demonstrate pain (lower anchors) or degree of pain relief (upper anchors).

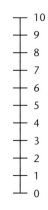

Figure 11.2 Example of an NRS for pain assessment. The 10 cm line is anchored at either end, but also features descriptive information (in this case in the form of numbers, not words) along its length. This scale has demonstrated both consistency and internal validity.

- Secondary features associated with pain in all body systems, e.g. signs of:
  - Disuse, e.g. muscle wasting, chest infection.
  - Sympathetic overdrive, e.g. tachycardia, tachypnoea, sweating.
- Associated features of conditions known to cause pain. This will involve all systems, but should particularly include:
  - Neurological system – motor, sensory and autonomic alterations indicative of nerve damage should be examined for.
  - Skin, for example changes associated with complex regional pain syndrome (CRPS).

Special tests

Quantitative sensory testing

This is the quantification of responses to specific stimuli of known type and degree (Chapter 10). Most commonly used in the research setting, but may helpfully document status in complex patients.

Behavioural testing

The most commonly used example of this is the facial action coding system (FACS). This is most likely to be useful where there are difficulties with achieving patient self-reporting. Unfortunately cultural differences in responses to pain are common and frequently complicate the picture in patients whose mother tongue is not the same as the examiner.

Physiological and neurological measures

Vital signs

Vital signs (e.g. pulse rate, blood pressure) have traditionally been used to confirm or exclude the presence of pain. However, they have very poor sensitivity (falsely fail to identify real pain) and specificity (identify many causative conditions in addition to pain). They should therefore only be used as a last resort.

Electromyography

This can provide objective documentation and assessment of neuromuscular function in the clinical setting. A fine needle electrode is placed in the muscle under examination and action potentials from it are recorded under conditions of rest, passive contraction and active contraction against resistance. Under normal conditions this results in no activity with the muscle at rest and smooth waves during contraction (the frequency and amplitude of which depend upon muscle bulk and force of contraction). Radiculopathy, neuropathy and myopathy result in differing patterns of activity at rest and altered activity during contraction. Since anti-cholinergic agents may influence the findings and anti-coagulants may result in excessive bleeding from the electrode site, patients should always contact the department prior to their arrival to check any necessary alterations in drug therapy.

Following electromyography (EMG) studies, patients have reported both a reduction and an increase in pain. Despite this, the technique is finding increased use in the context of biofeedback programmes. This rests upon the premise that increased abnormal muscle activity may itself result in pain. By using visual cues of muscle activity, patients may be actively taught to relax muscles.

Nerve conduction studies

Objective studies to determine the speed of neuronal transmission are usually performed in conjunction with EMG. Two skin surface electrodes are utilized; one placed over the nerve under test (stimulating) and the other over the muscle it supplies (recording). The time taken from nerve stimulation to muscle contraction can then be recorded and compared to nomograms. Some patients find this procedure, with the associated discomfort and tingling, unpleasant. However, since it may be helpful in the diagnosis of radiculopathy, entrapment and peripheral neuropathy, it is important to support patients through the procedure.

Positron emission tomography (PET)

This technique can provide information regarding cerebral metabolic activity. Labelled chemicals and drugs highlight areas where synaptic or cellular activity is high. As regards the brain, this is not necessarily analogous to neuronal activity, since non-neuronal support elements will also light up positively (May et al., 1999). Particular compounds will localize to particular areas (hydrogen ions label water and demonstrate blood flow) and provide information related to that area. A further problem with the current generation of scanners is the relatively poor spatial and temporal resolution possible (when compared to functional magnetic resonance imaging (fMRI)). The scan is performed by administering a radioactive tracer, with a very short half-life. This produces positively charged electrons (positrons) that can be detected by a specialized scanner. Numerous functionally distinct areas have been shown to exhibit activation in association with painful stimuli (including the thalamus, anterior cingulate and primary and secondary somatosensory cortical areas). Some groups have demonstrated that such activation occurs bilaterally when the perceived pain intensity is high. Others have reported alterations during hypnosis. Currently the meaning of such findings is under debate and the technique remains in the research arena.

Single photon emission computerized tomography (SPECT)

Like the PET scan this investigation depends upon intravenous administration of a radionucleotide. The radiation is detected during its passage in the blood vessels, providing information about blood flow.

Functional magnetic resonance imaging(fMRI)

This technique detects blood flow in an organ under examination (in the case of pain, usually the brain). It depends upon the tissue magnetic susceptibility of the iron component being much greater for deoxygenated than oxygenated haemoglobin. Thus alterations in cerebral blood flow will be clearly visualized. The spatial (1–2 mm) and temporal (~500 ms) resolution provided is more precise than that provided by PET scanning, but brain activity is not directly measured (only inferred from alterations in blood flow). A single high-resolution scan provides anatomical information (Davis *et al.*, 1998). In the research setting this can be followed by multiple low-resolution scans in the presence and absence of painful stimuli.

Key points

- Pain evaluation allows measurement and monitoring over time. It documents responses to treatment and provides a tool for analysis of both individual patients and general audit data.
- Patient self-report is the most important feature of pain evaluation. Wherever possible all areas of the painful experience are identified including intensity, but also affective and cognitive components.
- Physical examination may support diagnoses associated with pain.
- Special investigations cannot replace adequate history taking, but may provide objective documentation of tissue damage – both neuronal and other tissue.

References

Davis, K.D., Kwan, C.L., Crawley, A.P. & Mikulis, D.J. (1998). Event-related fMRI of pain: entering a new era in imaging pain. *Neuroreport*, **9**: 3019–3023.

JCAHO (2003). Improving the quality of pain management through measurement and action (available through www.jcaho.org).

Katz, J. & Melzack, R. (1999). Measurement of pain. *Surg. Clin. North Am.*, **79**: 231–252.

May, A., Buchel, C., Bahra, A., Goadsby, P.J. & Frackowiak, R.S. (1999). Intracranial vessels in trigeminal neuralgia transmitted pain: a PET study. Neuroimage, **9**: 453–460.

Melzack, R. (1975). The McGill Pain Questionnaire: major properties and scoring methods. *Pain*, **3**: 277–299.

12

PAIN HISTORY

A. Holdcroft

The key elements of a pain evaluation include a structured record of the:

1 History
  • Pain complaint.
  • Medical disease.
  • Psychological and social factors.
  • Degree of disability.
  • Medication history.
  • Treatment history.
2 Physical examination.
3 Laboratory, electrophysiological and radiological tests.
4 Diagnosis and management.

The pain complaint

A pain history is often time consuming, but can be diagnostic. During the history both the words used by the patient and their body language should be recorded. Another person may accompany the patient and their relationship should be noted. Where possible the history should be taken directly from the patient, but responses of the other person/people (verbal, etc.) can be valuable. A brief pain history mnemonic is PQRST:

  • **P**osition,
  • **Q**uality,
  • **R**adiation,
  • **S**everity,
  • **T**emporal relationship.

The expanded version is shown in Table 12.1.

The triggering event

Questions to explore this event are as follows:

  • How did it happen?
  • Where did it happen?
  • Who was involved?
  • Who may have been responsible?

Table 12.1 A structured pain history with examples of questioning

What the history should include	Examples of questions to elicit in the history
Position (location)	Where is the pain? NB. Providing a picture is useful
Quality (character/description)	What does it feel like?
Radiation	Does it go anywhere?
Severity	How bad is it?
Temporal (frequency)	Does it come and go? If so, does it occur: rapidly, daily, weekly, monthly
Onset	When did the pain start?
Multiple sites	Do you have pain anywhere else?
Aggravating factors	Does anything make it worse?
Alleviating factors	Does anything make it better?
Symptoms	Are there any associated symptoms or complaints?
Cause	What do you think the pain is due to?
Affect	What do you feel about the pain? What are your fears?
Depression	Do you feel depressed or even suicidal?
Expectations	What do you think can help the pain?
Past health	Have you managed pain/sickness before?
Activity	Does the pain limit your activity?
Therapies	What treatments have you tried? What effect did they have?

Interpretation of words used

During the description of the pain the words used should be recorded. Many of the words used will depend on the patient's vocabulary, but they can usually be classified into the categories described in the Magill pain questionnaire (MPQ) (Chapter 10 & 13):

- Sensory.
- Affective.
- Evaluative.
- Others.

Thus words such as 'dull' and 'sharp' will indicate sensory differences that may relate to the type of afferent input (C- or Aδ-fibre activity, respectively). Words such as 'fearful' may be expressing an emotive component to the pain, with words such as 'slight' indicating the amount of pain. In the chronic pain setting, where patients generally record a visual analogue score of 7 or above, these additional descriptive words are further clues to pain assessment. A formal MPQ score may be measured later in the consultation, but during the history it is better to let the patient be less structured and allow a listening process to evolve.

If sensory words are used, their timing in relation to the pain may be important (e.g. the pain of trauma is often sharp at first and then becomes duller). Words used to describe location are often helpful. Superficial or deep pain may distinguish between somatic or visceral pain. Sensory changes should be elicited – the type of clothes worn may provide a clue about allodynia (pain to touch) leading to sensory testing. Tenderness is also a valuable symptom and may be associated with muscle pain. Pain radiation is another indicator and is usually associated with a visceral component (e.g. angina radiating into the arm).

If affective words are used, the interviewer may wish to explore the reasons behind the use of these words (e.g. ask about relationships or feelings in general). The general health of the patient may reveal the cause of the use of these words (e.g. tiredness is associated with pregnancy or anaemia).

Past pain history

It is recognised that a previous history of pain may influence pain reports at a later date. Therefore, common problems should be specifically questioned for. In women a menstrual and reproductive history should be taken. All hospitalisations, trauma and surgical procedures should be documented, and for each episode a brief pain history taken. Remember, trauma includes sexual abuse of either sex at any age. This

approach may elicit additional symptoms. Moreover, it should also indicate general health and provide evidence of somatisation should it exist (i.e. symptoms are described that are real to the patient but have no pathological basis. For further information see Chapter 45). The interviewer should be attempting to assess whether the present situation is new, or part of an ongoing disorder.

Pain diary

It may not be possible in a pain history for the patient to remember the details required by the clinician. A pain diary is a useful adjunct and may reveal potential problems. It can be used to record medication and activities, as well as the amount of pain experienced.

Psychological and social factors

The patient's social situation may relate not only to the pain complaint, but also to the expected response to therapies. Social questions will include:

- Current family situation.
- Deaths.
- Employment.
- Education.
- Childhood.

It is not uncommon for pain symptoms to be related to a life event (either made worse by or start in relation to it). Questions such as 'Have you suffered a personal loss?' are part of a pain history. Death, disease and divorce are commonly described. Patients may look sad, or have difficulty concentrating and are difficult to communicate with. A tearful interview may follow such questions as 'Do you feel sad?' A referral to support services and other professional groups may be necessary. If the patient is accompanied, additional positive or negative factors may be revealed.

Where trauma is the initiating event a history of legal activity should be taken. Financial rewards may be maintaining pain – a history of disability payments, compensation awards, etc. should be included in the history.

Behavioural assessment during history taking

The patient may be willing to describe their daily function, or may find it quite difficult to develop this theme. If the patient is depressed and withdrawn very little response to questioning may result. A starting question is to ask directly how the patient reached hospital. If the history is copious and full of complaints, more specific questions are needed to reduce the time spent eliciting the basic information. Directed questions can be made about: exercise, work, housework, driving, sitting, leisure, shopping, social functioning, sexual function and sleep (e.g. 'When do you rest?', 'Do you wake up in the night?', 'How often do you drive?', 'How much time have you had off work in the last month?'). If goal setting is required, or to examine realism among the pain complaints, the patient can be asked what they would like to do that they cannot do at present because of the pain. A ranked order (from easy to hard to achieve) may be a suitable target for treatments.

A baseline assessment of behaviour is useful and its relation to factors, such as diurnal variation, response to analgesics and location during activity. Activity can be quantified (unlike subjective assessments, such as pain intensity) and may be recorded in a pain diary as time 'up' and time 'down'.

Aggravating/relieving factors may indicate the types of behaviour that are avoided or sought. Questions may relate to many different experiences:

- Local sensations (heat, cold, vibration).
- Climate (wet, dry, hot cold).
- Massage (physiotherapy, alternative practitioners).
- Daily activity (straining, getting up, lying down, sitting, standing, coughing, drinking).
- Exercise (running, walking).
- Feelings (anxiety, tiredness, anger).
- Environment (noise).

Medication

A full medication history includes the following questions:

- What drugs are you taking now?
- What drugs have you taken before?
  - Including: name, dose, duration of use and effect.
- Why was the medication stopped?
  - Did this relate to effectiveness or poor tolerance?
- How do you use medication?
  - Regularly, on demand (i.e. only when in pain).
  - Non-compliant (prescribed drugs but avoids them).
- Do you use recreational drugs?
  - Alcohol, tobacco, others.
- Do you take drugs to help mood or sleeping?
- Do you take medications that are over the counter/ not prescribed/homeopathic, etc.?
- Who is prescribing your medications?
  - Ask about drug problems/drug abuse (see Chapter 46).

A good history should confirm any drug problem; for example, multiple therapies for the same condition, allergies, abuse. It should also identify if drugs have been used in appropriate dosage and for a reasonable period to test their efficacy. It may be necessary to ask the patient's general practitioner for more details; for example, if a patient is unaware of the drugs they have tried or are taking.

Previous pain therapies other than medication

A review of previous pain therapies may reveal patient preferences, beliefs, cognition and potential compliance. The list of therapies may include:

- *Physical therapies* – for example, acupuncture, braces, casts, trigger point injections, exercises, trans-cutaneous nerve stimulation, chiropractic, homeopathy and physiotherapy.
- *Situational therapies* – for example, hypnosis, relaxation and behavioural therapy.

The choice of therapies selected by a patient may reflect economic circumstances or social pressures. History elicited from a patient may usefully start a dialogue with the patient about causes of pain and their relevant therapies.

Interview of 'significant other'

All questions should be directed at investigating the patient and occur with the patient's permission:

- What changes have you observed in the patient?
- How do you know when the patient is in pain?
- Do you think the pain has been getting worse?
- How do you cope with the pain?

Key points

A structured history will include:

- The pain complaint in relation to present and past history, medications and therapies.
- Medical and psychiatric disorders.
- Social and physical disability assessment.
- Identification of reinforcing factors, cognition and behavioural responses to pain.

Further reading

Fields, H.L. (1987). *Pain*. McGraw-Hill Book Company, New York.

PSYCHOLOGICAL ASSESSMENT

13

E. Keogh

Overview

Our current understanding of pain is that it is not just a sensory experience but also has a psychological component. What we think, what we feel and how we behave can all influence the experience of pain. Indeed, such cognitive, emotional and behavioural processes are believed to moderate pain sensation by inhibiting or facilitating noxious signals. The fact that pain experiences can have little to do with nociception or tissue damage and much more to do with how patients respond to pain has important implications for pain management. The primary objectives of this chapter are therefore to:

- Provide readers with an overview of the contribution that psychology has made to our understanding of the experience of pain.
- Outline some of the main methods used to evaluate such psychological processes.

Role of psychology in the experience of pain

Emotions and moods

One of the main psychological responses to pain is an emotional one. When in pain, patients often report feeling anxious, depressed, angry and/or frustrated. Although the terms emotion and mood are often (and confusingly) used interchangeably they should be considered conceptually distinct. Emotions are discrete states, relatively short in duration (seconds, minutes), have a rapid onset and are usually caused by specific events. Moods are of longer duration (days, months), relatively stable, gradual and often non-specific. Although the casual link between emotions and moods its not always clear, the two are certainly related. For example, someone with a stable negative mood is more likely to experience extreme (emotional) fear when they perceive themselves to be in a painful situation. Furthermore, over time negative emotions can become relatively stable moods, and if extreme may also become the focus for treatment.

Although there are many different types of emotion and mood, the greatest focus has been on those with a negative tone. Few investigations have examined positive emotions, such as joy and contentment. Most studies have examined anxiety and depression, which is not surprising given that both can indicate serious mental illness. Depression is defined as a tendency towards experiencing negative thoughts and feelings about past events. It is associated with a lack of positive affect (anhedonia), greater hopelessness and withdrawal. Anxiety, also has a strong negativity component, but is generally associated with extreme concerns, worries, and fears about potential future events. Clinically, there are a number of different types of anxiety, including generalised anxiety disorder, phobias (social events, spiders, etc.), panic disorder, obsessive-compulsive disorder and post-traumatic stress disorder. Although this means that it is difficult to determine exact prevalence rates among pain patients, chronic pain patients seem to experience greater depression and anxiety when compared to the general population.

In terms of the effects that such negative emotions and moods have on chronic pain patients, depression and anxiety predict a range of negative outcomes, including greater pain, disability, health care utilisation and longer time to get back to work. Among acute pain patients it has been shown that pre-operative anxiety and depression are good predictors of post-operative pain, analgesic use, length of hospital stay and recovery. Finally, within non-clinical healthy individuals, anxiety and depression are associated with sensitivity to experimentally induced pain, for example lower pain threshold and tolerance levels. Understandably therefore, the role that emotions have in the experience of pain seems critical to our ability to provide effective pain management interventions (Summary 13.1).

Cognitive factors

Alongside understanding how people in pain feel, psychologists have also been interested in how people think about their pain. Particular focus has been placed on patients' information processing systems,

---

Summary 13.1 Emotions, moods and pain

- Emotions and moods are important psychological constructs that change in response to pain.
- Negative emotions, such as anxiety and depression, can maintain chronicity.
- Such negative emotions are often targeted in pain management interventions.

Summary 13.2 Cognition and pain

- How people think affects pain sensitivity.
- Cognitive biases exist in attention and memory for pain material.
- Appraisals, judgements and decision-making can influence pain behaviours.

---

examining: perceptual, attentional and memory processes, as well as appraisal, decision-making and reasoning. Such processes are thought to directly influence how successful people are in being able to manage their pain.

Investigations into the perception of pain involve basic psychophysics. They specifically focus on the way in which different types and intensities of noxious information are processed in normal and clinical pain states. For example, distinctions have been made between different types of threshold, e.g. sensation and pain thresholds. The perceptual heat threshold of most C-fibre heat-sensitive nociceptors ranges between 39°C and 41°C, whereas thermal heat pain threshold is around 45°C.

Attention involves the selective processing of incoming sensory information. Investigations have included assessment of the stage at which such selection occurs, for example pre-conscious or conscious levels. Hyper-vigilance for pain-relevant material has not only been found in pain patients, but also within healthy individuals who fear pain sensations, suggesting that such biases may form part of shared (latent) vulnerability triggered by pain.

Memory is also affected by pain. Not only do pain patients selectively recall more negative information than healthy controls, but also depression seems to increase such biases. These cognitive biases are believed to reinforce and maintain negative emotional states, such as post-traumatic stress disorder and depression. They are therefore relevant to our understanding of chronicity.

Cognitions (and emotions) are also thought to influence appraisal processes, judgements and decision-making. For example, applying Lazarus and Folkman's (1984) model of stress and coping to pain, it is believed that in a pain-related situation, they are initially appraised as to whether they are irrelevant, positive, or negative. Secondary appraisals then occur, which influence emotional responses to the event, including which coping strategies will be attempted, as well as subsequent behaviours. What we think and feel about pain, therefore influences how we act (Summary 13.2).

Pain behaviours

When in pain it is believed that patients engage in a wide range of pain-related behaviours, such as taking medication, careful movement and avoidance behaviours. Such 'pain behaviours' are often considered to be maladaptive since they not only result in negative avoidance and increased passivity (e.g. bed rest, complaining), but also reduce more positive adaptive behaviours, such as exercising and socialising. It is believed that such maladaptive pain behaviours are positively reinforced by patients (and sometimes their family members), increasing the likelihood of reoccurrence. Conversely, positive behaviours are negatively reinforced (i.e. punished through pain sensations) and so are less likely to be repeated. This leads to the interesting, yet counter-intuitive scenario, in which allowing oneself to experience pain might be instrumental in leading towards better outcome.

Coping behaviours have been conceptualised as either *avoidant* (e.g. denial, distraction, repression and suppression) or *non-avoidant* (e.g. attention, focused problem solving). However, others have argued such coping behaviours should be considered as either *active* (e.g. exercise, activity) or *passive* (e.g. withdrawal, rest, medication use). Whichever description is used however, the typical finding is that in the long-term, avoidant, passive coping behaviours are associated with less positive outcomes, such as poorer functioning and greater disability. Treatment-outcome studies confirm this view. They reveal that the teaching of positive pain coping strategies is associated with greater psychological adjustment, as well as improvements in pain reports and disabilities.

Although we have separated emotions, cognitions and behaviours, it is clear that there is some overlap between them. Two coping behaviours that have strong emotional and cognitive components are catastrophising and fear avoidance. Catastrophising is viewed as a negative cognitive process, associated with exaggerated negative rumination and worry. It is related to a wide range of different pain behaviours, such as increased pain reports, higher analgesic use, as well as poorer adjustment, greater disability and psychosocial

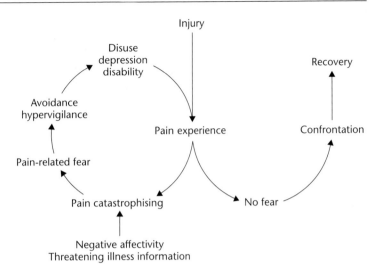

Figure 13.1 Vlaeyen, J.W.S. & Linton, S.J. (2000). Fear avoidance model of pain. Fear avoidance and its consequences in chronic musculoskeletal pain: a state of the art. *Pain*, **85**: 317–332. Copyright 2000 by International Association for the Study of Pain. Reprinted by permission.

dysfunction. Fear avoidance refers to avoidance of movement or activity based on fear of injury, which some have labelled as the irrational fear of movement. Pain-related fear is also related to avoidance, disability and impairment, so much so that fear of pain has been found to be more disabling that the pain itself. An example of how fear avoidance behaviours, emotions and negative cognitions have all been considered together in the conceptualisation of pain can be found in Vlaeyen and Linton's (2001) fear avoidance model of pain (see Figure 13.1 and Summary 13.3).

Summary 13.3 Behaviour and pain

- Patients engage in a variety of 'pain' and 'well' behaviours.
- Psychological therapy promotes well behaviours, such as exercise, and reduces negative pain behaviours.
- Catastrophising and fear avoidance are important psychological coping constructs associated with greater disability.

Psychological evaluation

Although pain is almost universal (excluding those with some form of congenital insensitivity), it is also a very personal and private experience. The subjective multidimensional nature of pain means that reliable and valid methods of assessment are vital to the management of pain. This next section will outline the main methods used to evaluate the emotional, cognitive and behavioural components thought to be important in the experience of pain.

Self-report measures

Perhaps one of the most obvious methods of ascertaining pain and its psychological correlates is to simply ask patients to indicate how much pain they experience. For example, patients are often administrated scales using single items, e.g. on a scale of 0–10, indicate the level of pain you are experiencing; with 0 indicating 'no pain', and 10 indicating the 'worst possible pain ever'. Visual analogue scales have also been used (see Figure 13.2 – lower section). These follow a similar format but seem to be more sensitive than verbal scales. Unfortunately, such scales fail to reflect the multidimensional nature of pain; therefore alternative measures have been developed. The McGill Pain Questionnaire (MPQ) comprises a number of descriptor words that reflect the sensory (e.g. sharp, pinching, burning) and affective (e.g. punishing, frightening) components of pain. The short-form version of the MPQ is presented in Figure 13.2. Self-report methods have also been used more specifically to examine the thoughts, feelings and behaviours associated with pain.

The clinical assessment

Psychological assessment can be conducted (using a clinical interview) when the therapist wants to ascertain the complex emotional, cognitive and behavioural interactions that occur within the patient. Clinical interviews may also use psychiatric assessment tools in order to ascertain the suspected existence of an emotional and/or behavioural disorder.

Perhaps one of the most common diagnostic tools used in clinical assessment is the Diagnostic and Statistical Manual of Mental Disorders – Fourth

Please rate each of the following qualities of pain experienced on the scale of 'none', 'mild', 'moderate', or 'severe'.

	None	Mild	Moderate	Severe
Throbbing	————	————	————	————
Shooting	————	————	————	————
Stabbing	————	————	————	————
Sharp	————	————	————	————
Cramping	————	————	————	————
Gnawing	————	————	————	————
Hot burning	————	————	————	————
Aching	————	————	————	————
Heavy	————	————	————	————
Tender	————	————	————	————
Splitting	————	————	————	————
Tiring exhausting	————	————	————	————
Sickening	————	————	————	————
Fearful	————	————	————	————
Punishing cruel	————	————	————	————

Visual analogue scale
Please mark on the line below which best reflects the severity of pain that you perceive at present.

No pain   Worst possible pain

Figure 13.2 Melzack, R. (1987). The short-form McGill Pain Questionnaire. *Pain*, **30**: 191–197. Copyright 1987 by Elsevier Science Ltd. Reprinted by permission.

Edition (DSM-IV, 1994), which is published by the American Psychiatric Association. The DSM-IV is a collection of standard definitions and classifications of mental disorders used by mental health professionals. For each disorder a set of diagnostic criteria are included which indicate what symptoms must be present (and absent) in order to meet the criteria for diagnosis. Other more specific measures that are often used as part of the clinical assessment process include the Beck Depression Inventory (BDI), the Hospital Anxiety and Depression Scale (HADS) and the General Health Questionnaire (GHQ). The BDI, HADS and GHQ can be used as self-report measures, and all have standardised cut-off points that can be used to indicate a possible clinical (psychiatric) state.

The clinical interview can take either a structured or semi-structured format. With structured interviews, a set number of questions are asked, which assess core elements of interest. With semi-structured interviews, the clinician usually has a set of specific objectives (e.g. ascertain pain behaviours), but also has much greater flexibility to develop areas of particular relevance to the patient's condition. Clinical interviews can also focus specifically on certain areas of interest. For example,

behavioural interviews are used to gain a description of current patterns of pain and well behaviours, as well as identify any factors that may control behaviour. Such interviews are often conducted with family members, in order to ascertain whether they are positively reinforcing pain behaviours. This method helps target pain behaviours for intervention.

Diaries

One problem associated with self-report measures (and the clinical interview) is that they are usually conducted on one day and require the patient to generalise about the frequency of specific behaviours and feelings. A method that allows the clinician to assess the temporal relationship between pain and psychological factors is a pain diary. Diaries allow the assessment of the actual occurrence of target behaviours, in addition to helping reduce response bias and error in reporting. Information is collated and used to produce simple frequency data of behaviour use. For example, diaries are used to help ascertain uptime/downtime. Moreover, the clinician can ask the patient to complete such diaries on more than one occasion during the day. More recently hand-held computer notebooks

Summary 13.4 Pain assessment

- Emotions, behaviour and cognition should be included in the evaluation of pain patients.
- Subjective measures of pain evaluation include self-report, clinical interview and diary methods.
- Objective measures include behavioural observation and psychophysiological methods.

have been used. These are programmed to request key information at specified times during the day.

Observational methods

One of the most basic methods of measuring pain behaviours is to observe what people actually do. People in pain will often communicate their pain experiences in a non-verbal manner, whether this is through body postures or via facial expressions. Such non-verbal behaviours are particularly useful for the clinician working with groups that are unable to easily verbally communicate their experiences, such as the elderly or children. However, observation can be a time-consuming exercise, in that some effort is needed to develop naturalistic settings. There are also important issues associated with measurement; in an ideal situation patients are videotaped engaging in various behaviours, which are then rated by trained observers. Observer responses are collated and checked for consistency. Although time consuming, such observational methods can provide valuable insight into the context-specific behaviours exhibited by pain patients.

Psychophysiological measures

The final method to be considered here are psychophysiological assessment tools. The underlying assumption is that changes in the internal psychological make-up (especially emotional and cognitive) of the individual can be measured via objective physiological changes. One of the most commonly used measures is skin conductance, which varies wit changes in sweat gland activity in response to emotional stimuli. For example, increases in skin conductance have been found in acute pain patients, suggesting greater emotional arousal. Cardiovascular events, such as heart rate and blood pressure, are also believed to reflect changes in underlying emotional states. Interestingly, blood pressure is inversely related to pain sensitivity, in that hypertensives and normotensives that have high resting blood pressure, exhibit a decrease in pain sensitivity, which some believe reflects a neural overlap in the pain control (opioid) and blood pressure systems. Other cardiovascular-related indices that seem to change in response to pain include blood flow and skin temperature (e.g. vasoconstriction) (Summary 13.4).

Key points

- Pain is a subjective multidimensional construct.
- Psychological processes, such as emotions, cognition and behaviour, influence the perception and experience of pain.
- The measurement and evaluation of such psychological processes is critical to our understanding and ultimate management of pain.

Further reading

Gatchel, R.J. & Turk, D.C. (eds) (1999). *Psychosocial Factors in Pain*. Guilford Press, Edinburgh.

Keogh, E. & Herdenfeldt, M. (2002). Gender coping and the perception of pain. *Pain*, **97**: 195–201.

Lazarus, R.S. & Folkman, S. (1984). Stress, appraisal, and coping. New York: Springer.

Pincus, T. & Morley, S. (2001). Cognitive-processing bias in chronic pain: a review and integration. *Psychol. Bull.*, **127**: 599–617.

Price, D.D. (1999). *Psychological Mechanisms of Pain and Analgesia*. IASP Press, Seattle, WA.

Vlaeyen, J.W.S. & Linton, S.J. (2000). Fear-avoidance and its consequences in chronic musculoskeletal pain: a state of the art. *Pain*, **85**: 317–332.

PAIN IN THE CLINICAL SETTING

14

W.A. Macrae

Introduction

Epidemiology is the study of the distribution and determinants of diseases and the application of the findings to the control of health problems. By studying the distribution of a disease we can learn about:

- How many people are affected.
- Who is at risk.
- Causes.
- Risk factors.

Epidemiology has various applications:

- Understanding the natural history of a disease.
- Planning and evaluating services.
- Disease prevention:
  - Primary: stopping the problem from arising.
  - Secondary: early detection and treatment.
  - Tertiary: minimising impairment and disability.

Epidemiological studies of pain

The first step in the study of a disease is to define the population group and develop a valid set of diagnostic criteria. This has been a major problem in studies both on the general problem of pain as a whole and of specific conditions.

- *Prevalence* is the number of cases of a given disease in a given population at a designated time (e.g. 'point', 'period' and 'lifetime' prevalence).
- *Incidence* is the number of new cases arising during a given period in a specified population.

There have been many studies published on the prevalence of chronic pain. The results of these studies vary widely, because they used different:

- Study populations.
- Diagnostic criteria.

Studies of pain clinic patients are limited by the difference in referral patterns between clinics and an inability to define the population from which the patients are drawn. Surveys based in general practice give a better indication of the size of the problem, but have been hampered by an inability to agree standard definitions. One study showed that 63% of patients who attended general practitioners (GPs) for whatever reason had pain. Another study, which only counted those who attended because of pain, found an incidence of 22%. Studies conducted on the general population should give the best estimation of the prevalence of pain. However, the results vary from 7% to 82%, mainly because different definitions were used.

The problem of pain suffered by patients in hospital has changed little from the early studies in the 1970s. In one study of over 5000 patients (from a cross section of wards, in several different hospitals) over 60% suffered pain. In a third of these the pain was present all or most of the time, being moderate to severe in 87%. In over 40% of cases, patients had to request analgesia and the drugs did not arrive immediately.

Gender, age and pain

There is no simple relationship between gender and pain. Not only does the pattern vary across different conditions, but also across different age groups.

Pain in children received little attention prior to the 1970s (Chapter 27). Surgery and other painful procedures were routinely performed on neonates and infants without adequate analgesia. There was a widespread and erroneous belief that the immature nervous system could not appreciate pain. Post-operative pain was often inadequately treated. Thanks to the tireless efforts of a small group of basic scientists and clinicians the position has improved in recent years.

Epidemiological data on pain in children is still scarce. Although some conditions associated with pain have been studied (e.g. juvenile rheumatoid arthritis) data on pain is usually absent. Cancer in children is thankfully less common than in adults. The common types of cancer are also different (e.g. leukaemia) and are associated with less pain than the common cancers found in adults. However, the few studies in this area have shown that children do suffer pain, not only from the disease, but also from the treatment and procedures. Chronic pain syndromes in children often follow a course of remission and relapse, rather than the continuous pain usually suffered by adults. Examples include abdominal pain and limb pain, often referred to as growing pains.

Evidence concerning the prevalence of pain in older people must be interpreted with caution, as few studies have specifically addressed this problem. General population studies may miss older citizens, who may be sequestered in institutions or unable to complete questionnaires or answer telephone surveys. Studies focusing exclusively on older people find higher pain prevalence than general cross-sectional studies. As 73% of those over the age of 85 are women, gender differences obviously influence age-specific prevalence studies.

Acute pain probably has a similar incidence across all age groups, but chronic pain increases with age (up to about 65 years of age). Several painful conditions which are more likely to occur in older people (e.g. pain caused by cancer or post-herpetic neuralgia) are relatively uncommon, and so tend to be underestimated in general surveys. The most common problem is joint pains and this reflects an increasing pathological load with advancing age. The prevalence of hip and knee pain in patients over 65 is more than double that found in young adults. However, several pain syndromes actually decrease in frequency with age (e.g. headache, facial pain and abdominal pain) with chest pain being most prevalent in middle age.

Back pain

Back pain is a description rather than a diagnosis. The aetiology of back pain remains illusive, although it is clearly multifactorial involving a complex interaction of many factors: physical, psychological and social. What is clear is that it is common and that it causes much disability and work loss. The estimated days of work loss caused by back pain in Britain in 1993 was 52 million days, at a cost to the National Health Service (NHS) of £481 million.

Most people will experience back pain at some time in their life. Studies show a point prevalence of 14–30%, with a period prevalence over a year of about 40%. The lifetime prevalence is between 60% and 80%. Lifetime prevalence for sciatica is around 3–5%. Back pain however is a 'soft' measure; disability and work loss being more reliable measures, with more utility.

However, work loss is subject to several limitations, in that it:

- Only applies to the working population.
- Correlates poorly with biomedical measures of pain and clinical outcomes.
- Is also strongly influenced by the socio-economic climate.

Despite these shortcomings work loss is one of the most important consequences of back pain and, therefore, a major outcome measure of health care.

Most episodes of back pain are short lived. About 50% of acute episodes will settle in 4 weeks, but in 15–29% the problem will continue for at least a year. A fifth of back pain sufferers will continue to have back pain for long periods of their life. Disability caused by back pain is a major problem. A typical study in 1993 showed that 8% of those with back pain (or 3% of the general population) had to lie down all or most of the day, for at least 1 day in a 4-week study period, because of back pain. In this period, 6% lost at least 1 day off work, with 1% off work for the entire 4-week period. In a year, 8–20% of the population will have some time off due to back pain. The lifetime prevalence of work loss from back pain is 25–30%. About half of the lost working days are in short spells (averaging 6 days) and half in longer spells (of at least 4 weeks). The longer a person is off work with back pain, the less likely they are to return to work.

Studies on risk factors for back pain have shown that there is little difference between men and women. The problem usually starts between the late teens and early forties, with the prevalence increasing until the age of about 50 when it plateaus. Work loss due to low back pain is commoner in lower social classes; however, this may be related to manual work. Heavy manual work and perhaps driving and jobs involving exposure to whole body vibration, are risk factors for work loss due to back pain. There is an increased prevalence of low back pain in smokers.

Pain caused by cancer

Cancer is not a single disease and the prevalence of pain varies widely between different types of cancer. Cancer causes pain by various mechanisms, including involvement of bone, viscera or nerves. Pain is more prevalent in later stages of the disease and may be modified by treatment. The complexity of the problem is compounded by the fact that treatment may sometimes cause pain, or make existing pain worse. It is clear then that in any individual patient, whether they suffer pain or not depends on many factors and in practice most patients have more than one type of pain. There is evidence that pain from cancer is often inadequately treated.

The prevalence of pain in cancer varies according to how the data is collected. A study of all stages of the disease in a cancer hospital found a prevalence of 38%. However, studies of advanced cancer in hospices have found prevalences of 60–80%. The cancers that most commonly cause pain are: bone, cervix, oral cavity, stomach, lung, genitourinary, pancreas and breast. The incidence is lower in cancers such as lymphoma and leukaemia.

Pain in acquired immune deficiency syndrome

Pain is a major problem in patients with acquired immune deficiency syndrome (AIDS), particularly in the later stages of the disease. The problem is comparable to, or worse than, that found in patients with cancer. In human immunodeficiency virus (HIV)-infected patients in the early stages of the disease, the incidence of clinically significant pain has been reported at about 30%. But, in patients with AIDS the prevalence gradually increases as the disease progresses. In the early stages pain occurs in around 45% of patients, rising to almost 70% in later stages of the disease. In a hospice study, 93% of patients experienced pain in the last 2 weeks of life.

There is evidence of under-treatment of pain in patients with AIDS. Studies have shown that:

• Many patients with severe pain are not prescribed opioid analgesics.
• Adjuvant analgesics are under-utilised.
• In some cases, no analgesia at all is prescribed.

Women, less well-educated people and drug abusers are more likely to be under-treated.

Headache

Headache is the most common pain complaint. It may be secondary to other disease or a primary problem. Primary headache divides broadly into:

• The migraines.
• Cluster headache.
• Tension-type headache.

Migraine affects about 15% of the population. It is two to three times more common in women, although in children the prevalence is the same in both sexes. The peak onset in females is between 14 and 16 years,

for males it is 10 and 12 years. It rarely starts after age 50. The median frequency of attack is 1.5 per month, but 10% of migraineurs have weekly attacks. There is clear evidence for genetic factors, which are complex.

Cluster headache by contrast is rare, and five times more common in males than females. The onset is normally between the ages of 20 and 40.

There are several forms of tension-type headache. It is probably commoner than migraine, with a lifetime prevalence of around 80%, but prevalence decreases with age. It is commoner in women than men.

Tension-type headache and migraine may occur in the same patient.

Neuropathic pain

Neuropathic pain is a mechanism-based diagnosis that cuts across anatomical and pathological criteria. One of the unanswered questions is why some patients with diabetes, shingles, trauma or surgery, will develop pain, but others will not. Recent work in mice suggests there may be a genetic predisposition. The prevalence of neuropathic pain in the population has been quoted as 1%, but it varies with aetiology and across different age groups. For example, in post-herpetic neuralgia the overall incidence in patients who have had shingles is 9–34%. The incidence increases with age, and by age 60 years 50% of patients will be affected. In diabetics, about 45% will develop neuropathy over a 25 year course. The incidence of chronic post-surgical pain varies according to the type of operation. For example, for breast reduction the quoted incidence is 22% but for mastectomy and reconstruction it is 49%.

Pain after amputation

Following amputation almost all patients will experience phantom sensations, and for about 70% of lower limb amputees these will be painful at some time. Many amputees also experience stump pain and back pain. The natural history of phantom pain is variable; in some patients it seems to improve with time, but in others it can stay the same or get worse. In a population of amputees, the prevalence of phantom pain will remain fairly constant. It can arise immediately after amputation but has been reported to start as late as 2 years after amputation. Risk factors have been extensively investigated: sex, age, site of amputation, reason for amputation, ethnicity and educational level are not predictive. Severity of pain prior to amputation seems to be a positive risk factor. There is some evidence that early use of a prosthesis decreases the incidence of phantom pain and may prevent the remapping that occurs in the primary sensory cortex after amputation. From the point of view of primary prevention, as most amputations are caused by vascular disease, stopping smoking would be a major contribution.

Chronic widespread pain and fibromyalgia (Chapter 19)

Many patients who attend GPs and pain clinics complain of widespread musculoskeletal pain. Fibromyalgia, where muscular tenderness predominates, may represent one end of a spectrum of syndromes of widespread pain. Many have other symptoms as well, including: headache, bowel and bladder dysfunction, circulation problems, sleep disorder and fatigue. Prevalence rates vary (as usual) according to diagnostic criteria, but also with age and sex. Two large surveys of over 4000 people in Britain and the USA found a prevalence for chronic widespread pain of about 10%, higher in women than men and increasing with age. Studies on fibromyalgia, with more specific criteria, showed a lower prevalence, around 1–3%.

Key points

- Pain is a common complaint.
- Studying distribution and natural history of disease may help formulate new treatments.
- Prevalence rates vary with diagnostic criteria.

Further reading

Breitbart, W. (1998). Pain in AIDS: an overview. *Pain Rev.*, 5: 247–272.

Clinical Standards Advisory Group (1994). *Epidemiology Review: The Epidemiology and Cost of Back Pain*. HMSO, London.

Crombie, I.K., Croft, P.R., Linton, S.J., LeResche, L. & Von Korff, M. (1999). *Epidemiology of Pain*. IASP Press, Seattle.

Last John, M. (2001). *A Dictionary of Epidemiology*, 4th edition. Oxford University Press, New York.

B.J. Collett

Epidemiological studies

Epidemiological studies have shown wide variation in their estimates of chronic pain in the community ranging from 7% to 54%. Most of these studies are cross sectional; that is, they provide information at only one point of time. However, a recent longitudinal study reported pain prevalence in the same community over a 4-year period. There was no significant difference in pain reports between men and women at baseline. The proportion of the population reporting chronic pain significantly increased with age. The overall prevalence of pain increased from 45.5% of the population at baseline to 53.8% at follow-up; that is, an increase of 8.3% over the 4 years. There was a larger increase in prevalence among women than men and the increase was highest in the youngest age group (25–34 years). Of those who had pain at baseline, the pain persisted in 78.5% and resolved in 21.5%. Health factors (as measured by the SF-36) appeared to be better predictors of chronic pain rather than measured socio-demographic factors (such as level of education, marital status, housing or employment status). Individuals who were in the lowest quartile of SF-36 domains – physical functioning, social functioning and bodily pain at baseline – were more likely to develop chronic pain at follow-up and less likely to recover from chronic pain. This study reinforces previous work that has shown chronic pain to be a common and persistent problem in the community. In this study, health factors appeared to be better predictors of onset or recovery from chronic pain than socio-demographic factors.

Prevention

Primary prevention is intended to prevent a disease or symptom from occurring. Secondary prevention is aimed at early detection so that treatment begins before it becomes chronic. In the pain context, strategies to prevent acute back pain from becoming chronic, or antiviral treatment of acute herpes zoster infection to prevent post-herpetic neuralgia would be

good examples. Tertiary prevention seeks not to prevent disease or symptoms, but to minimise disability and handicap arising from it. Illness behaviour and psychological morbidity can develop following the onset of chronic pain and tertiary prevention would be aimed at reducing these sequelae.

Epidemiologists describe a web of causation and group aetiological factors under three headings: agent, host and environment. These factors do not act in isolation but interact and are often represented as the triangular web of causation (Figure 15.1).

Causative agents include physical trauma (such as surgery, heavy lifting and accidents) and infective agents (including herpes zoster). Host factors can modify the impact of these physical factors. For example, the likelihood that herpes zoster will lead to post-herpetic neuralgia will depend on the age of the patient. Potential host influences, such as psychological, immunological, physiological and anatomical factors, are also important. Environmental factors comprising

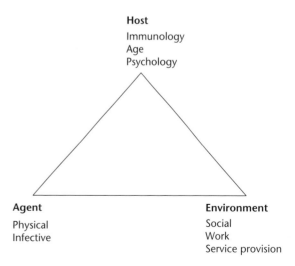

Host
Immunology
Age
Psychology

Agent
Physical
Infective

Environment
Social
Work
Service provision

Figure 15.1 The web of causation. With permission from Crombie, I.K. (1997). Epidemiology of persistent pain. In: Jensen, T.S., Turner, J.A. & Wiesenfeld-Hallin, Z. (eds). *Proceedings of the 8th World Congress on Pain, Progress in Pain Research and Management*, Vol. 8. IASP Press, Seattle.

the social context in which the patient lives and works are a significant influence. For example, the concept of a solicitous spouse reinforcing pain behaviour is well established. Environmental factors relating to work, such as compensation for work injury or work dissatisfaction may be relevant.

Pain progression

One of the greatest puzzles in our understanding of pain is why some injuries lead to pain that continues for months or years, whereas other acute pains come and go as expected. The concept that chronic pain is multifactorial in origin has evolved to explain this. The endogenous mechanisms that modulate and control pain may be genetically determined. The balance between the extent of tissue injury and the body's defence system against it determines whether acute pain can be controlled or will lead to chronicity. In this transition, psychosocial factors may act as a catalyst and then maintain chronic pain. These factors need to be understood when attempting to prevent acute pain becoming chronic.

Common causes of chronic pain

Surgery and trauma

Surgery and trauma are two of the commonest causes of chronic pain. In a survey of 5130 patients attending pain clinics in North Britain, surgery was assessed as contributing to pain in 22.5% of all patients seen. It was second only to degenerative disease in the causation of pain. Surgery was commonly responsible for pain in the abdomen, perineum, anal and genital regions, but was also implicated in lower limb pain. Trauma was the third commonest cause with 18.7% of patients citing this as the cause of their pain. Patients with pain due to trauma tended to be younger and male.

Nerves can be injured during medical interventions. Pain following interventions and anaesthesia can result from: direct trauma, peri-operative ischaemia, compression of nerves, scar entrapment and post-injury chronic neuralgia. The nerves most often injured are as follows:

(a) Brachial plexus.
(b) Palmar cutaneous branch of median nerve.
(c) Infra-patellar branch of saphenous nerve.
(d) Ilio-inguinal, iliohypogastric, genitofemoral and femoral nerves.
(e) Accessory and greater auricular nerves.
(f) Long thoracic nerve.

(g) Intercostobrachial nerve (following breast surgery).
(h) Saphenous and sural nerves (after varicose vein stripping).

There is a strong correlation between the severity of post-operative pain and chronic pain following breast cancer surgery and thoracotomy. Minimising pre- and post-operative pain may reduce the incidence of long-term pain.

Traumatic or surgery amputation is a frequent cause of chronic pain. In assessing pain post-amputation, it is useful to distinguish between phantom sensation, phantom pain and stump pain (Figure 15.2).

Phantom sensation	Any sensation of the missing limb except pain
Phantom pain	Painful sensations referred to the missing limb
Stump pain	Pain referred to the stump

Figure 15.2 Assessing symptoms after amputation.

Back pain

Back pain is a common complaint. Rare but serious diseases need to be identified in medical examinations, such as signs and symptoms related to fracture, tumours, neurological damage and infections. However, cognitive, behavioural and emotional factors appear to play an important role in the transition from acute to chronic back pain (Figure 15.3).

Cognitive	Pain and fear-avoidance beliefs, catastrophising
Emotional	Depression, distress, anxiety, stress
Behavioural	Passive coping strategies, alcohol
Psychosocial	Workplace factors

Figure 15.3 Risk factors for back pain.

Risk factors involved in the onset and development of back pain

Current guidelines stress the need for early preventive intervention for patients with back pain who are likely to develop persistent pain problems. Psychological factors are related to back pain from its inception to the development of a persistent problem. They seem to be pivotal in the transition from acute to chronic pain. Clinicians need to be wary of inadvertently reinforcing 'sick behaviour' by avoiding these psychological factors.

Psychological

Psychological factors, such as stress, distress, anxiety, mood and depression, appear to be more important in the development of pain and disability than most biomedical or biomechanical variables. Fear-avoidance beliefs have a particularly significant relationship with the development of dysfunction. Pain is often linked with injury and the central fear in patients with chronic pain is the fear that pain is a sign of injury or illness. Several studies have confirmed the findings among patients with chronic back pain that 'hurt means harm'. Full and explicit explanation regarding the results of patients' investigations is vital if miscommunication and misunderstanding of symptoms is to be avoided. Pain catastrophising is an exaggerated negative misinterpretation and reaction towards a noxious stimulus. Volunteers with a high frequency of catastrophic thinking about pain become more fearful when threatened with the possibility of intense pain than do volunteers with a low frequency of catastrophic thinking. Catastrophic thoughts regarding the pain are strongly associated with fearful responses. Chronic pain patients hesitate to exercise because of increased pain. Many patients have stopped attending physiotherapy because it made their pain worse. Longstanding physical inactivity can have a detrimental effect on the musculoskeletal system, leading to increased muscle and joint stiffness and a 'disuse syndrome'. Highly anxious individuals demonstrate hypervigilance; that is, a propensity to attend to a stimulus being presented to the body. This may amplify the pain experience. Thus, fear of the pain itself, fear of potential re-injury and fear of physical activity, all contribute to a misinterpretation of the chronic pain experience. This can cause a cascade of psychological and physical events including muscle spasm, avoidance of activity, guarding behaviours and physical disuse. These in turn aggravate and perpetuate the pain and the functional impairment. In addition, adverse psychosocial workplace factors and inappropriate family support can promote the development of persistent back pain. Cognitive variables, such as beliefs about the pain and catastrophising, are related to outcome.

Pain severity

Pain severity is an important predictor. However, because pain severity is subjective, it is influenced by numerous factors other than physical pathology.

Alcohol and substance abuse

A history of alcohol and substance abuse has consistently been shown to be predictive of chronicity. Prior or current use of alcohol or illicit drugs indicates a relatively poor prognosis for those who suffer an acute episode of back pain (particularly if related to a work-related injury).

Perceived stress and coping responses

Perceptions of stress and the occurrence of numerous stressful life events have been identified as predictors of chronicity. The extent of stress identified during the acute phase of an injury, along with inadequate or maladaptive coping, will affect the transition to chronic pain.

Health perceptions

Patients' general somatic preoccupations, their own health perceptions and their beliefs about the severity of their current medical condition are important factors during periods of acute pain.

Litigation and availability of wage replacement

In many countries, persons who experience work-related injuries are eligible for disability compensation. Expectation of compensation may contribute to delayed recovery and reinforce the sick role. More severe pain symptoms, greater distress and functional impairment have been reported in those patients involved in compensation, although other studies have refuted this. Longer duration or higher incidence of disabilities has been reported in areas with high unemployment. Therefore duration of disability may be sensitive to the prospects of employment in the immediate area.

Pain across lifespan

The pain symptoms of many conditions and diseases vary with: age, reproductive status and hormonal variations, including phase of the menstrual cycle, pregnancy, immediately post-partum and during the menopause and andropause.

Adulthood

Social roles and lifestyle become entrenched in individuals during adulthood. Women predominate as caregivers. Men participate in physically demanding occupations and risk-taking recreational activities (such as smoking and alcohol). Peri-menstrually (and during pregnancy) fluid retention can increase tissue pressure around nerves, thereby precipitating or exacerbating painful neuropathies (such as carpal tunnel syndrome or meralgia paraesthetica).

Pregnancy

Musculoskeletal pain, particularly back pain, is a common occurrence during pregnancy. During pregnancy the female body undergoes significant hormonal, postural, musculoskeletal and biomedical changes. Increases in oestrogen and progesterone concentrations produce visceral and smooth muscle changes. An increase in serum relaxin increases collagen synthesis. Changes in the connective tissue of the pubic symphysis during pregnancy have been described. These include an increase in total collagen, increased water uptake and a decrease in viscosity of the ground substance. This remodelled collagen has greater pliability and extensibility predisposing the ligaments of the musculoskeletal system to laxity and compromising joint stability.

The incidence of low back pain during pregnancy is high at 48–59%. One-third of women report their back pain is severe, interferes with daily life and compromises their ability to work. This back pain can also continue into the post-natal period and subsequent pregnancies. Advice and education to prevent back and pelvic pain should be available to pregnant women. Encouragement to undertake general fitness will aid behavioural rehabilitation and aims to decrease disability levels.

Several recent studies have shown no association between epidural anaesthesia and chronic backache. During labour and delivery women should adopt the most comfortable position for them. Guidelines from the Association of Chartered Physiotherapists in Women's Health stress awareness of the masking effect of epidural and spinal anaesthesia in relation to excessive abduction of hips.

In pregnancy, symphysis pubis dysfunction is a relatively common condition with reported figures of 1:300–1:800. The normal gap of 4–5 mm of the symphysis pubis may increase and the level of separation cause severe pain. Patients find walking difficult and tend to shuffle without lifting their feet. Re-education of the pelvic floor musculature plays an important part in rehabilitation. Early referral for physiotherapy is vital.

Sexual and physical abuse

At least 20% of American women and 15% of boys have been sexually abused as children. Men perpetrate 90% of sexual abuse; 70–90% of perpetrators are known to the child, while 33–50% of girl victims are assaulted by family members. Over 50% of women presenting to a chronic pain clinic report histories of sexual and physical abuse. Abused women report greater pain intensity, more medical problems and more lifetime operations than non-abused controls. There is also a higher incidence of sexual abuse reported in patients with functional bowel disorders and pelvic pain.

Studies have shown links between a history of abuse and a variety of psychiatric and psychosocial difficulties for both boys and girls. However, no one set of symptoms has been uniquely characteristic. There is a greater than chance association between a history of abuse and the following diagnoses:

- Depression.
- Generalised anxiety disorder.
- Panic disorder.
- Phobias.
- Obsessive-compulsive disorder.
- Post-traumatic disorder.
- Somatoform disorders.
- Eating disorders.
- Substance abuse.

Mood disorders are commonly identified in abuse victims and this may be related to low self-esteem and feelings of loss of control. Community studies support the notion that victims of sexual abuse feel stigmatised and isolated as adults. Women sexually abused in childhood report difficulties relating to men and women, ongoing problems in relationships with their parents and difficulties in being parents themselves. Abusing others is another expression of feeling powerless and about one-third of abused children become perpetrators. Physical abuse has been linked to aggression towards others and this may be pertinent in pain patients, since there is evidence that anger intensity contributes to predictions of pain intensity and activity levels.

An awareness of the impact that previous or present sexual and physical abuse may have on the patient with pain is important when taking an integrated approach to pain management. Despite the increasing attention paid to abuse in recent years, many patients have not previously revealed their abuse or have ongoing problems relating to these incidents.

Key points

- The transition from acute to chronic pain is multifactorial.
- Chronic pain, once established, is persistent and resistant to treatment.

- Progression from acute to chronic pain is an important area for further research.
- Increasing our understanding of the relevance of physical, psychological and psychosocial influences in this process is important.

Further reading

Crombie, I.K., Davies, H.T.O. & Macrae, W.A. (1998). Cut and thrust: antecedent surgery among patients attending a chronic pain clinic. *Pain*, **76**: 167–171.

Elliot, A.M., Smith, B.H., Hannaford, P.C., Smith, W.C. & Chambers, W.A. (2002). The course of chronic pain in the community: results of a 4-year follow-up study. *Pain*, **99**: 299–307.

Jacob, M.C. & DeNardis, M.C. (1998). Sexual and physical abuse and chronic pelvic pain. In: Steege, J.F., Metzger, D.A. & Levy, B.S. (eds) *Chronic Pelvic Pain: An Integrated Approach*. WB Saunders, Philadelphia.

Kendall, N.A.S., Linton, S.J. & Main, C.J. (1997). *Guide to Assessing Psychosocial Yellow Flags in Acute Low Back Pain: Risk Factors for Long-Term Disability and Work Loss*. Accident Rehabilitation and Compensation Insurance Corporation of New Zealand and the National Health Committee, Wellington, New Zealand.

Main, C.J. & Watson, P.J. (1995). Screening for patients at risk of developing chronic incapacity. *J. Occup. Rehabil.*, **5**: 207–217.

U. Waheed

Pain in the ICU is commonly multi-factorial, arising from:

1 Pre-existing disease (e.g. recent surgery and myeloma).
2 Therapeutic devices (e.g. drains, non-invasive ventilation masks and endotracheal tubes).
3 Invasive procedures (e.g. intravenous access).
4 Routine nursing care (e.g. airway suctioning, physiotherapy, mobilization and dressing changes).
5 Monitoring (e.g. oesophageal Doppler).

In order to avoid patient suffering, these nociceptive stimuli require suitable analgesia, using adequate dosages and appropriate regimens.

Why are patients in pain?

1 Staff fear of potent analgesics, particularly with regard to the potential:
   – Obscuring of diagnosis.
   – Occurrence of adverse side effects (cardiovascular system (CVS), respiratory, gastrointestinal (GIT) system).
   – For drug addiction.
2 Staff difficulties with pain assessment.
3 The multi-factorial nature of influences affecting the patients' perception of pain, specifically:
   – Expectation of pain.
   – Prior pain experiences.
   – Emotional state.
   – Cognitive processes.

What are the complications of inadequate pain relief?

Inadequate analgesia contributes to:

1 Exhaustion, disorientation and agitation, consequent upon insomnia.
2 An enhanced stress response, characterized by tachycardia, increased myocardial oxygen consumption, hypercoagulability, immunosuppression and persistent catabolism.

3 Pulmonary dysfunction, with guarding of muscles around painful areas leading to restrictive movements of the chest wall and diaphragm.

How can pain be assessed in the intensive care unit?

Clinical pain assessment relies heavily on subjective patient reports (Table 16.1). However, critically ill patients are often unable to communicate their level of pain (particularly if sedated, anaesthetized or paralysed). This does not negate the need for accurate and systematic pain assessment. In such cases, the use of behavioural and physiological indicators (to infer the presence of pain) has been advocated.

Pain therapy can be divided into non-pharmacological and pharmacological methods as follows.

Non-pharmacological methods

Simple measures are important to maintain patient comfort and should include:

1 Attention to positioning (i.e. ensure comfortable posture and take care when moving patient).

Table 16.1 Assessment of pain in the intensive care unit (ICU)

Verbal report
Numerical rating scale (NRS)/verbal rating scale (VRS)

Pain-related behaviours

Movements	Facial indicators	Posturing
None	Grimacing	Rigid
Slow/decreased	Frowning	Splinting
Restlessness	Tears	Tense
Attention seeking	Wrinkling of forehead	
Vocalization		

Physiological indicators
Hypertension/hypotension
Tachypnoea/hypoventilation
Perspiration
Pallor

2 Stabilization of fractures.

3 Eliminating irritating physical stimuli (e.g. ventilator tubing pulling on endotracheal tubes and catheter blockage causing urinary retention).

4 Generalized environmental factors (e.g. ensure maintenance of diurnal rhythm, institute appropriate lighting, avoid unpleasant auditory stimuli, etc.).

Pharmacological methods

Desirable characteristics of pharmacological agents include physical, pharmacokinetic and pharmacodynamic attributes.

Physical

- Easy to administer (multiple formulations).
- Long shelf life.
- Low cost.

Pharmacokinetics

- Rapidity of onset and offset, easy to titrate (short context sensitivity half life).
- Metabolized in the circulation.
- No active metabolites/accumulation of metabolites.
- Not renally excreted.
- Reversible effects and availability of a recognized antagonist.
- Removed by dialysis.

Routes

Agents may be given orally, per rectum and via a nasogastric tube when absorption is unaffected by GIT motility, nausea, vomiting or first pass metabolism. However, these routes are of limited use in the presence of gastric stasis or diarrhoea (which may be secondary to infection, medication and feed types).

Due to altered perfusion (and thus variable absorption) intra-muscular administration is not recommended in haemodynamically unstable patients. Moreover, if patients are anticoagulated (a common event in ICU), intra-muscular injections may lead to the development of haematomas. Therefore, the intravenous route should be used if enteral administration is not possible. In non-critically ill patients, patient controlled analgesia (PCA) has been shown to result in stable drug concentrations, less sedation, less opioid consumption and reduced adverse effects (e.g. respiratory depression) in comparison to standard therapy (i.e. intravenous infusions). Some drugs (e.g. fentanyl) are also presented as transdermal patches. However, the extent of absorption depends upon multiple skin factors: permeability, temperature, perfusion and thickness. Patient selection is very important since many ICU patients have poor peripheral perfusion and soft tissue oedema (significantly affecting drug delivery).

The use of epidurals and local anaesthetics in the intensive care setting has not been well described in the literature, although many units accept patients in whom such analgesic techniques are in use. The major problem is failure to recognize important adverse events, because patient sedation prevents complaints. These include haematomas causing neural compression in cavities including the epidural space or the brachial plexus sheath.

Regimens

If continuous pain is likely (or observed), analgesics should be administered on a continuous or scheduled basis. Supplemental rescue doses should be provided as required.

Pharmacodynamics

The ideal analgesic for ICU patients would have the following pharmacodynamic activity:

- Nervous system:
  - No effect on intracranial pressure (ICP).
  - No effect on neuro-muscular junction activity.
- Minimal cardiovascular effects, which may be:
  - Primary effects on the myocardium or vascular resistance.
  - Secondary effects, consequent upon chemical release (e.g. histamine causing vasodilatation and hypotension).
- No effects on the respiratory tract, which may be:
  - Central (depressed respiratory drive).
  - Peripheral (bronchconstriction).
- No effects on renal system consequent upon:
  - Inadequate perfusion.
  - Altered cellular function.
- No adverse gastrointestinal effects, including:
  - Abnormal smooth muscle peristalsis.
  - Muscle sphincter contraction.
  - Deranged hepatic/pancreatic function.

Pharmacological therapies (alone or in combination) include:

- Opioids.
- Non-steroidal anti-inflammatory drugs (NSAIDs).
- Paracetamol (acetaminophen).
- α_2 adrenergic agonists.

Disease states, such as renal or hepatic insufficiency, may alter drug and metabolite elimination and are common in the ICU setting. Therefore, titration against effect, to reach the desired response, is necessary in all patients.

Opioids

Opioid analgesics are the drugs of choice for pain relief in the critically ill (see Table 16.2). Routes of administration vary, but opioids are most commonly given intravenously, by either intermittent bolus or continuous infusion. This route is preferred because drug absorption may vary with other routes. The choice of specific agent depends upon the patient, drug pharmacology and potential for adverse effects.

Important adverse effects of the opioid drugs in the ICU setting relate to the following.

- *Nervous system*: Sedation is a well-documented side effect of opioid use, which may be important when weaning from the ventilator, or endotracheal tube, is commenced. It may of course be advantageous, while intubation or ventilation is required.
- *Cardiovascular system*: Hypotension is particularly likely to occur in response to opioid use if the

patient is hypovolaemic. It may be secondary to sympatholysis, vagally mediated bradycardia or histamine release.

- *Respiratory system*: Adverse effects may relate to central or peripheral properties. Central respiratory depression may be a particular problem when weaning is commenced. One component of this is depression of the cough reflex. While this may be a problem during weaning, it may be helpful when deep suctioning is required.

Bronchoconstriction, secondary to histamine release, may be problematic during both spontaneous and controlled ventilation, since gas trapping will adversely affect lung mechanics. Furthermore, chest wall rigidity has been observed (particularly in neonates) when high doses are used.

- *Renal system*: Sphincter dysfunction may be important if the urinary catheter is removed in an effort to reduce infection risk. Retention may result in cardiovascular instability (secondary to

Table 16.2 Opioids commonly used in the ICU

Drug	Metabolism	Excretion	Active metabolites	$t_{1/2}$	Caution
Morphine	Glucuronidation; high first pass metabolism (60–80%)	Renal (90%), faeces (10%); not removed by dialysis	Morphine–3–glucuronide. Morphine–6–glucuronide is up to 20x *more* potent than morphine and is not cleared by dialysis	1.7–4.5 h	
Fentanyl	Hydroxylation, N-dealkylation	Renal (10%); not removed by dialysis	No	1.5–6.0 h	Parent drug accumulates
Alfentanil	N-dealkylation, glucuronidation	Renal (90%); not removed by dialysis	No	1.5 h	
Sufentanil	Unknown	Renal (60%), bile (10%); not removed by dialysis	No	2.0–3.0 h	
Remifentanil	Ester hydrolysis by non-specific and plasma esterases; N-dealkylation is a very minor pathway	Independent of renal and hepatic clearance	Carboxylic acid derivative; 300–1000x *less* potent than the parent drug	10–21 min	Prepared in glycine and hence should not be used in the epidural space
Pethidine	N-demethylation, hydrolysis	Renal (1–25%) depending on urinary pH; not removed by dialysis	Norpethidine has 50% the analgesic potency of pethidine; not removed by dialysis	2.4–7 h	Hypertensive crises with Monoamine Oxidase Inhibitors (MAOIs). Accumulation of norpethidine in renal failure; this compound has marked proconvulsant properties

parasympathetic overdrive) or pressure damage to renal parenchyma.

- *Reduced gastrointestinal tract motility*: Nausea and vomiting are generally unpleasant. However, if a non-cuffed tracheostomy tube is in use, potential for aspiration is a serious problem. This may result from central stimulation of the chemoreceptor trigger zone, but peripheral receptor effects also occur. These may result in:
  - Gastric hypomotility (possibly requiring the use of jejunal feeding tubes).
  - Ileus.
  - Constipation – potentially compromising respiratory function due to abdominal distension.
- *General*:
  - Pruritus may lead to significant patient discomfort.
  - Remifentanil is an ultra-short-acting agent that is well established for use during anaesthesia. When compared to the other opioids it has a unique pharmacokinetic profile, with a short duration of action. Of all the opioids mentioned, remifentanil is the nearest to the ideal agent and a promising step forward in optimizing the provision of analgesia in ICU patients.

Should opioids be used long-term in ICU?

Patients exposed to high doses of opioids (e.g. 5 mg/day of fentanyl) during a prolonged length of stay (>7 days) may develop physiological dependence. Thus, rapid discontinuation may be associated with evidence of withdrawal (see Table 16.3). The clinical picture in adult ICU patients is complex and other medical conditions may mimic withdrawal. It is vital to consider all the potential diagnoses when determining the cause of such symptoms and signs. Such diagnoses may include those in Table 16.4.

Table 16.3 Signs and symptoms of opioid withdrawal

Symptoms	Signs
Restlessness	Sweating
Irritability	Tachycardia/hypertension
Nausea	Vomiting/diarrhoea
Muscle cramps/aches	Fever
Anxiety	Tachypnoea

Withdrawal problems are most likely to be avoided by the use of careful unit protocols. These should include the following features:

- Gradually reducing doses.
  For example, 5–10% daily dose decrements or an initial 20–40% reduction followed by 10% reductions every 12–24 h.
- Conversion to a longer-acting agent to facilitate intermittent administration. For example, controlled released morphine preparations as used in patients suffering with chronic or terminal pain.
- Use of alternative agents, for example clonidine, which has rarely been associated with dependence.

NSAIDs

In addition to having analgesic and anti-inflammatory activity, NSAIDs are anti-pyretic and inhibit platelet aggregation. In contrast to opioids, they do not cause sedation, respiratory depression or hypotension. NSAIDs can reduce opioid requirements by

Table 16.4 Differential diagnoses of opioid withdrawal (ARDS = Adult Respiratory Distress Syndrome)

System	Example of condition mimicking withdrawal
Central nervous system (CNS)	Meningitis/encephalitis Intracerebral haemorrhage/infarct Epilepsy/seizures
Respiratory system	Hypoxia (e.g. ARDS, pneumonia, pneumothorax, pulmonary infarct)
Cardiovascular system	Myocarditis/pericarditis
Gastrointestinal system	Hepatic encephalopathy Uraemia
Metabolic	Dehydration Hypoglycaemia Hypocalcaemia Hyponatraemia
Drug induced	Neuroleptic malignant syndrome

30–50%, particularly when used in combination with paracetamol. However, their analgesic benefit has not been systemically studied in ICU patients. The main reason for this is their potential to cause significant adverse effects including:

- Gastrointestinal bleeding, secondary to mucosal ulceration and platelet inhibition.
- Bleeding from other sites, consequent upon platelet inhibition.
- Bronchoconstriction, which may be particularly problematic in patients with respiratory compromise or those requiring mechanical ventilation.
- Development of renal impairment. Known risk factors for this include:
  - Age >65 years.
  - Hypotension (mean arterial blood pressure (MAP) <65 mmHg).
  - Hypovolemia and oliguria.
  - Circulatory failure (hypotensive and/or cardiac failure).
  - Chronic renal disease.
  - Severe hepatic failure (associated with portal hypertension).
  - Hypertension associated with widespread vascular disease.
  - Diabetes with known nephropathy or renal vascular disease.

Clearly, many of these factors are present in ICU patients.

When using NSAIDs prophylactic treatment for gastric ulceration should be given (proton pump inhibitors being more effective than antihistamines and sucrulfate).

The use of cyclo-oxygenase (COX)-2 inhibitors in the critically ill warrants caution. It was hypothesized that they may have a lower risk of gastrointestinal complications (bleeding, perforation or obstruction) than traditional NSAIDs because the COX-2 isoform inhibitors have no effect on thromboxane adenosine type 2 receptors (A_2) production. The CLASS and VIGOR studies (non-ICU patients) both showed unequivocal benefit over traditional NSAIDs. However, COX-2 inhibitors are not ideal ICU agents. By decreasing prostaglandin I_2 (PGI_2) production they may tip the natural balance between prothrombotic thromboxane A_2 and anti-thrombotic PGI_2, thus potentially increasing thrombotic cardiovascular events.

Paracetamol (acetaminophen)

Paracetamol is a non-narcotic analgesic and antipyretic, used to manage mild to moderate pain or discomfort. The mechanisms of its analgesic and antipyretic effects are contentious, but inhibition of prostaglandin (PG) formation within the CNS appears to be important. Unlike NSAIDs, it has no anti-inflammatory effects. Its use is associated with few adverse effects, although post-administration hypotension has been noted. As a single agent paracetamol lacks potency; however, when used in combination with NSAIDs it is known to be opioid sparing. In combination with an opioid, paracetamol produces an analgesic effect comparable to higher doses of opioid alone (i.e. an additive effect). When compared with NSAIDs (as analgesic adjuncts to opioids) paracetamol is more effective and avoids the potential adverse effects of NSAIDs.

Paracetamol is rapidly absorbed from the upper gastrointestinal tract (bioavailability 70–90%) and peak concentrations occur within 1–2 h. Metabolism occurs in the liver by glucuronidation and sulphation (with 20% first pass metabolism) to an inactive metabolite that is excreted in the urine ($t_{1/2} = 1.9$ h). Rectal administration, however popular, is known to be slow, erratic and incomplete. Several factors may account for this variability including the placement of the suppository, the degree of lipophilicity of the vehicle and the pH of the rectum. Studies have shown that higher doses are required to achieve adequate plasma levels via this route (40 mg/kg rather than 20 mg/kg), but it is not possible with current data to set dosing standards. Care must be taken to avoid excessive and potentially hepatotoxic doses. In normal individuals 10 g in one 24-h period may exceed the ability of hepatic glutathione to conjugate the toxic metabolite. Patients in ICU with depleted glutathione stores (resulting from hepatic dysfunction or malnutrition) are more susceptible and should be maintained on a reduced dose.

α_2 adrenergic agonists

The α_2 adrenergic agonist clonidine has been used for many years as an adjunct to sedation and analgesia in ICU. It can augment the effects of opioids and treat drug withdrawal syndromes.

Epidural clonidine produces analgesia by action at α_2 adrenoceptors located on the dorsal horn (DH) neurones of the spinal cord. Local effects may include:

- Inhibition of the release of nociceptive neurotransmitters (e.g. substance P (SP)) from pre-synaptic first-order neurones.
- Decrease in the rate of depolarization of post-synaptic second-order neurones.

Parenteral, epidural and intra-thecal administration provides analgesia, with synergistic enhancement of opioid effects (in combination, less opioid is required to achieve a desired analgesic effect). The reasons for synergism remain controversial, with theories including:

- Interactions mediated at delta opioid receptor (DOP) and α_2 receptor subtypes.
- Alterations in N-type calcium channels.
- Altered G-protein function.

Dexmedetomidine is a highly selective α_2 adrenergic agonist, with receptor affinity eight times that of clonidine. Along with analgesic and sedative effects, it has been shown to produce anxiolytic effects comparable to benzodiazepines. Rapid administration is associated with a biphasic cardiovascular response. A transient rise in blood pressure is followed by a reduction, which is exaggerated in the presence of intravascular volume depletion or high sympathetic tone. Its role in ICU remains to be determined.

Analgesic drug interactions

For details on important drug interactions in the ICU, refer Table 16.5.

Specific conditions

Neurosurgery

An important objective in the medical treatment of neurosurgical patients is to maintain adequate cerebral perfusion pressure (CPP):

$$CPP = MAP - (ICP + jugular\ venous\ pressure)$$

Therefore, controlling intracranial pressure (ICP) and maintaining adequate mean arterial pressure (MAP) are critical. Since the skull is a fixed volume box, ICP will depend upon the volume of intracranial blood, cerebrospinal fluid (CSF) and brain tissue.

Nociceptive stimulation is associated with a rise in ICP (and therefore a reduction in CPP). Opioids are

Table 16.5 Important drug interactions in the ICU

Class	Drug	Effect
Opioids		
Antibiotics	Erythromycin, ketoconazole	Increased plasma concentration of alfentanil (because of reduced clearance)
	Ciprofloxacin	Reduced plasma levels of ciprofloxacin
Antidepressants	MAOIs	CNS excitation/depression; hypertension/hypotension; most common with pethidine
	Selective serotonin reuptake inhibitors (SSRIs)/tricyclic anti-depressants (TCA)	CNS toxicity with tramadol causing drowsiness/hallucinations/convulsions
Cardiovascular	Esmolol	Increase plasma concentrations of esmolol
NSAIDs		
Cardiovascular	Angiotensin converting enzyme inhibitors (ACEI); anti-angiotensin II	Reduction of hypotensive effect; increased risk of renal impairment; hyperkalaemia, (especially with ketorolac)
	Diuretics: loop/thiazide	Increased risk of nephrotoxicity
Antibiotics	Quinolones	Convulsions
Anticoagulants	Clopidogrel/ticlopidine/warfarin	Enhanced effects and bleeding
Antipsychotics	Haloperidol	Severe drowsiness, (especially with indomethacin)
Bronchodilators	Theophylline	Possible association of rofecoxib with increased levels of theophylline
Paracetamol		
Anticoagulants	Warfarin	Enhanced effects – causing bleeding
Anion exchange resins	Cholestyramine	Reduces oral absorption of paracetamol – therefore reduced analgesic efficacy
α_2 adrengenic agonists		
Cardiovascular	ACEI	Enhanced hypotensive effects requiring smaller incremental doses of ACEI
	β-adrenergic blockers	Rebound hypertension on withdrawal of clonidine

frequently used to prevent this. However, controversy persists regarding the effects of opioids on ICP and CPP. Studies have demonstrated opioid-related vasodilatation (and hence an increase in cerebral blood flow), which may lead to an increase in ICP – especially in the presence of intracranial pathology. The mechanism is unclear, but an autoregulatory, vasodilation phenomenon, secondary to reduction in MAP is a likely explanation. Other studies have shown rises in CSF pressure with sufentanil, alfentanil and fentanyl (and hence a reduction in CPP). Most studies agree that significant, but transient, increases in ICP are observed after bolus injections of opioids. Continuous infusions are therefore preferable for analgesia and sedation in such patients.

Remifentanil is the drug of choice in many neurosurgical ICUs because it is:

- Safe and easy to administer intravenously.
- Of ultra-short duration (allowing frequent neurological examination).
- Associated with minimal changes in ICP and CPP, even with endotracheal suctioning.
- Associated with minimal cardiovascular effects – although bradycardia may be problematic.
- Unaffected by hepatic and renal failure ($t_{1/2}$ is unchanged).
- Cost efficient (as a sole agent) when compared to propofol + opioid in this patient group.
- Useful in non-intubated patients (0.1 μg/kg/min) in units familiar with its use (although profound respiratory depression is a risk).

Key points

- Pain assessment is difficult in the ICU patient, but attempts should be made to undertake this in all patients.
- Critical illness may affect the pharmacokinetics of analgesics. This should be considered when administering drugs. However, it should not be used as an excuse to avoid provision of analgesia.
- Pain can be physiologically detrimental to ICU patients – in addition to being unpleasant.
- ICU patients are frequently administered a wide range of drugs: pharmacokinetics and dynamics of both analgesics and other agents may be altered by interactions.

Further reading

Boldt, J., Thaler, E., Lehmann, A., *et al.* (1998). Pain management in cardiac surgery patients: comparison between standard therapy and patient controlled analgesia regimen. *J. Cardiothor. Vascul. Anesthesiol.* **12**: 654–658.

Jacobi, J., Fraser, G.L., Coursin, D.B., *et al.* (2002). Task force of the American College of Critical Care Medicine (ACCM) of the Society of Critical Care Medicine (SCCM), American Society of Health-system Pharmacists (ASHP), American college of chest physicians. Clinical practice guidelines for the sustained use of sedatives and analgesics in the critically ill adult. *Crit. Care Med.* **30**: 119–141.

Markowitz, J.S., Myrick, H. & Hiott, W. (1997). Clonidine dependence. *J. Clin. Pharmacol.* **17**: 137–138.

Mukherjee, D., Nissen, S.E., Topol, E.J., *et al.* (2001). Risk of cardiovascular events associated with selective cox-2 inhibitors. *J. Am. Med. Assoc.* **286**: 954–959.

Puntillo, K.A., Miaskowski, C., Kehrle, K., *et al.* (1997). Relationship between behavioral and physiological indicators of pain, critical care patients' self reports of pain, and opioid administration. *Crit. Care Med.* **25**: 1159–1166.

Silverstein, F.E., Faich, G., Goldstein, J.L., *et al.* (2000). Gastrointestinal toxicity with celecoxib versus non steroidal anti-inflammatory drugs for osteoarthritis and rheumatoid arthritis. The CLASS study: a randomized control trial. *J. Am. Med. Assoc.* **284**: 1247–1255.

Zimmermann, H.J. & Maddrey, W. (1995). Acetaminophen hepatotoxicity with regular intake of alcohol. Analysis of instances of therapeutic misadventure. *Hepatology* **22**: 767–773.

17

A. Howarth

Chronic pain is defined by the International Association for the Study of Pain (IASP), as pain that persists for longer than the time expected for healing, or pain associated with progressive, non-malignant disease. Often chronic pain persists long after the tissue damage that initially triggered its onset has resolved; it may present without any identified ongoing tissue damage or antecedent injury.

Chronic pain serves no purpose and often makes no sense. It is often unrelated to tissue damage and does not warn the individual of injury or disease. Overall the experience is distressing and frustrating, as the pain does not respond to the usual treatments for acute pain, such as analgesics, rest, taking time off work and seeking medical advice.

Different people respond differently to the experience of pain. How an individual responds depends upon their gender, age, culture and previous experience of pain. Some chronic pain patients who present with specific nerve damage or disease may be able to cope with their pain, however, others may go on and develop characteristics that are referred to as the 'chronic pain syndrome' (Hanson and Gerber, 1990).

Chronic pain includes the following:

- A history of unsuccessful treatments.
- A level of physical disability exceeding that expected.
- Psychosocial problems, such as depression, anxiety, anger, sleep loss, loss of pleasure from normal activities and a preoccupation with pain.

Over time patients often become withdrawn, isolated and dissatisfied with their abilities and role in society. When these patients present in a pain clinic they may have had their pain for a prolonged time. It is common for them to have been seen and investigated by a variety of specialists including: neurologists, orthopaedic surgeons, rheumatologists and gynaecologists, in addition to their general practitioner. Some have sought second opinions and changed their general practitioner due to dissatisfaction.

The impact that chronic pain has on individuals varies considerably and changes as the pain problem

Table 17.1 Impact of chronic pain

Unemployment	Sleep difficulties
Financial worries/litigation	Poor concentration
Less able to do things	Preoccupied with pain
Less satisfaction	Dissatisfaction with
Frustration	state health care
Less contact with others	Uncertainty
'Not belonging'	Irritability
Not 'the person I used to be'	Anger
Difficulties with relationships	Upset
Difficulties with sex life	Depression
Being misunderstood	Worry
Less self-confidence	Guilt
	Negative and unpleasant
	thoughts

progresses. The main issues that impact upon peoples' lives are listed in Table 17.1.

Unemployment

Patients with chronic pain may either be made unemployed or not feel in a position to be able to apply for jobs. This results from the unpredictable nature of the pain, leading to them being perceived as unreliable and requiring regular periods of time 'off-sick'. Employers vary in their response to this. Some are supportive and attempt to find ergonomic adaptations to help people stay at work. This might include altering workstations and purchasing specialist seating, or offering flexible working times and practices. Others however, are less sympathetic and view the unpredictability of their employee as a burden. People who are not employed and wish to return to work often find that they are not considered for posts due to their medical history and employers' unease about taking on someone with a chronic condition. Moreover, patients who have been injured while at work often find themselves in dispute with employers over returning to work, sick pay and compensation issues.

Financial worries

Due to difficulties with employment, patients often face financial concerns, especially if they are/were the main salary earner. Patients with chronic pain are in some instances entitled to benefits and allowances from the state, but the complex and lengthy process of obtaining these is often problematic. Some patients assessed for benefits are turned down as being fit to work, while they feel that their pain precludes this. Issues around patients who feel the need to maintain pain behaviours in order to justify their benefits are complex. These should be taken into consideration, but not used as justification to assume that patients are making their pain up, or exaggerating it so as to claim benefits.

Pending litigation is sometimes cited as a reason why patients experience ongoing pain. It may be perceived that they 'do not want to get better or improve' in case this reduces their chance of winning a court case or receiving compensation. Evidence for this is sketchy and many people have been found to have ongoing pain after the completion of litigation even if they have been successful.

Less able to do things

The majority of patients attending pain clinics will report that their level of activity has reduced, including activities viewed as both a pleasure and a chore.

Less satisfaction and more frustration

As the patient's physical abilities are reduced, they experience less satisfaction. This leads to frustration at their own inabilities and at other people's reactions to and expectations of them.

Less contact with others

People with chronic pain often find themselves withdrawing socially and subsequently have less contact with friends and family. This occurs because their ability to do things has reduced, thus limiting their range of activities. Patients may maintain activities regardless of their pain, but this is hard work and tiring, leading to bad temper. If patients are aware of this they may consciously decide to withdraw, not wishing people to see them in this position, or feeling that they are no longer any fun, or pleasant to be with. Relatives and friends will often express how difficult a person has become. Bad moods, unpredictability and preoccupation with the pain, may lead them to withdraw from the patient, causing further social withdrawal.

'Not the person I used to be' and 'not belonging'

Not belonging or feeling different to before, relates to patients inability to perform and fulfil the role that they have been used to. This can include being a partner, mother/father, son/daughter, good employee, team member, husband/wife, breadwinner or housewife/husband. Patients often feel that they do not belong in their social group, as they cannot be the reliant and dependable person that people were used to. They feel a great sense of failure that they cannot do what may normally be expected of them in their family unit. These aspects all contribute to the patient's sense of frustration and loss of satisfaction.

Difficulties with relationships and sex life

When people feel that they do not belong and cannot fulfil the role expected of them, it is bound to affect their relationship with others. Partners, relatives and friends are usually very sympathetic when a person initially has problems. However, sympathy and understanding often wane, as they fail to understand the nature of chronic pain. Withdrawal leads to breakdown in communication and can affect patients, family and friends.

Patients with chronic pain may find that they are no longer able to have a sexual relationship, or that sexual contact with a partner is reduced. This may be due to the sensory changes, physical positioning, flare-up of pain following activity or the result of pharmaceutical interventions (e.g. guanethidine blocks). Patients may also feel less desirable, or lose the urge to maintain a sexual relationship, due to changes in the dynamics of their relationship.

Being misunderstood

Many patients with chronic pain express their frustration that nobody understands them; including health care providers, partners, family and friends. The unpredictability of chronic pain means the patients abilities will vary quite considerably on a day-to-day basis. One day they may be able to go shopping and clean the house, whereas the next day the best they can manage is to get up and out of bed. If people observe such behaviour and do not understand that chronic pain is often cyclical and linked to levels of activity, then a patient's actions may be misconstrued as: 'swinging the lead', avoiding things they do not want to do, or being 'poorly' when it suits them. Of course, all these things are possibilities in our society, but it does not mean that people with chronic pain do not have genuine limitations that vary in relatively short time scales.

Health care professionals used to dealing with acute pain may not understand why patients do not get better, or why when investigations are negative the patients still complain of pain. Their expectation is often expressed as disbelief, with patients being sent away without an explanation and made to feel they are imagining their pain.

Less self-confidence

The culmination of these issues often undermines a person's self-confidence. As they are not able to be the person they used to be and are not believed by people they care about and respect, patients may start to doubt themselves and their abilities to contribute anything to society. Patients often have low self-esteem and self-worth, which makes adaptation to ongoing pain difficult.

Sleep difficulties

Sleep problems are commonplace because of pain, inactivity and an over active mind. Pain itself will stop a person sleeping. They may experience initial insomnia (i.e. they cannot get to sleep due to the pain) or maintenance insomnia (i.e. the pain wakes them up and then does not allow a return to sleep). Maintenance insomnia often results from lying in particular positions for prolonged periods causing an increase in pain. Additionally, the efficacy of analgesics may have worn off.

Night is the classic time for worry and rumination. The quiet of the night, with no one to talk to or distract them, allows individuals to become wrapped up in their thoughts, preventing sleep.

Insomnia is unpleasant leaving people feeling groggy and tired in the morning; this can be problematic, if people need to get up for work or to care for their families. It also makes a person less capable of coping with their pain during the day. Things they would normally take in their stride may upset or anger them. A vicious circle is set up, as their inability to cope

with the pain due to lack of sleep makes their perception of pain worsen. This in turn may prevent sleep on subsequent nights.

Poor concentration and preoccupation

Pain and lack of sleep often leads to problems with concentration and attention. The mind is only able to deal with information selectively. If pain is occupying a high proportion of the individual's attention other incoming information may be filtered out. Patients often say they cannot concentrate on anything else because their pain is the focus of their attention and they become preoccupied with what they can do about it.

Dissatisfaction with state health care

Patients have often seen a multitude of health care professionals from different specialities before they come to the pain clinic. They may have had to wait a long time to see these professionals and at the end of their wait, their pain has still not resolved. If so called 'experts' cannot cure them, or even in some instances give them a reason why they are experiencing prolonged pain, people become disillusioned and frustrated. Often people feel that the state owes them a cure or at least an explanation. They cannot understand why, in an age of modern technology, when we can transplant hearts and reattach limbs, we cannot cure their pain. Patients also become dissatisfied, feeling that they have been lied to, not listened to and misled. This results from people being told that their pain 'will go away', that it 'should have gone away' or from them receiving mixed messages from professionals. Different clinicians may have diverse ideas about what is causing an individual's pain and these conflicting ideas provide mixed and confusing messages for patients. Patients who are dissatisfied often present showing signs of anger and frustration that is not directed at the clinician in the clinic, but at the establishment and health service in general. Others may opt for 'alternative' health care.

Uncertainty

The unpleasant and unpredictable nature of chronic pain leads to a lot of uncertainty in an individual's life. Their concerns often centre on issues such as: 'What is the cause of the pain?', 'Is it going to go away?', 'When is it going to go?' and 'How am I going to be in

5, 10 or 20 years time?'. No one can give honest and truthful answers to these questions. Even if they could, patients may be reluctant to believe them after past experiences of being told things that subsequently proved to be incorrect.

Irritability, anger and upset

Patients' anger and/or irritability in clinic may be due to lack of sleep, or having to cope with the persistent pain, frustration and fear of the unknown for the future. The direction of their anger may be to the situation, themselves or others. People become upset at the prospect of the future with ongoing pain and do not see how they are possibly going to manage.

Depression

Depression is a problem commonly experienced by patients with chronic pain. It is often difficult to establish if patients are depressed because of their pain, or if their perception of pain is heightened by pre-existing depression. Depression often becomes part of the vicious circle, intensifying preoccupations with pain and an inability to cope with pain on a daily basis. If the patient is withdrawn this presentation may be difficult to assess without expert help.

Negative and unpleasant thoughts

Patients, who are depressed, worried and angry about reduced abilities to function normally in society quite understandably experience negative and unpleasant thoughts. These may be on a regular or intermittent basis and are often a problem at night. Thoughts such as 'what if its cancer and they have not found it or told me?' or 'there is no point carrying on because I have no future' may predominate but are counter productive.

The whole picture presented here may appear quite desperate. However, many patients attending a pain clinic will not be affected by all factors. Even when an individual is only affected by a few of the problems, it is easy to see why their chronic pain is so difficult to deal with and manage. Their treatment has to be comprehensive and consistent and if possible without prejudice. Thus, it is now accepted that the most appropriate form of treatment for patients with chronic pain is through the bio-psychosocial approach in a multidisciplinary pain clinic.

Key points

- Contacts with health care professionals have usually not produced the results or answers patients had hoped for.
- Ongoing pain impacts on physical abilities, psychological state and social interactions.
- The complex nature of chronic pain is best approached through multidisciplinary care.

Further reading

Gatchel, R.J. & Turk, D.C. (1996). *Psychological Approaches to Pain Management*. The Guildford Press, London.

Hanson, R.W & Gerber K.E. (1990). *Coping with Chronic Pain*. Guildford Press, London.

18

POST-OPERATIVE PAIN MANAGEMENT IN DAY CASE SURGERY

T. Schreyer & O.H.G. Wilder-Smith

Introduction

Day case surgery (DCS) forms an increasingly large part of all surgery performed in the developed world. In fact, it was an American anaesthesiologist who opened the first 'Downtown Anaesthesia Clinic' in Iowa in the early 1900s. Today about 60% of all surgery in the US is performed in day case units and about 50% of surgery in UK is ambulatory. In this context, the UK Department of Health (2002) has recently published a 'Basket of 25' of the most important procedures to be performed as DCS.

Advantages of DCS

- *Better patient satisfaction*: Patients may choose their admission date, leading to greater satisfaction and a substantial decrease in appointment cancellations. Furthermore, patients subsequently go home; in fact, to much more agreeable and convenient surroundings for their recovery.
- *Greater cost effectiveness*: Procedures in DCS can be performed in a much more cost- and time-effective fashion, thus increasing the numbers of patients that can be treated, resulting in shorter waiting lists.

Disadvantages of and differences between DCS and inpatient surgery

- Quality standards must be set higher for DCS than inpatient surgery because complications have a greater overall impact and the opportunity and time for correcting problems is much more limited.
- DCS has a narrower range of analgesic drugs/regimens/techniques available because of higher security and quality standards.
- DCS is highly dependent on *well-organised, efficient and forward-looking workflows*. Thus, qualitatively different and quantitatively greater demands are placed on ancillary and supporting systems than with inpatient surgery.
- Most pain after DCS occurs (and becomes a problem!) when the patient has gone home, where

no immediate medical advice or observation are available.
- 66% of elderly patients suffer from pain on the first morning after DCS.
- 83% of children undergoing hernia repair experience pain at home.

Thus DCS post-operative pain management has to be safely organised in advance, taking into account the post-operative period in a home setting.

Effective peri-operative pain therapy and DCS

- Pain therapy is not only a humanitarian obligation, it also has a positive impact on the immune system, wound healing and complication rates.
- Satisfactory pain therapy after DCS helps to avoid unanticipated and unplanned hospital admission. It is therefore an important factor in cost effectiveness.

Goals for peri-operative pain therapy in DCS

Goals for peri-operative pain therapy are as follows:

- Effective.
- Reliable.
- Safety and low rate of adverse effects.
- Comfortable and simple application.
- Cost and resource effective (money and time!).
- Patient satisfaction – patients dissatisfied with anaesthesia and post-operative pain management are more likely to be dissatisfied with ambulatory surgery in general.

Background

DCS and factors increasing the risk of post-operative pain

- Type of intervention (see Figure 18.1).
- Unplanned prolongation of operation.
- Post-operative nausea and vomiting (PONV) precipitates pain (e.g. increased movement, autonomic activity, lack of absorption of oral analgesics).

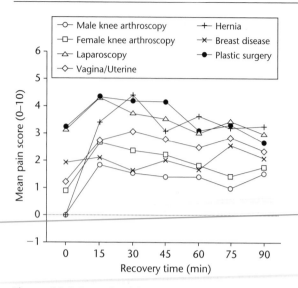

Figure 18.1 Example of how post-operative pain scores differ, depending on the type of surgery performed (Pavlin *et al.*, 2002).

Consequences of pain management failure in DCS

- Pain is a major reason for unplanned hospital admission (0.3–1.4% of DCS).
- Workflow impairment, lowering effectiveness and increasing costs.
- Increased numbers of complications.
- Less patient acceptance of the whole procedure.
- After pain, PONV and anaesthesia lasting longer than 2 h are the next most important risk factors for unplanned hospital admission.

Basic principles

Both organisational and therapeutic aspects of post-operative pain management must be carefully considered for DCS. In each of these categories some very important basic principles must be followed.

Organisational principles and their implementation

- Clearly defined patient selection criteria and adherence to these!
  - For example, fitness for anaesthesia, good home circumstances, compliance (Department of Health, 2002).
- Clear, comprehensible and complete patient information:
  - Preferably provided before day of intervention.
  - Preferably written, but provide for phone contact in case of problems.

- Structured and easy to understand advice and rules covering analgesia during the first days at home:
  - Useful: pre-packed, standardised take-home medication packs.
  - Provide for regular baseline analgesia at defined intervals and for defined minimum durations.
  - Provide for adequate rescue ('patient controlled') analgesia.
- Provide a 24-h contact phone number for advice and troubleshooting.
- Institute formal quality management procedures – the best way to improve and maintain effectiveness and outcome of DCS procedures:
  - Institution of information feedback systems.
  - Regular meetings to present, review and act on quality management information.
  - Further goal: better standardisation of the workflow.

Therapeutic principles

- *Use a multimodal approach*: By focussing on more than one possible site and mechanism of anti-nociceptive action, one can achieve greater overall analgesic efficacy (including synergistic effects) and reduced adverse effects.
  - Cyclo-oxygenase (COX) inhibitors (e.g. non-steroidal anti-inflammatory drugs (NSAIDs)).
  - Opioid receptor agonists (e.g. short-acting opioids: remifentanil, alfentanil, fentanyl during surgery (Table 18.1)). These short-acting opioids provide only *very short* post-operative effects and have to be replaced by regular post-operative longer lasting analgesics (e.g. codeine and paracetamol).
  - N-methyl-D-aspartate (NMDA)-receptor antagonists (e.g. ketamine: in low doses to avoid psychotomimetic effects).
  - Local anaesthetics (LAs) (locally infiltrated, next to specific peripheral nerves, or intrathecal or epidural) are particularly suited to DCS and provide excellent post-operative analgesia (Table 18.2).
- *Consider pre-emptive use of analgesia*: Although evidence is still limited in human studies, analgesia commenced prior to surgical incision and continued into the post-operative period seems to improve post-operative pain (and perhaps other) outcomes (Wilder-Smith, 2000).
- *Control the therapeutic effect of analgesia*: Follow the patient's quality of analgesia; please ask your patient about his or her pain regularly! Nurses and doctors systematically *underestimate* patients' pain levels, and patients often accept pain unnecessarily. Ensure the best possible standard of analgesic care

Table 18.1 Pharmacokinetic data for LAs available for infiltration. All times and amounts are dependent on site of application (e.g. infiltration or axillary block) and on presence of vasoconstrictors

	Onset (min)	Duration (min)	Maximum mg/kg (plain)	Maximum mg/kg (with epinephrine)
Lidocaine	2–4	30–60	4.3	7
Prilocaine	2–4	30–90	7	8.5
Mepivacaine	2–4	45–90	4.3	7
Etidocaine	2–4	120–180	4.3	5.7
Bupivacaine	5–8	120–240	2.5	3.2
Chloroprocaine	14–18	15–30	11.4	14.3

Table 18.2 Pharmacokinetic data pertaining to anaesthetics and analgesics in common use for DCS

	Time to maximum effect (min)	Vd_{ss}(l/kg)	Clearance (ml/kg/min)	Duration of effect (min)	Plasma protein binding
Fentanyl	4–5	3–6	10–20	30–60	80%
Alfentanil	1–2	0.4–1.0	4–9	5–10	90%
Sufentanil	2–3	3–4	10–15	10–15	93%
Remifentanil	1–2	0.2–0.4	30–40	1–2	70%
Morphine	15–30	3–4	15–30	200–300	20–40%

for the patient by making sure that rescue analgesics are taken *promptly*.

Practical application of methods available

Regional anaesthesia

Intravenous (i.v.) regional analgesia (Bier's block) is the most commonly used regional anaesthesia procedure in DCS. However, it provides little post-operative analgesia. Other regional techniques (such as brachial plexus block, spinal and epidural anaesthesia) provide for analgesia lasting well into the post-operative period. When performed properly, regional anaesthesia provides quick, safe, cost-effective and long-lasting analgesia for DCS. Patient-controlled analgesia (PCA) catheter techniques may be developed in the future (as single-use infusion devices become cheaper and more reliable).

The intravenous regional analgesia

- Using a proximal tourniquet, the LA is injected in a distal vein of the arm or leg. Relatively large volumes of LA (40 ml) are needed, resulting in

higher risks of systemic side effects of the LA. Commonly used drugs include: lidocaine 0.5%, prilocaine 0.5% and mepivacaine 0.5%. The tourniquet must remain inflated for at least 20 min after LA injection, to allow for tissue fixation, thus lowering the risk of systemic toxic effects. These include: dizziness, convulsions, myocardial depression, bradycardia, asystole and ventricular fibrillation.

Infiltration of the operation field (Table 18.1)

- Can be sub-cutaneous, sub-fascial, intra-articular.
- Performed before or after surgery.
- Addition of adrenaline prolongs duration of analgesia.
- Future: long-acting formulations of LA:
  - Microspheres for 24-h effects are under clinical evaluation.

Nerve blocks

- Digital nerves.
- Peripheral nerve blockade (e.g. median, ulnar, radial, femoral, posterior tibial nerve).

Plexus blocks

- Best performed with electric nerve stimulator.
- Brachial plexus nerve block:
  - Potential approaches: axillary, inter-scalene, supra-/infra-clavicular.
  - Axillary approach is safest.
  - Supra-/infra-clavicular approach risks pneumothorax.
  - Future: catheter techniques will probably play a role when cheap single-use infusion pumps are available.

Neuraxial blocks

- *Spinal anaesthesia* (e.g. heavy bupivacaine 0.5%, 2–3 ml): The most common side effects of spinal anaesthesia are urinary retention and headache.
- *Epidural anaesthesia* (e.g. lidocaine 2%): Lumbar epidural anaesthesia has a higher risk of motor blockade when compared with thoracic epidural anaesthesia.
- *Caudal anaesthesia* (especially children) (e.g. 0.5 ml/kg bupivacaine 0.25%).
- For all *neuraxial blocks*, motor block must have fully regressed before discharge home. There is a risk of urinary retention even without motor block. In principle, a patient who can get up and go to the toilet can go home.

Systemic analgesia

In most of the cases, anaesthesia should be performed with a *combination* of one or more systemic analgesics, or together with regional analgesia:

- *Opioids*: These are most commonly used pre- and intra-operatively. Short-acting opioids (e.g. remifentanil, alfentanil and fentanyl) are used intra-operatively, if no post-operative need is anticipated. Long-acting opioids in low doses (e.g. morphine) may be used in the immediate post-operative period in the recovery ward.
- *NSAIDs, paracetamol*: These are suitable for use pre- and post-operatively, in the recovery unit and at home:
  - Paracetamol (oral).
  - Diclofenac (oral).
  - Parecoxib (parenteral).
  - Ketorolac (parenteral).
- *Ketamine*: It is a non-competitive NMDA receptor antagonist. It has distinct suppression effects on central nervous system (CNS) sensitisation. Furthermore, it acts synergistically with opioids, inhibiting tolerance and rebound hyperalgesia.
  - Bolus: *s*-ketamine.

In the context of DCS, opioids are more useful for the treatment of early post-operative pain, while NSAIDs have a particular role to play during ambulation.

Example of a peri-anaesthetic pain management algorithm for a normal adult

- Consider regional analgesia whenever possible – pre- or post-operatively.
- Patients should be starved but may drink water until 2–3 h pre-operatively (no fatty fluids).
- Give NSAID p.o. (*per os*, by mouth) on the morning of the operation.
- Give an opioid (or *s*-ketamine) *before* the stress of intubation and incision (e.g. fentanyl 0.15–0.25 mg i.v., alfentanil 1–2 mg i.v. or remifentanil infusion).
- Try to maintain constant plasma levels of the opioid during surgery, (e.g. continuous infusion of remifentanil or alfentanil).
- Provide pre-emptive antiemetic (e.g. cyclizine 50 mg i.v. slowly).
- Early escape analgesia in the recovery ward can be morphine (titrated i.v.). Nurses and doctors should ask their patients *early* on about pain – *before* it becomes a problem.
- Pre-packed pain medication for 3 days is handed out to the patient in the day case ward before discharge with instructions on their use. Such pre-packed pain medication systems are useful when integrated in a quality management system (e.g. diclofenac 2–3 × 50 mg p.o. or ibuprofen 3 × 400 mg p.o. as basic, plus codeine as escape opioid).
- If possible, ask your patients to bring back the unused part of the pre-packed set after 3 days for quality control and to build up your own database about the efficacy of your peri-operative analgesic management.
- Establish a 24-h phone line for your patients and their general practitioners (GPs) to offer help with subsequent acute (pain) problems.
- Audit re-admissions.

Key points

- The early bird gets the worm:
  - Start analgesia *pre*-operatively and continue well into the post-operative period ('extended pre-emptive analgesia').
- Work multimodally:
  - Use several different drugs/techniques to block pain using different pathways.
- Check the results of analgesia:
  - *Speak* to your patients regularly, *ask* them about pain, then evaluate their satisfaction.

- Document pain scores and treatment outcomes.
- Remember, patients often will not tell you spontaneously about pain.

Further reading

Department of Health (2002). *Day Surgery: Operational Guide*, August. http://www.doh.gov.uk/daysurgery/daysurgery.pdf

Dolin, S.J., Cashman, J.N. & Bland, J.M. (2002). Effectiveness of acute postoperative pain management. I. Evidence from published data. *Br. J. Anaesth.*, **89**: 409–423.

McQuay, H. & Moore, A. (1998). An evidence-based resource for pain relief. Oxford University Press, Oxford, UK, p. 187.

Pavlin, D.J., Chen, C., Penaloza, D.A., Polissar, N.L. & Buckley, F.P. (2002). Pain as a factor complicating recovery and discharge after ambulatory surgery. *Anesth. Analg.*, **95**: 627–634.

Wilder-Smith, O.H. (2000). Changes in sensory processing after surgical nociception. *Curr. Rev. Pain*, **4**: 234–241.

PAIN SYNDROMES

G. Carli & G. Biasi

Neural mechanisms of muscle pain

Action potentials originating from nociceptors carry information about noxious stimuli, but the perception of pain from muscles is the end product of information processing in the central nervous system (CNS).

Nociceptors

In skeletal muscles, there are three types of nociceptors that encode the intensity of noxious stimuli:

(a) Specific mechanical nociceptors responding only to high-intensity stimuli.
(b) Polymodal nociceptors encoding innocuous and nociceptive, mechanical and chemical stimuli.
(c) The free nerve endings in muscle tissue concentrated around small arterioles and capillaries between the muscle fibres and not activated by normal muscle movement or increasing muscle tension.

As in other tissues, nociceptor information in muscles is transduced and carried to the CNS by $A\delta$- and C-afferent fibres. C-fibres are mainly excited during ischaemic contractions and are sensitized following tissue lesion and inflammation.

Dorsal horn neurones

When muscles are healthy, most dorsal horn (DH) neurones receive projections from $A\delta$-afferent fibres, sometimes in combination with C-fibres. DH neurones receiving exclusive projections from C-afferent fibres are quite rare. The effect of C-afferent fibres on DH neurones increases greatly following inflammation. Thus, it has been suggested that, in the absence of peripheral muscle pathology, acute pain is mainly due to $A\delta$-fibres, while chronic muscle pain is related to C-fibres.

In models of experimental muscle pain (Mense *et al.*, 1997), myositis-induced hyperexcitability of DH neurones involves the activation of neurokinin 1 (NK-1) and *N*-methyl-D-aspartate (NMDA) receptors, whereas spontaneous hyperactivity appears to be due to reduction of nitric oxide (NO) synthesis. This has led to the suggestion that in patients with chronic muscle pain, increased background activity could account for ongoing pain, while increased DH neurone excitability could be responsible for hyperalgesia.

Tonically active inhibition originates in supra-spinal centres and affects both superficial and deep peripheral nociceptive input to DH neurones. Therefore, a malfunction of this inhibitory system could also lead to widespread pain.

Pain localization

In both clinical and experimental scenarios, focal stimuli to muscle tissue may be clearly associated with muscular pain that is: localized, poorly localized or referred. It has been suggested that mechanisms of temporal summation contribute to pain diffusion, while referred pain is related to the intensity of the stimuli. The fact that pain and hyperalgesia can spread to areas far removed from the injured region implies that central changes (i.e. central sensitization) as opposed to convergence, are involved. Sensitization of neurones in the DH and other areas of somatosensory pathways follows a peripheral injury. This is reflected by:

- Increased spontaneous activity.
- Reduced thresholds.
- Increased response to afferent inputs.
- Prolonged after-discharges to repeated stimulation.
- Expansion of the peripheral receptive fields of central neurones.

Pain measurement

Clinical inspection

In examining the muscular system, one should not only observe the volume, contour, power and tone of the muscle, but also evaluate the strength and function of muscle groups. This can be performed by:

- Observing movements.
- Applying passive resistance to the movement.
- Having the patient resist the examiner's active attempt to move fixed parts.

Scales and questionnaires

The subjective experience of muscle pain intensity can be expressed unidimensionally with categorical rating scales, numerical rating scales and visual analogue scales. Multiple dimensions may be expressed using the McGill pain questionnaire (MPQ) and a diagram allowing patients to mark the areas of pain.

Referred pain and hyperalgesia

Muscle pain is frequently associated with:

- Deep hyperalgesia (which may occur independently of pain).
- Tenderness.
- Referred pain – most frequently manifested as secondary hyperalgesia, in dermatomes and myotomes connected to the same spinal segments innervating the stimulated muscle.

Clinical syndromes

Muscle pain is not synonymous with muscle disease. Musculoskeletal aches and pains are extremely common in everyday life and transient types may not be associated with a definable aetiology. Muscle tissue represents a large amount of body weight (up to 30% of overall body mass in young athletes) and is provided with a rich innervation. Some 'rheumatic complaints' that cannot be attributed to diseases of the spine, joints or connective tissues have their source in muscles. This chapter will cover two examples of musculoskeletal syndromes:

1 Myofascial pain syndrome, with regional localized pain.
2 Fibromyalgia syndrome (FMS), with diffuse pain.

According to the Committee on Taxonomy of the International Association for the Study of Pain (IASP), myofascial pain syndromes should be separated from the FMS:

- *Myofascial pain syndromes*: Characterized by specific trigger points (TP) in one of several muscles.
- *Fibromyalgia*: Characterized by local tenderness at 11 or more specified sites of tenderness (tender points (TeP)), with widespread aching lasting more than 3 months.

Myofascial pain syndromes

These syndromes occur frequently, may cause severe disabling pain and once recognized, are relatively simple to manage. They have been described using a variety of terms including: myalgia, myositis, myofascitis, fibromyositis, muscular rheumatism and muscular strain. They constitute a large group of muscle disorders characterized by hypersensitive sites (called TP) within: one or more muscles, the underlying connective tissue or both. Symptoms include:

- Pain.
- Muscle spasm.
- Tenderness.
- Stiffness.
- Limitation of motion.
- Weakness.
- Autonomic dysfunction (occasional).

Although local pain may also be present, the symptoms are usually referred to a deep area in muscle distant from the TP.

Symptoms

Trigger Points (TP)

A TP (also known as a trigger area, trigger zone or myalgic spot) is so named because its stimulation, by pressure or muscle activation, produces effects at another place, called the reference zone or area of reference.

During a physical examination, systematic palpation of muscles may cause the patient to jump, wince, or cry out, because of pressure on the extremely tender TP. TPs can develop in any muscle of the body, but occur most frequently in:

- Neck.
- Shoulder girdle.
- Lower back.
- Extremities.

They are usually located in the mid-portion of the muscle belly, but may also be found at the muscle attachment to the bone, or at other points along the muscle (Figure 19.1).

TPs may be active or latent as follows:

- An *active* TP is associated with pain at rest, or following a movement that stretches or overloads the muscle. Only active TPs are responsible for clinical pain complaints.
- A *latent* TP is diagnosed when pain is elicited locally and in the area of reference by discrete pressure on a muscle spot. A latent TP may cause limitation of range of movement and weakness in the affected muscle.

Taut band

According to Travell and Simons (1983), a palpable taut band associated with a TP is a critically important

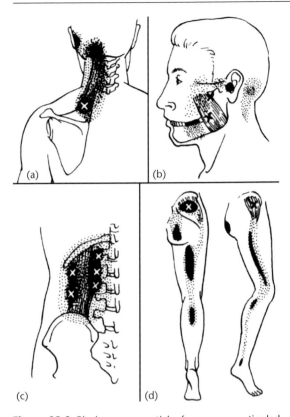

Figure 19.1 Black areas: essential reference zone; stippled areas: spillover reference zone; TP (from Sola and Bonica, 2001). (a) TP and associated pain patterns of levator scapulae muscle. (b) Masseter muscle demonstrating some of its characteristic pain reference sites. (c) Quadratus lumborum muscle with common TP and local pain reference pattern. (d) Gluteus medius TP (one of the most powerful TP in the body) with its local pain and reference zones in the thigh and leg. Also tensor fasciae lata TP and characteristic hip pain and lateral thigh and leg reference zones.

objective finding. A rope-like taut band can be palpated whenever a muscle is sufficiently close to the skin, with the TP being the point of maximum tenderness along the course of a taut band. When the muscle is gently stretched until the onset of resistance (but not beyond) the band's tense fibres can be distinguished from the normally lax fibres surrounding it.

Referred pain

Referred pain patterns are the key to identifying the muscle responsible for myofascial pain. They are relatively constant and predictable, indicating the use of fixed neural pathways. However, the constant distribution of referred somatic pain does not correspond to a dermatomal organization or nerve root distribution. The essential reference zone is present in all patients and can be associated with a much larger

area. This is the spillover reference zone, in which pain is felt only in some patients (Figure 19.1).

The clinician can use the predictability of pain patterns as a reference to locate the source of myofascial pain (i.e. the TP). Deep (often continuous) hyperalgesia or tenderness are associated with pain in the reference zone.

Local twitch response

Snapping palpation across the TP elicits a local twitch response, due to transient contraction of the taut band fibres. This is an objective physical sign that occurs only after this type of mechanical stimulation. Therefore, it represents the most reliable technique to systematically search for a TP. The greater the local twitch response, the more active or sensitive the TP.

Restricted motion

On examination, muscles with a TP display:

- Reduced range of movement.
- Pain upon passive lengthening of the muscle beyond the onset of resistance.
- Weakness.
- Decreased maximal tension.
- Pain upon vigorous voluntary contraction.
- Delayed development of the tendon reflex.

Aetiology and physiopathology

The most identifiable causes of the development of TPs or activation of latent TPs are:

- Trauma to myofascial structures.
- Overload of muscles.
- Microtraumas, from daily activities or repetitive movements while working.
- Overuse of unconditioned muscles.

The initial area of stress or injury can spread to several muscles, which may contain clusters of hypersensitive TP. The initial dysfunction phase of myofascial TP formation can be explained by local vicious circles related to muscle contraction, release of algogenic substances, sensitization of muscle nociceptors and activation of sympathetic vasoactive responses (Simons and Travell, 1981) (Figure 19.2). Although not experimentally proved, this hypothesis is supported by the efficacy of three main treatments that interrupt the pain cycle and eliminate the TPs.

Treatment

The management of myofascial pain syndromes is simple and successful.

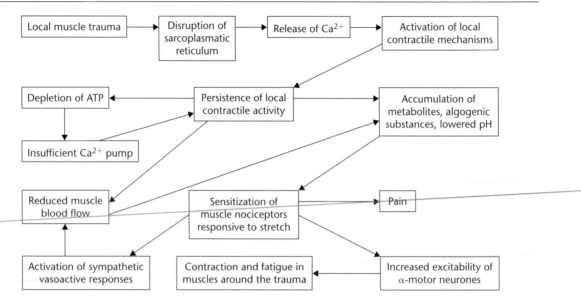

Figure 19.2 Development of myofascial pain syndrome. An initial local muscle trauma can be followed by disruption of the sarcoplasmic reticulum, which releases Ca^{2+} ions that activate contractile mechanisms. This local contraction occurs in the absence of action potentials and is responsible for the taut band. The persistence of local contractile activity results in two synergistic vicious circles. One is related to: depletion of muscle ATP causing an insufficient Ca^{2+} ion pump, thus maintaining the muscle contraction, and the other to contraction sensitizing muscle nociceptors (particularly the mechanoceptors sensitive to stretch): (a) directly through reduction of blood flow and (b) indirectly through local accumulation of algogenic substances, metabolites and lowered pH. Nociceptor sensitization may also be responsible for local pain and increased excitability of α motor neurones. This in turn may elicit contraction and fatigue in muscles around the trauma.

Stretch and spray

This very effective procedure consists of spraying the skin overlying the muscle of the trigger area with a jet or stream of vapocoolant and subsequently stretching the muscle. It has been suggested that the spray facilitates the stretching by suppressing nerve conduction (and thus pain and stretch reflexes). Stretching the shortened sarcomeres should separate the actin and myosin filaments, breaking the vicious circle. Stopping the uncontrolled contractile activity terminates the increased metabolic activity permitting adenosine triphosphate (ATP) accumulation (an essential step for activation of the calcium pump) with ensuing muscle relaxation.

Pressure

This procedure is effective mainly as an initial approach to reassure the patient. Sustained firm pressure on the TP probably causes ischaemic compression and elicits local stretching of the shortened sarcomere filaments, nerve block and emptying of the capillaries. This is followed by rebound hyperaemia. The nerve block may be responsible for pain suppression and interruption of sympathetically mediated local reflex ischaemia. It is postulated that rebound hyperaemia flushes away contraction metabolites and algogenic substances.

TP injection

This treatment consists of simple penetration of the TP by a needle, with or without injection of saline or local anaesthetic (LA). Needle insertion and LA elicits tenderness and pain (locally and in the reference zone) and could block nerve conduction. Injection of saline may 'wash away' the contraction metabolites and algogenic substances. All these methods have been reported to give good results. Pain relief and related phenomena persist for several hours or days.

Fibromyalgia syndrome (FMS)

The FMS is a controversial chronic condition of unknown aetiology that affects all ages, ethnic groups and cultures. It occurs in about 2% of the general population and (in adults) is more common in women. Nevertheless, the concept of fibromyalgia is not universally accepted. The diagnosis is based on the 1990 American College of Rheumatology (ACR) classification criteria. These guidelines, an important milestone

Sodium valproate

Common problems include: nausea (number needed to harm (NNH) 3.3), tremor (NNH 6.2), drowsiness (NNH 6.3) and dizziness (NNH 6.5).

More serious, but less frequent problems include: hepatic dysfunction, acute pancreatitis and increased bleeding times (associated with both thrombocytopenia and altered coagulation profiles). The teratogenic nature of this compound makes it less useful in young women.

$\alpha2-\delta$ compounds – gabapentin and pregabalin (Chapter 42)

These compounds have a unique mechanism of action that differs from other anticonvulsants. Their pharmacological activity appears to be related to their ability to bind to the $\alpha2-\delta$ protein, associated with voltage-gated calcium channels. These subunits may play a major role in hyperalgesia and allodynia, via actions in the spinal cord and dorsal root ganglion (DRG). Both reduce the release of several neurotransmitters (e.g. glutamate, NE, 5-HT, dopamine, SP and calcitonin gene related peptide (CGRP)) from spinal cord slices after paw inflammation or spinal nerve ligation. Neither compounds show activity at opioid or gamma amino butyric acid (GABA) receptor sites.

Pharmacokinetic features of these drugs are:

- Rapid absorption following oral administration.
- Ready penetration of the blood brain barrier.
- Negligible metabolism in man.
- Elimination almost unchanged in the urine.

Both drugs decrease pain behaviour in models of neuropathic and inflammatory pain. Studies in surrogate human neuropathic pain models (e.g. the heat-capsaicin model) show gabapentin reducing the area of secondary hyperalgesia. This suggests an effect on central sensitisation, manifesting as neuropathic pain. Clinical studies (in PHN, PDN and mixed neuropathic pain syndromes) support the pre-clinical findings of efficacy. Though pain scores are significantly reduced against placebo, the overall responder rate is still under 50% of patients. Moreover, even among patients who respond to the treatment, significant numbers still have residual pain.

Reported studies document only mild to moderate adverse effects. These are mainly dizziness (NNH 9), ataxia (NNH 12), fatigue (NNH 14) and somnolence (NNH 9), reported by 6–16% of patients. No serious adverse effects have been reported (including effects on the cardiovascular system). This relatively benign side-effect profile may make it a more appropriate choice than the older agents. However, it appears to demonstrate no additional efficacy in comparison to older agents.

NMDA antagonists

Ketamine and other NMDA antagonists have anti-neuropathic effects in both the pre-clinical and clinical settings. They have been administered by numerous routes, including oral, i.v. and subdural. In animal models of neuropathic pain their use has been demonstrated to inhibit central sensitisation and wind up. The WHO recognises ketamine as an essential adjuvant drug for the management of neuropathic pain (last updated April 2002) and acknowledges its opioid potentiating effect. However, the evidence supporting use of these compounds is only level four (Chapter 31). Indeed, randomised controlled trials (RCTs) with agents such as dextrometorphan and memantine have failed to demonstrate any advantage over placebo. Despite the paucity of supporting data, many patients have been reported to benefit from these drugs, with the major limiting factor being the adverse effect profile. The major side effects are behavioural disturbances, including: nightmares, hyperactivity and alterations in memory and learning.

Non-steroidal anti-inflammatory drugs (Chapter 41)

Studies using non-steroidal anti-inflammatory drugs (NSAIDs) in neuropathic pain states have produced mixed results. Small studies in PDN have produced some useful effects, but in PHN no effect is seen. The likelihood of a significant effect from these drugs is small, as they do not target central sensitisation. Nonetheless, in combination with other drugs (e.g. anticonvulsants) they may produce an additive, or even synergistic, effect in neuropathic pain.

Opioids (Chapter 40)

Opioid analgesic efficacy in neuropathic pain is accepted to occur through effects on opioid receptors (μ opioid (MOP), κ opioid (KOP), δ opioid (DOP)). The use of opioids in neuropathic pain is still strongly debated and controversial. In pre-clinical neuropathic pain models, morphine produces very little effect. The dose required to produce any effect is also considerably higher than in nociceptive and inflammatory pain models. In surrogate human pain models, opioids produce modest results and are associated with significant side effects. In clinical studies of neuropathic pain syndromes, the results are mixed.

Tramadol (Chapter 40)

Tramadol is centrally acting producing analgesic effect through the combination of:

- Weak opioid effect on MOP (1/60 of morphine).
- Inhibition of 5-HT and NE uptake.

Results of studies in neuropathic pain have been contradictory. Where tramadol is effective in comparison to placebo, it also has significantly higher rates of side effects. These include nausea, dizziness, sedation and constipation.

Nerve growth factor (NGF)

A reduction in the retrograde transport of NGF to the cell body may be a factor in the development of neuropathic pain; for example, PDN. NGF is critical in maintaining cellular balance of neuropeptides and NGF antagonists have been investigated in clinical conditions of neuronal death. In animal models, responses to NGF are complex. Peripheral NGF may induce pain, yet NGF given intrathecally may alleviate neuropathic pain. Unfortunately, the results of clinical trials in PDN and in HIV-related neuropathy have failed to demonstrate any substantial effect of treatment. A major limitation of these has been that systemic administration provides poor bioavailability of nerve factor (NF) due to a short half-life.

Future trends

Combination therapy

Recently, strong pre-clinical evidence has emerged that a combination of different classes of drugs may result in additive effects, synergy or strong dose sparing effects. Some examples, where improved efficacy for fewer side effects are observed, include:

- Opioids + Gabapentin.
- NSAIDs + Gabapentin.
- Opioids + Clonidine.

If these findings are translated into the clinic, a greater number of patients achieving significant pain relief and improved quality of life should result.

Prevention of neuropathic pain

The principle of pre-emptive analgesia (i.e. analgesia given prior to the nociceptive stimulus) is one of the most attractive ideas arising from our increased understanding of the mechanisms involved in persistent neuropathic pain. The emphasis lies in inhibiting both wind up phenomena and peripheral and central sensitisation. Early reports of reduction in the incidence of 'phantom limb pain' with effective pre-surgical administration of opioids via the epidural route were promising. However, adequately powered studies have failed to reproduce these effects.

Recently, the use of novel drugs (e.g. gabapentin) has been reported to reduce secondary hyperalgesia in human surrogate neuropathic pain models. Moreover, administration prior to major surgery has been associated with a significant reduction in post-operative morphine consumption. It remains to be seen whether these effects are translated into an effective pre-emptive therapy for neuropathic pain.

Key points

- Neuropathic pain may result from a variety of conditions, including surgical trauma.
- The characteristics of neuropathic pain differ from those of nociceptive or inflammatory pain – these may need to be specifically questioned for.
- Analgesia is currently less efficacious in neuropathic pain when compared with pain from nociceptive stimuli.
- Compounds developed initially for use in non-painful conditions may be useful in the management of neuropathic pain (Tables 20.2–20.4).

Further reading

Jensen, T.S. (2002). Anticonvulsants in neuropathic pain: rationale and clinical evidence. *Eur. J. Pain*, **6 (suppl. A)**: 61–68.

Jensen, T.S. & Baron, R. (2003). Translation of symptoms and signs into mechanism in neuropathic pain. *Pain*, **102**: 1–8.

Woolf, C.J. & Mannion, R.J. (1999). Neuropathic pain: aetiology. Symptoms, mechanisms, and management. *Lancet*, **353**: 1959–1964.

K.J. Berkley

Pain mechanisms

From pathway

Current conceptualizations of pain mechanisms derive from Descartes' familiar drawing, in which fire on the foot activates a pathway to brain that interacts via the pineal gland with the soul-mind. This derivation is evident in a 1948 diagram concerning abdominal pain (Figure 21.1(a)). Interesting features in this diagram are as follows:

- Focus on visceral afferent nerve fibres (then just discovered).

- Depiction of convergence on spinal neurones of input from viscera, skin and muscles.
- Emphasis on how the 'mind' (cloud above the brain) influences perceptions by somehow activating descending paths from cortex to spinal cord (SC).

Modern traditional views have barely changed (Figure 21.1(b)). The 'mind' is now the brain. Reciprocal SC to brain and brain to SC pathways for pain and pain modulation involve multiple rather than single routes. And there are separate pathways for pain, touch and visceral control. To account for variations in reported pain experience despite similar noxious stimuli, 'pain

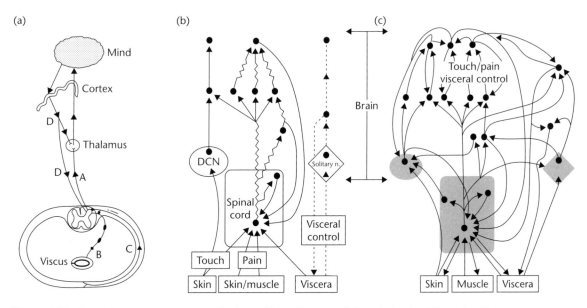

Figure 21.1 These diagrams are conceptualizations of how the transmission of stimulus information (from sensory receptors in skin, muscles and viscera) to and through various central neural pathways might give rise to pain perception, touch perception and visceral control. (a) Adapted from Kinsella's 1948 diagram. Note two features important for understanding visceral pain: (1) the existence of visceral afferents and (2) the influence of the 'mind' (cloud above the brain). A: output from spinal cord to thalamus; B: sensory afferents from viscus to spinal cord; C: sensor afferents from somatic structures (skin, muscle) to spinal cord; D: descending projections from cortex to spinal cord. (b) The currently popular, traditional pathway view. Different information-processing pathways are invested with different perceptual functions. (c) A *dynamic distributed ensemble* view in which the many perceptions of pain and touch arise from an overall balance of activity in distributed portions of the brain. This distributed network may be unique to each individual and change over that individual's lifespan as experiences dictate. (From Berkley, 2001, with permission.) DCN: dorsal column nuclei.

modulating' descending controls, which can increase or decrease spinal activity are included. Although this traditional view is useful, it requires noxious bodily stimulation for pain to occur. Thus, problems arise when painful conditions occur in the absence of appropriately located bodily pathophysiology.

Via modulation

Prompted by this clinical problem and recent research findings, a different conceptualization of the mechanisms of pain is emerging.

Sensitization

Although the response properties of sensory afferent fibres are precise (small receptive fields, and organ and modality specific), these properties can change. Thus, afferent sensitivity can be altered (by trauma, injury or inflammation – see Chapter 6) or fluctuate with hormonal variations – see Chapter 29 (e.g. the ovarian cycle). Nevertheless, response properties still remain precise, for example sensitized fibres responsive to vaginal stimulation do not respond to direct bladder stimulation. Similar (central) sensitization can occur at SC level (see Chapter 5).

Divergence and convergence

Despite the response specificity of sensory afferents, information conveyed by them is delivered to widespread regions in the SC (divergence). This arriving information then converges with information arriving from other tissues. Thus, it is common to find a neurone located in, say, an upper lumbar spinal segment responsive to brushing the foot, pressing on a leg muscle, distension of the vaginal canal *and* distension of the colon. We now know that this multisystem convergence also occurs in the *dorsal column nuclei* (DCN) and the *solitary nucleus* (SN, parasympathetic). This newer information is surprising, because, as depicted in Figure 21.1(b), DCN neurones were thought to receive input *only* from afferents responsive to gentle skin stimulation, while the SN neurones supposedly received information *only* from viscera. We now know that DCN neurones can convey information about viscera as well as skin, and that SN neurones can convey information about skin as well as viscera.

Of relevance is that neurones in these three entry regions (SC, DCN and SN) convey information to each other as well as to a large array of interconnected brain areas. The consequences are considerable:

- Enormous potential for integration of information from bodily structures with others.

- Central sensitization is not limited to the SC, but also occurs throughout the brain (e.g. references to 'pain memories').
- Electrical stimulation within the thalamus can reproduce pains in patients who have recovered from their pain (e.g. toothache and angina).

To dynamic ensembles

These findings have led to a new conceptualization of pain mechanisms (Figure 21.1(c)). Instead of pathways, perceptual processes involve 'dynamic distributed ensemble networks' in the central nervous system (CNS). The components (and relative activity of these components) change continuously with experience across the lifespan, with molecular mechanisms underlying the changes being remarkably similar to those that underlie learning and memory.

Applied to visceral pain, this conceptualization means that all aspects of an individual's pain perception are a consequence of activity within a CNS network. At any moment, pain sensation is derived from the many co-operative controls being exerted on the flow of information about bodily stimuli (e.g. viscera into the active and dynamic brain). The controls are continually updated by experience. Thus, the CNS creates pain uniquely for each individual.

Visceral pain: diagnosis

The term 'visceral pain' has been used to refer to:

- Pain that arises from pathophysiology in an internal organ.
- Pain that an individual localizes in an internal organ and, therefore, attributes to pathophysiology there (e.g. 'stomachache').

But is visceral pain as so defined a perceptual entity different from musculo-skeletal or cutaneous pain in a way that is useful clinically for diagnosis and therapy?

Pathophysiology in an internal organ

Pathophysiology in an internal organ can produce:

- A vague, dull or cramp-like pain that is poorly localized 'internally' in the general vicinity of the organ.
- Pain referred to skin or muscles in the bodily segments associated with the organ ('referred pain').
- Tenderness in skin and muscle ('referred hyperalgesia').

Less well recognized is that such pathophysiology does not necessarily evoke pain ('silent pathophysiology'). Furthermore, visceral pathophysiology has long-term consequences. For example, referred tenderness

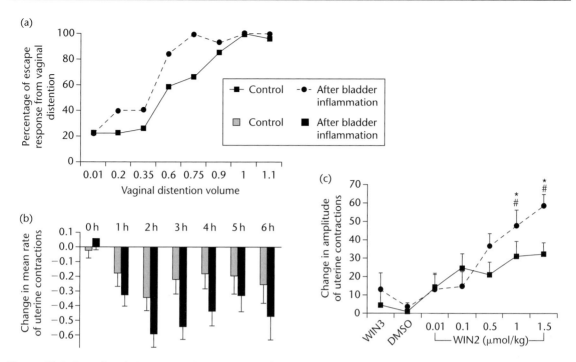

Figure 21.2 Examples of viscero-visceral interactions in laboratory rats: influence of bladder inflammation on: (a) *Vaginal sensitivity (increased)*: Percentage of trials that an awake rat escapes different volumes of vaginal distention increases when the rat is retested several days after the rat's bladder had been mildly inflamed with a solution of turpentine in olive oil. (b) *Uterine contractility (decreased)*: Mean rate of uterine contractions in urethane-anaesthetized rats (number of contractions/5 min) changes over a 6-h period after intra-vesical infusion of either saline or turpentine in olive oil. The rate of bladder contractions is decreased significantly more after the turpentine infusion than after the saline infusion. (c) The effects systemic delivery of the cannabinoid CB1-receptor agonist (WIN 55,212-2) on the uterus (reduces efficacy). Arterial injection of WIN 55,212-2 increases the amplitude of uterine contractions in urethane-anaesthetized rats in a dose-dependent manner, with bladder inflammation decreasing the effect. (a) and (b): from Berkley (2001), with permission; (c) modified, with permission from Dmitrieva, N. & Berkley, K.J. (2002). Contrasting effects of WIN 55,212-2 on motility of the rat bladder and uterus. *J. Neurosci.*, **22**: 7147–7153.

in muscles remains long after the pathophysiology has resolved.

Most investigators agree that convergence from viscera, muscles and skin on SC neurones probably explains the referred pain and hyperalgesia experienced during acute visceral pathophysiology. The pain is 'referred' because information from skin and muscle is conveyed to the SC by afferents (A alpha, beta, delta and C) whose influence on the dorsal horn neurones dominates over that conveyed from viscera (Aδ and C afferents). It is also generally agreed that central sensitization at least partly explains the long-term effects. What is not well understood is why some visceral pathologies:

- Produce more pain than seems to be warranted.
- Continue long after the pathophysiology has resolved.

- Fail to produce pain at all.
- Fail to respond to normally efficacious pharmacological agents.
- Occur concurrently, or with other pain conditions (e.g. dysmenorrhoea or endometriosis, interstitial cystitis, irritable bowel syndrome, migraine and tension headaches, temporomandibular disorder, fibromyalgia).

The widespread divergence and convergence of information from bodily afferents on CNS neurones is one mechanism. Besides providing a substrate for *viscero-somatic* interactions (between internal organs and muscle or skin), divergence–convergence mechanisms also provide a substrate for *viscero-visceral* interactions (between widespread internal organs). In health, such interactions are probably important for co-ordinating internal bodily functions with each other and external circumstances.

These co-ordination mechanisms may explain why pathophysiology in one internal organ influences functions in another. Furthermore, extensive co-ordination could give rise to central sensitization extending into neural regions associated with body segments remote from the original site. For example:

1 Pain associated with uterine dysfunction (dysmenorrhoea, endometriosis) can result in tender deltoid muscles.
2 Inflammation of the bladder can:
   – Produce vaginal hyperalgesia (Figure 21.2(a)).
   – Reduce the rate of uterine contractions (Figure 21.2(b)).
   – Decrease the efficacy of a drug's action on the amplitude of uterine contractions (Figure 21.2(c)).
3 Pain behaviours associated with artificial ureteral stones are increased in rats that are also subjected to surgical induction of endometriosis (Figure 21.3(a)). The ureteral stones also evoke uterine pain behaviours not evident with endometriosis alone, which is an effect called 'viscerovisceral referred pain'. Moreover, pain behaviours associated with the ureteral stones are *decreased* in rats subjected to a control surgery (Figure 21.3(a)), an effect called 'silent kidney stones'. Similarly, in women who suffer from repeated kidney stones, the presence of dysmenorrhoea or endometriosis is associated with an increase in the number of pain crises produced by stones and a vastly changed cyclical pattern of pain crises (Figure 21.3(b)).

When a patient reports 'visceral pain', what is the source of that pain?

The source of all pain is activity in the CNS (Figure 21.1(c)). When a patient complains of, say, a 'stomachache', potential reasons include:

- Pathophysiology in the stomach.
- Viscero-visceral interactions.
- 'Pain memories'.

Thus, 'stomachache' could be referred from some other organ, or be triggered by an environmental circumstance associated with prior stomach pathology. One known example of the former is the association of interstitial cystitis with endometriosis and endometriosis with interstitial cystitis. One known example of the latter is the recurrence following hormone replacement therapy in post-menopausal women of the cyclical pelvic pain they had experienced pre-menopausally.

When a patient reports 'muscle pain' or 'cutaneous pain', can it be visceral pain?

Viscero-visceral and viscero-somatic interactions force us to recognize and incorporate into clinical practice new knowledge that pain symptomatology

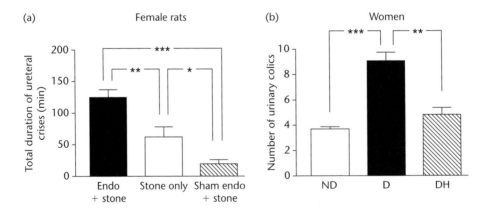

Figure 21.3 Example of viscero-visceral interactions: influence of endometriosis on pain behaviours. (a) The duration of ureteral pain crises in rats is significantly enhanced by a co-existing surgically induced endometriosis (partial hysterectomy and autotransplant of uterine tissue in the abdomen) and is significantly decreased by the control surgery (partial hysterectomy only). Adapted from Giamberardino, M.A., Berkley, K.J., Affaitati, G., Lerza, R., Centurione, L., Lapenna, D. & Vecchiet, L. (2002). Influence of endometriosis on pain behaviours and muscle hyperalgesia induced by a ureteral calculosis in female rats. *Pain*, **95**: 247–257. (b) The number of pain crises evoked by the passage of a kidney stone in women without dysmenorrhoea (ND) is significantly increased when compared with crises in women with dysmenorrhoea (D) or successfully treated (with hormones) dysmenorrhoea (DH). Adapted from Giamberardino, M.A., De Laurentis, S., Affaitati, G., Lerza, R., Lapenna, D. & Vecchiet, L. (2001). Modulation of pain and hyperalgesia from the urinary tract by algogenic conditions of the reproductive organs in women. *Neurosci. Lett.*, **304**: 61–64.

(and signs of visceral abnormality) may frequently reflect pathophysiology in organs remote in time and location from current complaints. Examples include:

- Sore back or shoulder consequent to prior uterine dysfunction.
- A tender left arm reflective of cardiovascular pathophysiology.

What about 'silent' visceral pain?

We now recognize that dysfunction in one organ may hide or exaggerate symptoms of dysfunction in another. This mechanism explains the existence of visceral pathophysiology that fails to produce symptoms.

For example, silent ischaemia, silent kidney stones, silent ovarian cancer, etc.

Thus, pathophysiology in organ X (e.g. uterus) may mask signs and symptoms in organ Y (e.g. bladder), or the differential diagnoses associated with organ X could be related to organ Y.

'Visceral nociception' versus 'visceral pain'

Effects of pathophysiology in an internal organ on responses of CNS neurones differ from the effects of pathophysiology in muscles or skin. This difference is mainly because information from viscera, muscles and skin to the CNS is conveyed by different complements of afferents. Moreover, visceral afferents are fewer than those from muscles and skin. Thus, visceral *nociception* (i.e. recognition by the CNS that a noxious event has occurred in an internal organ) differs from muscle and skin *nociception*.

When a patient reports the location of *pain* in an internal organ, the pain experience may reflect pathophysiology in one or several organs, the brain's trace of prior pathophysiology, or current pathophysiology. Furthermore, a report of pain or tenderness in a muscle or skin may reflect current, or prior, pathophysiology in an internal organ (sometimes even in an organ located in a segment remote from the tender area). Thus, the term 'visceral pain' has limited categorical validity. Awareness that pain in muscles can originate from viscera may be important in diagnosis.

Visceral pain: therapy

An obvious consideration for pain management is to adopt an approach that fits more with dynamic ensemble pain mechanisms than with a pathway view. Treatment for pathway mechanisms (Figure 21.1(a) or (b)) is

to target pathophysiology in discrete episodes. In contrast, if clinicians and patients adopt a dynamic conceptualization, it is likely that multiple therapies will be used simultaneously or in parallel with dynamic events (e.g. premenstrual exacerbation of somatic pains).

Research is beginning to answer the question: 'should the approach be any different for "visceral pain" as opposed to "musculo-skeletal" or "cutaneous" pain?' For chronic pain, the answer is likely 'No.' It is important, however, to recognize that pathophysiology in an internal organ can influence the efficacy of pharmaceutical agents acting not only on the diseased organ, but also on other organs. For example, animal studies have shown that bladder inflammation increases the efficacy of agents on the bladder but reduces their efficacy on the uterus.

Key points

- Information from internal organs conveyed by sensory afferents to the CNS converges with a denser input arriving from muscles and skin resulting in:
  - Vaguely localized internal pain.
  - Referred pain.
  - Tenderness in muscles and skin of the same bodily segment in which the organ is located.
- Such pathophysiology can sensitize CNS neurones for long periods, so that referred tenderness in muscles continues long after the visceral pathophysiology has resolved.
- As suggested by the dynamic ensemble mechanisms, divergence–convergence within the CNS together with the CNS's life-long learning mechanisms provides a substrate for:
  - Pathophysiology in one organ to influence functions of another.
  - Remote CNS sensitization.
  Thus, pathophysiology in one organ can either increase or decrease signs and symptoms associated with another organ, or result in referred muscle tenderness in remote bodily segments.
- Diagnostically, visceral pathophysiology can be:
  - Silent.
  - Present as musculo-skeletal pain.
  - Present as skin pain.
  - Mislocalized to another internal organ or remote body part.
- Therapeutically: pathophysiology in one organ may influence efficacy of therapies targeted at another.
- A polytherapeutic approach is likely to be more effective than a monotherapeutic one.

Further reading

Berkley, K.J. (2001). Multiple mechanisms of pelvic pain: lessons from basic research. In: MacLean, A.B., Stones, R.W. & Thornton, S. (eds) *Pain in Obstetrics and Gynaecology*. RCOG Press, London; pp. 26–39.

Berkley, K.J. & Holdcroft, A. (1999). Sex and gender differences in pain. In: Wall, P.D. & Melzack, R. (eds) *Textbook of Pain*, 4th edition. Churchill Livingstone, Edinburgh; pp. 951–965.

Deadwyler, S.A. & Hampson, E.R. (1997). The significance of neural ensemble codes during behavior and cognition. *Annu. Rev. Neurosci.*, **20**: 217–244.

Giamberardino, M.A. (1999). Recent and forgotten aspects of visceral pain. *Eur. J. Pain*, **3**: 77–92.

Kinsella, V.J. (1948). *The Mechanism of Abdominal Pain*. Australasian Medical Publishing Company, Sydney.

Lenz, R.A., Gracely, R.H., Hope, E.J. *et al.* (1994). The sensation of angina can be evoked by stimulation of the human thalamus. *Pain*, **59**: 119–126.

THE MANAGEMENT OF LOW BACK PAIN 22

C. Price

The key points covered in this chapter include:

- The size and nature of the problem.
- Work and disability issues.
- Treatment approaches.

for chronic low back pain.

Epidemiology

It is estimated that 60–80% of people will have low back pain (LBP) at some time in their life. The annual incidence of back pain in the UK is around 40%, with around 40% of sufferers visiting their general practitioner (GP) for help. Disability from back pain in people of working age is one of the most dramatic failures of health care in recent years. In 1998 the direct health care costs of LBP were estimated at 1.6 billion pounds to the UK. These are dwarfed by the indirect costs of LBP, related to lack of productivity and informal care services, estimated to be 10.7 billion pounds. This makes the so-called 'back pain epidemic' one of the costliest maladies in the Western world. Its greatest impact is on the lives of those affected and their families. However, it also has a major effect on industry through absenteeism and avoidable costs (the Confederation of British Industries estimate that back pain costs £208 for every employee each year) and at any one time 430,000 people in UK are receiving various social security benefits primarily for back pain. However, it is worth considering that although back pain is probably a universal complaint, its impact on suffers level of disability seems to be highest in the West, with sufferers in less developed areas of the world losing very little productivity. Only a societal approach to the problem is, therefore, likely to have significant impact on the reduction of these costs. Pain clinics play a small part in this.

Back pain accounts for 50% of an average pain clinic's workload. Pain clinics do not treat short-lived episodes of LBP, being generally referred patients who have developed chronic LBP and also suffer considerable disruption to their lives. The emphasis should be very much on management rather than cure and should follow a chronic disease framework. This represents a formidable challenge.

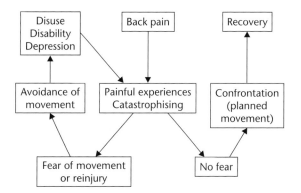

Figure 22.1 Mechanism of disability in low back pain – the fear avoidance model (after Vlaeyen, J.W. & Linton, S.J. (2000). Fear-avoidance and its consequences in chronic musculoskeletal pain: a state of the art. *Pain*, **85**: 317–332).

Aetiology

The aetiology of LBP is at best multi-factorial, at worst, unknown. Accurate diagnosis of the cause of LBP is only possible in about 15% of cases. Long-term pain can be highly disabling and costly. The aetiology of the pain itself is often obscure, but the mechanisms of disability are better understood.

The most powerful predictors of disability are the tendency to catastrophise regarding the ability to self-manage the episode of LBP and the level of fear engendered by that pain. Figure 22.1 shows how this translates into the common clinical picture encountered in pain clinics. Increasing disability leads to de-conditioning and more pain.

Patient assessment

Assessment of the patient should follow a bio-psychosocial approach. It begins with a full history, with particular attention paid to the patient's description of the pain in terms of the character and the chronology of symptoms, noting exacerbating and relieving

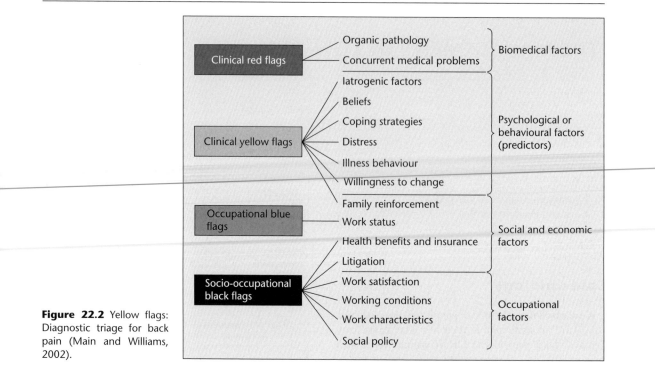

Figure 22.2 Yellow flags: Diagnostic triage for back pain (Main and Williams, 2002).

factors. The behavioural response to this pain should be noted. This includes downtime (rest time), beliefs, impact of pain on daily activities and goals of treatment. An examination with a focus on the musculoskeletal and nervous systems is mandatory.

The aim is to arrive at a shared understanding of the problem, show empathy and formulate together the appropriate way forwards for the individual.

The 1994 Clinical Standards Advisory Group report recommended that back pain be triaged as follows:

- Possible serious spinal pathology.
- Nerve root pain.
- Simple backache.

Pain clinics deal with the latter two scenarios. A diagnostic process that 'flags' areas for concern has been developed to aid this process (Figure 22.2).

Red flags

A red flag, that is, serious systemic disease associated with spinal pathology, is outside the scope of the pain clinic. A brief assessment to exclude these conditions is therefore necessary. It is important to have a good working relationship with other disciplines. Rapid referral for investigation, if required, is important if someone is struggling to manage their pain and may have a systemic disease. Figure 22.3 shows typical red flags.

- Presentation under age 20 or over 55
- Constant, progressive, non-mechanical pain
- Past history of cancer, steroids, human immunodeficiency virus (HIV)
- Weight loss, systemically unwell
- Violent trauma
- Thoracic pain
- Widespread neurological symptoms/signs
- Structural deformity
- Intravenous drug abuse with potential for spinal osteomyelitis
- Cauda equina syndrome requires immediate referral – suggested by sphincter disturbance, saddle anaesthesia and lower limb weakness

Figure 22.3 Red flags in LBP (indicative of potential major tissue pathology).

Nerve root pain is within the scope of a pain clinic. However, if there is major compression as evidenced by root signs or loss of bowel/bladder function this should be referred for surgical review.

One or more of the following features suggests nerve root pain:

- Unilateral leg pain that is worse than the back pain.
- Radiation below the knee.
- Numbness and/or paraesthesia.
- Reproduction of leg pain by straight leg raise or positive sciatic stretch test.
- Localised neurological signs.

Causes of acute radiculopathy include:

- Disc prolapse (95% at either L5/S1 or L4/L5).
- Foraminal stenosis secondary to degenerative changes.
- Hypertrophy of facet joint or ligament flavum.
- Abscess, haematoma and tumour.

Investigations have a very limited role. Nerve conduction studies or electromyography may confirm neuropathy. Magnetic resonance imaging (MRI) studies may be used to identify the pathological lesion if surgery is contemplated, but many people have prolapsed discs that are completely asymptomatic.

Most patients have 'simple' backache. Arriving at the diagnosis of 'simple backache' on clinical grounds could prevent a lot of unnecessary investigations and physical interventions, with both patient and clinician able to progress towards rehabilitation and return of function much sooner. Therefore, it is important to exclude the above conditions rapidly. However, by the time most people arrive at a pain clinic they are likely to have already spent considerable time in the referral loop in search of a diagnosis. They may also have had previous surgeries. From a biomedical perspective it is important to distinguish between nociceptive and neuropathic pain, and whether a radiculopathy is present. This can be achieved through careful history taking, looking for evidence of nerve injury and symptoms commensurate with this. For example, nociceptive pain will tend to be aching, worse on movement and helped by heat, massage, etc. Neuropathic pain tends to be present continuously, with the skin sensitive to touch and be burning, tingling or shooting in nature.

Yellow flags

Yellow flags are psychosocial barriers to recovery. Early identification and management of these yellow flag conditions may be helpful in limiting the chronicity of back pain and reducing the resulting disability. However, the majority of people referred with LBP to a pain clinic have become disabled by their pain. Thus, they will have one or more of these factors. It is important to elicit these in the history in a systematic fashion in order to plan treatment.

The following factors are important and consistently predict poor outcomes:

- Belief that back pain is harmful or potentially severely disabling.
- Fear-avoidance behaviour and reduced activity levels.

- Tendency to low mood and withdrawal from social interaction.
- Expectation of passive treatment(s) rather than a belief that active participation will help.

Figure 22.4 shows a useful mnemonic to elicit these areas.

• Attitudes and beliefs	• Diagnostic issues
• Behaviours	• Emotions
• Compensation issues	• Family and work

Figure 22.4 'Yellow flags' – psychosocial predictors of disability.

A specific behaviour that tends to lead to increased disability is the overactivity–underactivity cycle is shown in Figure 22.5.

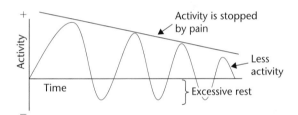

Figure 22.5 *Overactivity–underactivity cycle* – pushing through pain leads to doing less. 'Boom bust' is a common pattern of activity in anyone who is becoming disabled by their pain. It shows that someone is controlled by their pain rather than them managing it. A musculoskeletal pain sufferer is frustrated by an inability to carry out tasks as it hurts to move. Thus, when they hit a 'good day' they will try to carry on until the pain tells them to stop. If they rely on rest as the main way of dealing with their pain then they rest until the pain is better. During this time structures involved in movement become de-conditioned. The next time they come to do something these structures will ache more and the pain intensity will reach a higher pitch earlier. Thus, they will stop earlier. Gradually, disability worsens until the good day activity is a very small amount and a large amount of rest ensues. The amount of de-conditioning is dependent on how the individual views their pain. The only way out of this is by pacing up activities by a fixed quota every day. The therapist will work with the patient on establishing "baselines" for activity. This amount is done every day until the person is confident that they can do it no matter what the pain is like. Then that quota is slightly increased. In this fashion, disability decreases and the individual gains more confidence. Dealing with the frustration that comes with fixing baselines often requires careful handling. Managing the difficulties in setting baselines is usually a considerable challenge requiring a carefully planned psychological intervention.

Blue flags

Blue flags are occupational factors promoting work-related disability. The development of chronic pain and disability depends more on individual and work-related psychosocial issues than on physical or clinical features. People with physically or psychologically demanding jobs may have more difficulty working when they have LBP, and so lose more time from work. However, this can be the effect, rather than the cause, of their LBP. General disaffection with the work situation, attribution of blame, beliefs and attitudes about the relationship between work and symptoms, job dissatisfaction and poor employer–employee relationships may also constitute 'obstacles to recovery'.

Useful steps that a pain clinic team can undertake are as follows:

- Address the common misconception among workers and employers that you need to be pain free to return to work.
- Advise on ways in which the job can be adjusted to facilitate return to work.
- If reports are requested, then areas to work on should be highlighted rather than just a statement of current limitations.

Black flags

These are organisational or societal barriers to recovery eg no graded return to work, no incentives to losing benefits. Economic restructuring in the last 30 years has meant that a significant part of the population has drifted onto incapacity benefits. In addition, the support for these claimants has decreased, thus leaving them mired on this benefit. Musculoskeletal pain (mostly with spinal pain) accounts for 22% of this group. The main reasons given for remaining on benefits are: beliefs that there will not be appropriate work, lack of confidence in managing work and financial difficulties in coming off benefits. Yet being out of work is a significant health risk in itself, increasing the likelihood of depression and cardiovascular events. Joint working between benefits agencies and health care professionals, together with easier movement between benefits, is likely to be the only way to address these issues.

Overall, the assessment of 'red flags' will identify the small number of patients who need referral for an urgent surgical opinion. Similarly, patients with declared suicidal intent require immediate psychiatric referral. These two groups of patients need to be managed separately. For the vast majority of patients however, the identification of contributory psychological and social factors should be seen as an investigation of the normal range of reactions to pain, rather than the seeking of psychopathology.

Treatment options

A careful structured bio-psychosocial assessment as above will reveal the areas for treatment. As with any chronic disease, negotiation of treatment goals and an empathic approach are more likely to produce a satisfactory treatment outcome than a prescriptive approach. Treatments should, therefore, not be viewed in isolation, although the evidence for individual treatments is listed below. Figure 22.6 shows a summary of treatments generally available in pain clinics for the treatment of LBP.

Treatment	Example
Physical therapies	Graded exercise
Complementary	Acupuncture
Neuromodulation	TENS
Injection therapy	Epidural steroid injections
	Facet joint injection
	Radio frequency lesioning
Drug therapy	Paracetamol
Psychological	Cognitive-behavioural therapy

Figure 22.6 Groups of treatments for LBP commonly available in pain clinics.

Staying active compared with bed rest

Bed rest has consistently been shown to give worse outcomes in pain, functional status, recovery and sick leave, and cannot be recommended. All chronic LBP sufferers should be encouraged to keep fit. This reduces the risk of disabling flare-ups.

Behavioural treatments

Cognitive, operant and respondent treatments focus on the reduction of disability through the modification of environmental influences and cognitive processes. Treatments should address:

- The overactivity–underactivity cycle: through pacing techniques.
- Fear processes: through exposure techniques.
- Reduction of catastrophic thoughts: through cognitive challenging.

Systematic reviews have shown a moderate effect for cognitive-behavioural therapy in terms of improving functional outcomes. They do not aim to reduce pain, although pain reduction may occur. Recent works on specific behavioural treatments, which combine active rehabilitation with vocational training, suggest that high return to work rates from incapacity benefit are achievable.

Pharmacological interventions

As back pain is multi-factorial, so rational prescribing is difficult. Most pain will be nociceptive in mechanism and this would be expected to respond to conventional analgesia using stepwise increments. For all chronic pain, medication should be taken regularly. The role of antidepressant medication in back pain is uncertain.

Transcutaneous electrical nerve stimulation

Transcutaneous electrical nerve stimulation (TENS) is often used in pain clinics. It is non-invasive, safe and can be administered by trained nursing staff. It works by increasing Aβ signals into the spinal cord, which 'gates' pain messages. It can be helpful, although often practical problems in its application outweigh the benefits. Evidence for its benefit is not strong, but it remains popular with patients.

Acupuncture

Due to the problems of comparing acupuncture to an 'inert' control, there is not much quality research available. Some series have reported good results in the treatment of back pain. However, it must be viewed within the context of multidisciplinary treatments. High dependency on the therapist is a real risk.

Injection therapy

Epidural injections

Epidural steroid injections give short-lived pain relief for a minority of patients with radicular symptoms. This effect does not translate into improved functioning for most. They do not appear effective when there is significant disc prolapse. Providing a series of injections does not appear to improve outcome. There is an incidence of morbidity with epidural injections:

- Post-dural puncture headache.
- Intra-vascular injection.
- Epidural abscess and haematoma formation.
- A small risk of aseptic meningitis or arachnoiditis, if steroids are injected inadvertently into the sub-arachnoid space.

The risks and benefits of an injection need to be carefully discussed.

Facet joint injections

The facet (or zygapophyseal) joints are a potential source of back pain. Single photon emission computed tomography (SPECT) scans of hot spots correlate highly with certain types of back pain. They form the posterior articulations of the vertebrae and are paired. Innervation is complex. The medial branch of the posterior primary ramus innervates them. Each joint receives innervation from the dorsal ramus at the same level and also from the dorsal ramus of the vertebra above.

Pain secondary to lumbar facet joint problems may radiate into the hips, buttocks and thighs, and may be associated with spasm of the paraspinal muscles.

The joints themselves may be injected with 1.5–2 ml of local anaesthetic (for a 'diagnostic' block), possibly in combination with corticosteroid (for a 'therapeutic' block). Alternatively, the medial branch may be blocked, to denervate the joint. This may also be regarded as a diagnostic block, as success may be regarded as a prelude to a more lasting denervation with radio frequency lesioning or cryotherapy. However, diagnosis of facet joint dysfunction is impossible without blockade, which in itself may fail to be sufficiently specific to make a diagnosis. Thus, the utility of facet joint injections remains highly questionable. Again, pain relief is relatively short lived and usually requires concurrent other treatments.

Surgery

Surgery may be appropriate for some back pain sufferers. It is beyond the scope of a pain clinician, although it is important to recognise when to refer for surgery. Reasons for referral may include significant disc prolapse with neurological features and increasing neurological signs with spinal stenosis. Microdiscectomy, laminectomy and spinal fusion are examples of surgical interventions. Surgery for degenerative conditions affecting the lumbar spine has had disappointing results. There is no scientific evidence to show the long-term effectiveness of surgical interventions compared with placebo, or conservative management strategies. There is an appreciable incidence of persistent pain following back surgery. The 'failed back syndrome' affects up to 15% of back surgery patients. Recurrence of the original problem, an undiagnosed source of pain and post-surgical scarring are possible causes.

Key points

- Assessments needs to be structured systematically to look for biomedical, psychosocial and occupational barriers to recovery.

- There has been a paradigm shift in the management of chronic LBP presenting at pain clinics. The emphasis has moved from pain relief to improvement of psychophysical functioning.
- Assessment needs to take into account the known mechanisms for maintaining disability.
- The bio-psychosocial model has proved more successful than the biomedical one. Treatment should be directed through this model, often necessitating more than one approach.
- A multidisciplinary environment would seem the best way to deliver this sort of care for the needs of an average pain clinic attendee.
- A wide-ranging societal approach may, in the long term, be the most effective way of dealing with back pain.

Effective Health Care: Acute and Chronic Low Back Pain: 2000: 6:5. NHS Centre for Reviews and Dissemination: http://www.york.ac.uk/inst/crd/ehc65.htm

Main, C. & Williams, A. (2002). Musculoskeletal pain. *Br. Med. J.*, **325**: 534–537.

Topical Issues in Pain 2 (2000). In: Gifford, L. (ed.) *Biopsychosocial Assessment and Management*. CNS Press, Falmouth, Cornwall.

Von Korff, M., Glasgow, R.E. & Sharpe, M. (2002). Organising care for chronic illness. *Br. Med. J.*, **325**: 92–94.

Waddell, G. (1998). *The Back Pain Revolution*. Churchill Livingstone, London.

Waddell, G. & Burton, A.K. (2000). *Occupational Health Guidelines for the Management of Low Back Pain at Work – Evidence Review*. Faculty of Occupational Medicine, London.

Further reading

Department for Work and Pensions (2002). *Pathways to Work: Helping People into Employment*. HMSO, Norwich.

CANCER PAIN

23

S. Lund & S. Cox

Introduction

Pain is what many patients with active cancer fear and uncontrolled pain is associated with requests for euthanasia. Some consider such suffering inevitable and may expect that pain will increase in severity with disease progression. In fact up to 35% of patients with cancer will not experience pain. Research shows us that 95% of this pain is easily controlled using simple protocols. As ever, the successful relief of pain depends upon the careful evaluation of symptoms and constant review.

Aetiology and types of cancer pain

The experience and expression of pain in the context of active cancer may be affected, among other things, by the psychological state of the individual, their social circumstances, and support. The knowledge that prognosis is limited, or uncertain, gives pain heightened meaning.

Cancer patients can experience pain as a direct result of their disease, or indirectly from more general effects of illness, the treatment and unrelated causes (Table 23.1). Most disease-related pain is chronic, but patients also experience acute pains and accurate assessment is essential. It is important to recognize that most cancer patients with pain have multiple sites and causes for their pain. Every pain described by the patient must be evaluated and treated individually.

Assessment of cancer pain

The assessment of pain in patients with cancer can be misleading. As the pain is often chronic, the physiological signs we associate with acute pain (tachycardia, hypertension, etc.) are often absent. It may be difficult to link the severity of pain as reported by the patient with their physical appearance. In all cases it must be taken that 'pain is what the patient says hurts'.

Assessment includes a pain history (Chapter 12). Baseline visual analogue scale (VAS) or numerical

Table 23.1 Aetiology of cancer pain

Possible cause	Examples
Direct result of disease	Pancreatic pain from primary pancreatic cancer Back pain from bony metastases Nerve root compression pain
General effects of illness	Painful pressure areas Painful venous thrombosis (immobility and hypercoagulable state) Constipation
Treatment-related causes	Radiotherapy: mucositis/neuropathy Chemotherapy induced peripheral neuropathy Constipation Post-surgical pain
Unrelated causes	Ischaemic heart disease Osteoarthritis Cholecystitis Diverticular disease

rating scale (NRS) with follow-up monitoring may illustrate the response to treatment for individuals. In frail patients who may find pain difficult to describe, simpler pain scales, such as FACES or behavioural assessment (Chapter 27 & 28), may be more effective.

Management of cancer pain

Diagnosis of the cause of each cancer pain is important in order to direct management appropriately. Efforts should first be made to reverse the cause while symptomatic treatment is started (Table 23.2). Frequent reassessment of pain and its response to treatment is essential. Expression of pain will be affected by other symptoms, success or failure of oncological treatment, and the social and spiritual context. Failure to address such issues may result in poor pain control.

Table 23.2 Management of cancer pain

Assess pain	For example, multiple tender and painful bones
Diagnose cause	Bone pain from metastatic breast cancer
Reverse/treatment cause	Anticancer chemotherapy or hormonal therapy Radiotherapy to painful bones or bisphosphonate infusion
Symptomatic treatment	NSAIDs +/− WHO analgesic ladder
Frequent review and reassessment	

Table 23.3 Non-pharmacological measures for symptomatic treatment of cancer pain

- Explanation and information
- Heat/cold
- Rest/exercise
- Reflexology
- Relaxation techniques
- Aromatherapy
- Massage
- Acupuncture
- Anxiety management

Table 23.4 The WHO analgesic ladder

Step	Regular prescription	Plus 'as required' prescription
1	Non-opioid (paracetamol 1 g four times daily)	Weak opioid
2	Maximal dose weak opioid +/− paracetamol	Strong opioid
3	Strong opioid	Strong opioid

Symptomatic management of cancer pain

Symptomatic management of cancer pain may involve non-pharmacological measures in addition to drug treatment and interventional procedures.

Non-pharmacological measures for symptomatic treatment of cancer pain

Non-pharmacological measures including complementary therapies are important to many cancer patients (Table 23.3). Accessing such therapies gives individuals a feeling of control and helps them to cope with their illness. Explanation about their pain should be provided to the degree the patient requires. However, there is little evidence that these measures are effective in controlling cancer pain and other symptomatic measures are usually required.

Drug therapy for cancer pain

Symptomatic treatment of chronic cancer pain aims to render patients pain free. Since a patient may have progressive disease it must be anticipated that their pain will increase and provision should be made for this. Patients need regular analgesia to control their background pain with additional provision of equally strong analgesia for 'breakthrough' or extra pain. They must be reviewed sufficiently often to respond to changes in their disease, and therefore pain. Injectable routes for analgesia should only be used if patients cannot tolerate or absorb oral medication. A standardized approach should be used, but doses increased according to individual response. Finally, prescribers should be conscious of opioid fears in themselves and their patients.

In 1986 the World Health Organization (WHO) published international guidelines for the management of chronic cancer pain. These guidelines (the 'WHO analgesic ladder') comprise a step-wise approach to pain relief (Table 23.4). The WHO analgesic ladder represents a standard way of approaching a patient's cancer pain. Regardless of the severity of their pain, they should be started at the first rung that represents an increase in their analgesia. Therefore, if they have not been taking regular analgesia at all they should be prescribed regular paracetamol. At each step, review can be frequent and changes made daily with safety. If regular paracetamol has not controlled the pain after 24 h, the prescription is changed to regular weak opioids with or without paracetamol. Commonly used drugs at this step would be co-codamol 30/500 (codeine 30 mg and paracetamol 500 mg) two tablets six hourly, or tramadol 100 mg six hourly or 200 mg in the modified release form twice daily (but beware of confusion in the elderly). After about 24 h on this prescription the patient can be reviewed and changed to the third 'rung' of the ladder if they are still experiencing pain. In the context of chronic cancer pain the rotation or addition of alternate weak opioids is not recommended. Equally, it is felt that once cancer pain requires strong opioids, the weak opioids will add little of benefit and should be stopped.

The strong opioid of choice is immediate release oral morphine, prescribed four hourly at a standard starting dose of 5–10 mg *per* dose. This dose can be reviewed and increased each day until the pain is controlled. Accepted practice in specialist palliative care is to increase the dose of morphine by approximately 50% each time. Experience has shown that this is safe and effective. If a patient has required more than this increase in breakthrough medication it may be appropriate to use a larger increment. Once the pain is controlled on four-hourly dosing, a more convenient modified preparation of morphine, such as 'MST' (twice daily) or 'MXL' (once daily), may be substituted. At each rung of the ladder an 'as required' prescription of analgesia for breakthrough pain should be provided which is as strong or stronger than the regular prescription. The dose of strong opioid prescribed for breakthrough pain should be about a sixth of the daily regular prescription, or equal to a four-hourly dose. A regular laxative should be prescribed together with strong opioids unless the patient has diarrhoea.

Patients (and health professionals) may have commonly held misconceptions about prescribed morphine that need to be addressed. For example, patients with cancer pain may need reassurance that they will not become dependent on morphine or act like a 'zombie'. They are frequently concerned that starting morphine will leave them nothing 'strong' for 'when they need it'. They need to understand that being prescribed morphine does not imply they are close to death, although it may generate an important discussion about expectations and insight.

Side effects of strong opioids are many (Table 23.5), although the drugs are usually well tolerated in comparison to other analgesics. Individuals should be warned that they will experience drowsiness for the first few days, but it will usually wear off. Nausea is unusual in clinical practice – possibly as tolerance has developed to this side effect by the pre-prescription of weak opioids. For occasional patients the side effects of morphine may limit the dose or make it intolerable. There is some evidence that alternate strong opioids may be useful here, as the adverse effect profile may be better. This has been suggested for transdermal fentanyl and extrapolated to drugs like oxycodone, hydromorphone, transdermal buprenorphine and even methadone.

In situations where the oral route is inappropriate, transdermal or injectable analgesia should be substituted. Examples of this situation include patients unable to swallow, vomiting, or not absorbing through the gastrointestinal tract. The injectable opioid of choice is diamorphine and the route of choice in this event is subcutaneous. Diamorphine is preferred to morphine, as it is more soluble and therefore requires smaller volumes to be administered. The subcutaneous route can be managed by hospital or district nurses and allows for a combination of symptomatic drugs to be administered

Table 23.5 The more common adverse effects of opioids

- Constipation
- Drowsiness
- Nausea
- Dry mouth
- Itch
- Urinary retention

via a continuous infusion. Parenteral diamorphine is about three times as potent as oral morphine.

Other opioids can be given parenterally and may be required for those who develop intolerable side effects with diamorphine, or those who have renal failure. Fentanyl can be administered in a pump subcutaneously. The maximum concentration that can be used is $50\,\mu g/ml$ and therefore volume can limit the use of fentanyl in a syringe driver. Alfentanil is a synthetic opioid that is chemically related to fentanyl. It is metabolized by cytochrome P450 in the liver and therefore doses may need to be increased if it is prescribed with P450 enzyme-inducing drugs, or reduced if prescribed with P450 enzyme-inhibiting drugs. Dose reductions may also be required in those with liver failure and obese patients. Alfentanil is about 10 times as potent as diamorphine when given subcutaneously and about as potent as fentanyl.

Other routes of administration can be used in certain circumstances. Intra-nasal diamorphine has been used for breakthrough pain in a metered dose delivery system. Topical opioids can be applied to inert dressings for painful wounds.

Non-steroidal anti-inflammatory drugs

Although studies have shown that non-steroidal anti-inflammatory drugs (NSAIDs) are effective analgesics in many types of cancer pain, they are chiefly indicated for malignant bone pain or to reduce inflammation in pleuritic pain or liver capsular pain. They can be used preferentially or added to the analgesic ladder at any step.

Adjuvant analgesics

Adjuvant analgesics are drugs used to reduce pain whose primary indication is not analgesia (Table 23.6). Examples would be:

- Tricyclic antidepressants or antiepileptics in neuropathic pain.
- High dose steroids for raised intracranial pressure headache.

Table 23.6 Common adjuvant analgesics

Drugs	Symptom control
Tricyclic antidepressants Antiepileptics Ketamine	Neuropathic pain
Corticosteroids	Reduce pain associated with tumour oedema
Benzodiazepines Baclofen Buscopan	Muscle spasm
Bisphosphonates	Bone pain

The use of tricyclic antidepressants and antiepileptics in cancer pain is based on research in non-cancer neuropathy. Large randomized controlled trials in the cancer population have proved difficult to perform, although smaller studies support their use.

Interventional procedures

This incorporates physical ways of relieving pain, either by interfering with the physiological mechanisms of the disease, or by interfering with the neuronal pathways of pain. These processes can be used at all stages of the disease assuming that the patient is well enough to tolerate the intervention and that the potential side effects are acceptable to the patient. They include:

- *Radiotherapy*: especially useful in cases of pain secondary to bone metastases. It can also be used to reduce tumour bulk, so relieving visceral pain.
- *Surgery*: useful in reducing tumour bulk and may be necessary if acute situations arise (e.g. bowel obstruction).

- *Chemotherapy*: can be used to reduce primary tumour bulk and may have an effect on metastases.
- *Nerve blocks*: involves the injection of local anaesthetic with variable effect.

With all of these procedures, there are potential side effects that must be balanced against potential benefits for individual patients. For those patients with end stage cancer, physical debility may preclude several of the options.

Key points

- Cancer pain is not inevitable but can be devastating.
- The aim is to render the patient pain free.
- Accurate assessment is essential.
- Most cancer pain is easily treated using the WHO analgesic ladder.
- NSAIDs and adjuvant analgesics may be needed for inflammatory or neuropathic pains.

Further reading

Cancer Pain Relief and Palliative Care (1990). Report of a WHO expert committee: Geneva: World Health Organisation, 1990. *WHO Technical Report Series*, No. 804.

Foley, K.M. (1998). Pain assessment and cancer pain syndromes. *Oxford Textbook of Palliative Medicine*, 2nd edition. Oxford Medical Publications.

Hanks, G., Portenoy, R.K., MacDonald, N. & Forbes, K. (1998). Difficult pain problems. *Oxford Textbook of Palliative Medicine*, 2nd edition. Oxford Medical Publications.

O'Neill, B. & Fallon, M. (1997). ABC of palliative care. Principles of palliative care and pain control. *Br. Med. J.*, **315**: 801–804.

POST-OPERATIVE PAIN 24

T. Kirwan

Incidence

In 1990, The Royal College of Surgeons (RCS) report 'pain after surgery' found 30–70% patients with moderate or worse pain after surgery. A recent review finds that although the incidence of post-operative pain has reduced by ~2%/year for the last 30 years, 30% of patients still complain of moderate pain and 11% severe pain.

Factors affecting the severity of post-operative pain

Expected pain and analgesic requirements following surgery are extremely variable:

Type of surgery
- Size of the wound, amount of tissue damage.
- Muscle cutting or splitting incision.
- Technique, delicacy of dissection and retraction, type of stitch.

Site of surgery
- Movement of damaged tissues (e.g. chest and upper abdominal surgery).
- Oedema in a confined space (e.g. total knee replacement).

Patient factors
- Age, sex, medical condition and emotional state.
- Reason for/outcome of surgery.
- Other sources of distress: nausea, sleeplessness, noise.
- Home circumstances, anxiety about family, work.

Cultural background
- Attitudes to illness, treatment and pain.

Advantages of effective treatment

The fundamental imperative to treat post-operative pain is humanitarian; 'It is the basic duty of all health care professionals to relieve pain' RCS Report on Pain after Surgery 1990. We should not tolerate people suffering pain when effective treatment is readily available.

Other than the humanitarian, potential benefits may be:

1 *Physiological*: attenuating the stress response and reducing sympathetic stimulation.
2 *Clinical*: potentially reducing complications:
   - Effective analgesia promotes patient co-operation with physiotherapy, improved respiratory function, earlier feeding, better mobilisation with reduced risk of pressure sores and deep vein thrombosis. There is level 1 evidence (see Chapter 31) of improvement in respiratory, cardiovascular and overall outcome in with adequately treated pain.
   - Early and aggressive treatment of acute pain may prevent the development of chronic post-operative pain.
3 *Organizational*: following potential reductions in post-operative complications and improved mobility. Earlier discharge results in cost savings. The commonest cause of failure to discharge from day surgery is uncontrolled pain.

In Summary

- Post-operative pain can be controlled by optimal use of conventional analgesics.
- Analgesia fails because of organisational failures.
- There are major benefits from good pain control.

Reasons for failure

Post-operative pain can be treated effectively with appropriate combinations of local anaesthetic, morphine, non-steroidal anti-inflammatory drug (NSAID) and paracetamol. It is important to recognise that these drugs and their techniques of administration are well known. Sub-optimal use of conventional drugs is the commonest cause of failure of analgesia (Table 24.1).

Table 24.1 Causes and solutions for analgesia failure

Problem	Cause	Solution
Clinicians underestimate patients' pain	Staff do not ask patients about pain Patients do not report pain Patients expect to be in pain and do not want to be a bother	Regular pain assessment Self-scoring by patients
Doctors prescribe inadequate doses	Fear of adverse effects Fear of masking physical signs	Regular monitoring of vital signs Education: carefully titrated analgesia does not inhibit diagnosis
Nurses give drugs (particularly opioids) insufficiently frequently	Time needed to administer controlled drugs Fear of respiratory depression and over-sedation Fear of addiction	Patient controlled analgesia (PCA) Clear monitoring guidelines and procedures for managing adverse effects Education: addiction does not occur in patients taking opioids to treat acute pain
Patients fail to take analgesia	Side effects of drugs Fear of drugs/equipment	Regular prophylaxis for expected side effects Patient information, both as leaflet and personal discussion
Rigid traditional analgesic regimes	Doses too small, interval too long	Local evidence based analgesia guidelines
Analgesia which is prescribed pro re nata (prn)	Not given until the patient has pain therefore always fails to prevent pain	Regular administration

Management of post-operative pain

There is good evidence that three changes to practice have a major impact on post-operative pain control:

1 Introduction of local guidelines for simple analgesic techniques.
2 Education of patients, nurses and doctors to use the guidelines.
3 Regular pain assessment.

Guidelines (for more information see Chapter 50)

Implementation of local guidelines improves effectiveness and safety. Guidelines for each analgesic technique should include standard prescriptions, monitoring and procedure for adverse events. They allow each drug to be used to its optimal extent, while minimising the risk of complications.

Monitoring

Monitoring is essential for effective and safe pain management. Vital sign monitoring detects adverse effects of treatment, allowing the maximum safe dose of analgesia to be given. Thus, maximum benefit from each technique is provided (Figure 24.1).

Basic monitoring for every patient in hospital should include the pain score as the fifth vital sign recorded contemporaneously with: pulse rate, respiratory rate, blood pressure and temperature (Table 24.2).

Clinical assessment

Methodical assessment is key to successful analgesia. The cause and expected progress of post-operative pain are usually known. The primary concern is to measure intensity, changes with time and response to treatment. However, it is important not to overlook pain that may be a symptom of:

• Adverse effects of analgesia (e.g. gastric irritation).
• Complications of surgery (e.g. pleuritic pain).

PRE- AND POST-OPERATIVE OBSERVATION CHART

OPERATION DATE ....
OPERATION ....
....

PATIENT'S NAME ....   WARD ....
HOSPITAL NUMBER ....   CONSULTANT ....
NAMED NURSE ....

DATE														
TIME														
RGN Initials														

TEMPERATURE (°C)
41
40
39
38
37
36
35
34

BLOOD PRESSURE (mmHg) — PULSE (per minute)
250
240
230
220
210
200
190
180
170
160
150
140
130
120
110
100
90
80
70
60
50
40
30
20
10
0

Respiration rate (per minute)														
Oxygen delivery														
Oxygen saturation														
Sedation score (0–4)														
Pain score (0–4)														
Continuous analgesic (indicate route, type & dose)														
Intermittent analgesic (indicate route, type & dose)														
Nausea/vomiting Score (1–2)														
Antiemetic (indicate route, type & dose)														
Recovery Room Score (oxygen + sedation + pain + nausea/vomiting score)														

Analgesic route abbreviations: Intravenous (IV)   Epidural (EP)   Intramuscular (IM)   Subcutaneous (SC)   Oral (PO)   Rectal (PR)

Figure 24.1 Example of post-operative observation chart.

Table 24.2 Example of monitoring guidelines in a surgical ward

All patients	BP, HR, RR, pain, sedation and nausea scores check SpO_2 and monitor continuously if <95%	Hourly till stable, then 4 h
Additional monitoring requirements		
i.m. opioids	All scores before and 30 min after each i.m. injection	
PCA	Cumulative dose of morphine	Hourly till stable, then 4 h
Epidural	Continuous observation	Hourly for 12 h, 2 h when stable,
	Sensory level motor block	then 6 h
	Cumulative dose of epidural drugs, temperature	
	Inspection of pressure areas and catheter	
If there is any change in the patient's condition, increase frequency of observations to ¼h		

BP: blood pressure; HR: heart rate; RR: respiratory rate; SpO_2: oxygen saturation.

Table 24.3 CRIES neonatal pain assessment tool

	0	**1**	**2**
Crying	No	High pitched	Inconsolable
Requires O_2 for Sat >95%	No	<30%	>30%
Increased vital signs	HR and BP =/< pre-operative state	HR and BP increase <20% of pre-operative state	HR and BP increase >20% of pre-operative state
Expression	None	Grimace	Grimace/grunt
Sleepless	No	Wakes at frequent intervals	Constantly awake

Effective assessment

Self-reported
- Only the person suffering has real knowledge of the pain. Assessment should, whenever possible, be by the patient.

Specific
- Other causes of distress (such as nausea, anxiety, sleep disturbance) should be asked about, but not confused with pain.

Regular
- Assessment must be made frequently for patients with variable or poorly controlled pain and every time other routine observations are performed.

Quantitative
- A pain score must be recorded for comparison over time. This should be documented both at rest and moving (e.g. deep breathing, coughing, reaching the hand to the other side of the bed).

Methods of self-reporting in adults

- Categorical rating scales
  - Rating pain as: none, slight, moderate, severe, very severe.
  - Verbal score from 0 to 10 or 0 to 100.
- Visual analogue scale (VAS)

Marking a point to represent pain on a 10 cm line, where 0 cm represents no pain and 10 cm the worst imaginable pain. The scale needs explanation before surgery.

Methods of self-reporting in children and elderly patients

Children may evaluate their pain using pictures, toys and colours to represent intensity of pain. The Poker Chip Tool describes coloured counters representing bits of pain and the child picks some from the pile. The FACES scale is also useful (see Chapter 27).

Indirect pain scoring

When the patient is unable to report their own pain intensity (e.g. babies and toddlers, the very ill and demented) clinicians have to estimate pain indirectly. Methods include:

- *Professional judgement*: based on personal experience, previous professional experience, the appearance of patient and the vital signs.
- *Physiological and behavioural systems*: based on signs of sympathetic activity and behaviour usually associated with distress. Examples include:
  - FLACC (see Chapter 27).
  - CRIES system (Table 24.3).

0	1	2	3	3–4	3–4	3	2	1	0
Paracetamol prn	Paracetamol regular	Paracetamol regular	Paracetamol regular	Paracetamol regular	Paracetamol regular	Paracetamol regular	Paracetamol regular	Paracetamol regular	Paracetamol prn
		+NSAID regular	+NSAID regular	+NSAID regular	No NSAID with epidural catheter	+NSAID regular	+NSAID regular		
		+Codeine and laxative regular	+Morphine i.m./s.c. regular	+Morphine PCA and antiemetic	+Epidural infusion	+Morphine i.m./s.c. regular	+Codeine and laxative regular		
		or Morphine po regular					or Morphine po regular		
		or Tramadol regular					or Tramadol regular		

Pain score: 0 = no pain, 1 = slight pain, 2 = moderate pain, 3 = severe pain, 4 = very severe pain.

s.c.: sub-cutaneously; po: per OS.

Figure 24.2 Analgesia bridge (also known as Glyn's bridge).

In summary

- Effective pain control depends on education of staff and patients, use of local guidelines and regular pain assessment.
- Assessment of pain should be regular, specific, quantitative and recorded in the chart.
- Whenever possible pain assessments should be made by the patient.

Treatment of mild and moderate pain

Patient controlled analgesia (PCA) or epidural analgesia usually provides good pain control after major surgery. However, patients frequently have pain after intermediate surgery (or after stopping PCA or epidural) when treated with pro re nata (prn) oral/intramuscular (i.m.) analgesia. Appropriate analgesia should be provided throughout the post-operative period. A pain bridge, rather than a ladder, may help to emphasise the rising and falling nature of the analgesia requirement, and the need for appropriate step-down analgesia (Figure 24.2).

Use of the bridge

- Select a level of analgesia depending on severity of pain and patients condition.
- Regular administration: If more than one dose of analgesia is likely to be required it should be prescribed regularly, so that each dose is given before the effect of the previous one wears off.

- Combination of drugs of different types often gives better analgesia with fewer side effects. Drugs of the same type should not be combined.
- Prophylaxis against expected side effects.
- An 'insurance' analgesic regime should be prescribed prn for use if the first-line analgesic regime fails.
- Analgesics have adverse effects and contraindications to their use should be followed.
- It is prudent to use a small range of analgesics with which all staff are familiar.
- Regular opioids should be given only in compliance with a protocol, defining the standard of monitoring, and the range of physiological parameters which must be met for the dose to be given (Figure 24.3).

Treatment of severe pain

Opioids

Opioids are the gold standard of treatment for severe acute pain. Patients' requirements vary widely and effectiveness is increased by giving the dose that each patient needs, rather than using fixed dose regimes. If a dose has had its full effect (5 min after intravenous (i.v.), 1 h after i.m. and 90 min after oral) and the patient is still in pain, with stable vital signs, another dose can be given. Side-effects should be anticipated, watched for and prevented. For the sake of risk management hospitals should use one opioid as a regular first-line post-operative analgesic for severe pain, so that all staff are familiar with the standard regime. All

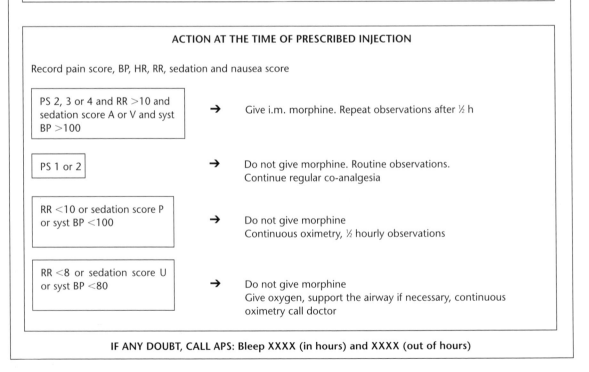

Regular IM morphine protocol chart

Patient's Name: ....

Ward: ......................D.O.B.................

Hospital Number:..............................

STANDARD PRESCRIPTION

Patients <70 years
>65 kg   10 mg morphine i.m./s.c.
<65 kg   7.5 mg morphine i.m./s.c.

Patient >70 years
>65 kg   7.5 mg morphine i.m./s.c.
<65 kg   5 mg morphine i.m./s.c.

MONITORING FOR PATIENTS ON OPIOIDS

BP, HR, RR, pain, sedation and nausea scores hourly till stable and then 4 hourly
BP, HR, RR, pain, sedation and nausea scores 30 min after each i.m. morphine injection
Check SpO_2 and monitor continuously if <95%

Pain score: 0 = no pain, 1 = slight pain, 2 = moderate pain, 3 = serve pain, 4 = very severe pain
Sedation score: A = alert, V = responds to voice, P = responds to pain, U = unresponsive

GENERAL INSTRUCTIONS

- Give oxygen as prescribed
- Regular co-analgesia and anti-emetics should be given as prescribed

ACTION AT THE TIME OF PRESCRIBED INJECTION

Record pain score, BP, HR, RR, sedation and nausea score

PS 2, 3 or 4 and RR >10 and sedation score A or V and syst BP >100	→ Give i.m. morphine. Repeat observations after ½ h
PS 1 or 2	→ Do not give morphine. Routine observations. Continue regular co-analgesia
RR <10 or sedation score P or syst BP <100	→ Do not give morphine. Continuous oximetry, ½ hourly observations
RR <8 or sedation score U or syst BP <80	→ Do not give morphine. Give oxygen, support the airway if necessary, continuous oximetry call doctor

IF ANY DOUBT, CALL APS: Bleep XXXX (in hours) and XXXX (out of hours)

Figure 24.3 Example of regular morphine protocol chart. APS: acute pain service; RR: respiratory rate; HR: heart rate; PS: pain score; sys BP: systolic blood pressure.

the opioids have similar and side effects. Which drug is chosen depends on local circumstances.

Administration

An i.v. bolus

An i.v. loading dose is usually required for uncontrolled severe pain. It should be used by slow i.v. injection while assessing its effect, until the patient is comfortable without excessive sedation or respiratory depression.

Oral

Morphine can be given by mouth. This route is suitable for patients whose gastrointestinal (GI) function is normal and whose requirement for analgesia is stable. However, bioavailability can be quite variable.

An i.m. injection

The traditional method of administration is safe and familiar. When used optimally it can be as effective as patient controlled analgesia (PCA). However, it often fails because it is given only when the patient is already in pain and then in inadequate doses after administrative delays. Plasma concentrations vary from excessive (with side effects) to sub-therapeutic (with breakthrough pain).

An i.v. infusion

A continuous infusion overcomes the problem of variable blood levels and the delays in administration of i.m. opioids. It requires a loading dose as a steady-state blood level is only obtained after about four half-lives. Infusion rate is adjusted according to response, but rapid changes in the need for analgesia are not accounted for. There is a risk of cumulation and overdose if the infusion continues at a steady rate regardless of the effect on the patient. Therefore, regular monitoring is crucial. This technique is especially suitable for intensive care unit (ICU), high dependency unit and terminal care.

Patient Controlled Analgesia (PCA)

PCA is a technique in which the patient self-administers a small dose of drug when necessary. This overcomes the practical problems of nurse administered intermittent i.m. analgesia. It has been shown to produce better analgesia and patient satisfaction with no greater incidence of adverse effects. However, The equipment is expensive, staff need to be trained in the technique, and the patient needs to be intellectually, emotionally and physically able to use the device.

When instituting PCA, the following parameters must be set:

Bolus
- The dose delivered when the patient presses the button.

Dose duration
- Some devices allow the bolus to be given over a variable period.
- Stat delivery allows the patient to feel the dose administered, but delivery over 2–3 min may reduce nausea.

Lock-out time
- Period within which the device will not give a subsequent dose Usually set at 5–10 min.
- Prevents multiple dosing and dosing prior to effect onset.

Background
- A continuous infusion used in addition to the bolus facility.
- Not used routinely for adults.
- There is no improvement in pain control but side effects are increased.

Loading dose
- A titrated dose of opioid given to establish analgesia before the patient takes over control.

Each patient can maintain the blood level of drug that gives the best pain control for the least side-effects, adjusting to the variable need for analgesia through the post-operative period.

The technique is intrinsically safe, in that the drug is only given on demand, so that if the patient becomes sedated administration stops. Respiratory depression and sedation may nevertheless occur and every hospital using PCA should have local guidelines for standard prescription, procedures and monitoring (Figure 24.4).

Other routes

- Intrathecal opioids may provide prolonged analgesia.
- Transdermal opioids and slow release preparations have a long half-life and are not suitable for treating acute pain.
- Newer routes of administration such as buccal and intranasal may be useful.

Local anaesthetics

Local anaesthesia provides total pain relief for the affected area. It is often used in the operating theatre and may be continued for post-operative analgesia. The duration of action of commonly used local anaesthetics ranges from 2 to 6 h. For longer-lasting

PATIENT WITH A PCA

ROUTINE CARE

Monitoring: On commencing infusion all observations are done 1/4 hourly for 1 hour, hourly for 4 hours, then 4 hourly if patient is stable. All observations 1/2 hourly if any instability.

4 hourly once stable	Oxygen saturation
(1/2 hourly if any instability)	Respiratory rate
	Sedation score
	Heart rate
	Blood pressure
	Pain score
	Nausea score
	Itch
Hourly	Volume administered via pump

Oxygen:
Use continuous oximetry and oxygen as required to keep saturation above 95% unless otherwise instructed.

Additional analgesia:
Additional opioids are not used
Other analgesics (e.g. Paracetamol, NSAIDs) should be given regularly if prescribed)

PROBLEMS

Pain is not controlled
Ensure maximum prescribed morphine is being used and maximum regular co-analgesia is given If this fails a re-loading dose should be given in increments intravenously by a doctor or the APS sister.

Respiratory depression or over-sedation
If: sedation score 2   ]   Suspend opioids
or: respiratory rate <10   ]   Administer oxygen. Measure oxygen saturation
or: syst BP <100   ]   Measure RR at least every 30 min
Opioids may be restarted, at a lower dose, once RR >10, syst BP >100 and sedation score <2.

If: sedation score 3   ]   Stop all opioids
or: respiratory rate <8   ]   Administer oxygen. Support airway if required. Measure oxygen saturation
or: syst BP <80   ]   Call doctor

Nausea and vomiting
All patients on PCA should have an anti-emetic (e.g. Cyclizine) given regularly If there is still nausea ondansetron is given as well. If this is unsuccessful call the APS

Itch
May be treated with a very low dose Naloxone IV (20–50 μg). Calamine lotion and Piriton can also be tried.

FULL GUIDELINES AVAILABLE ON INTRANET AND IN PAIN FOLDERS ON ALL SURGICAL WARDS.
IF IN ANY DOUBT, CALL APS: Bleep XXXX (in hours) and XXXX (out of hours)

OXYGEN SCORE		SEDATION SCORE		PAIN SCORE		NAUSEA/VOMITING SCORE	
0	Oxygen saturation >92% on air	0	Alert/awake	0	No pain	0	No nausea/vomiting
1	Oxygen saturation >90% on oxygen	1	Dozing/drowsy	1	Mild pain	1	Nausea
2	Oxygen saturation <90% on oxygen	2	Asleep / rousable	2	Moderate pain	2	Vomiting
		4	Asleep/unrousable	3	Severe pain		
				4	Unbearable pain		

DATE/TIME	COMMENTS

Figure 24.4 Example of PCA monitoring chart. APS: acute pain service.

analgesia repeated injections, or continuous infusion, is necessary.

Wound infiltration

Wound infiltration has been shown to be effective for most wounds. It is simple to perform, but likely to wear off before the pain abates. Therefore, other analgesia must be instituted early.

Topical

Local anaesthetic can be applied as a gel; for example, for venepuncture in children, or after surface, trans-urethral and eye surgery. This too is an easy method but short lasting.

Peripheral nerve and nerve plexus blocks

Peripheral nerve and nerve plexus blocks provide excellent pain control especially for limb surgery. A catheter can be used for extended post-operative pain relief, but catheters may become displaced and an alternative 'insurance' prescription is essential.

Epidural analgesia

Epidurals have major advantages but also carry significant risks. Effectiveness is increased and risk reduced by a high level of monitoring and skilled care. Staff must be trained in the technique and there must be sufficient throughput to maintain skills. Local guidelines should state a standard prescription, instructions for routine care and procedure for adverse effects. Levels of monitoring and facilities must be defined. Nursing requirements (general ward or in high dependency) depends on local circumstances.

Effects of epidural analgesia

- Sensory block provides high quality analgesia. Reduced risk of the sedation, respiratory depression and nausea associated with systemic opioids.
- Sympathetic block causes vasodilatation. This may result in hypotension if the block extends to levels involving sympathetic outflow (T1–L2) (particularly if there is co-existing hypovolaemia).
- Motor block may cause weakness.

Benefits of epidural analgesia

- Excellent analgesia can be achieved, without the use of systemic opioids, and the patient feels comfortable and well. Particularly useful for surgery involving chest, back, abdomen and legs.

- Combinations of opioids and local anaesthetics act synergistically to produce improved analgesia with fewer side effects.
- Mobilisation is improved, with patients able to cough and co-operate with physiotherapy. This is particularly useful for patients with respiratory disease, or following upper abdominal and thoracic surgery.
- A recent review of trials comparing patients with and without epidural in theatre found mortality reduced by one-third, pulmonary embolus by 55%, respiratory infection by 39%, and reductions in myocardial infarction and renal failure.

Disadvantages of epidural analgesia

- Analgesia fails if the catheter displaces.
- A high level of specialist care and monitoring are required.
- Complications include:

Needle
- Dural puncture (<1% of epidurals).
- Damage to nerves (about 1 in 5000) pleura, dura or viscus.
- Infection.
- Haematoma.

Local anaesthetic
- Hypotension.
- Excessive motor block.
- Urinary retention.
- Pressure sores.

Opioid
- Pruritus, nausea, sedation, urinary retention, respiratory depression.

Drug errors
- i.v. injection or overdose of local anaesthetic.

Non-drug analgesia

Non-drug analgesia should be used whenever possible and may be extremely effective. The painful stimulus may be reduced by immobilisation (e.g. a fracture) or careful mobilisation (e.g. low back pain). Inflammation and oedema may be reduced by elevation and ice packs. Non-painful stimulation, such as heat or trans-cutaneous nerve stimulation (TENS) is thought to reduce transmission of painful stimulation in the spinal cord. TENS is not effective as a sole treatment for moderate or severe pain. However, some trials have shown improved pain scores (or reduced opioid consumption) when used with conventional drug analgesia and some patients are very pleased with it. Psychological treatments may be very helpful. Some studies demonstrate that improvements in post-operative pain control can be achieved by:

– Patient information.
– Teaching skills, such as coughing, breathing exercises and relaxation.
– Formal programmes of psychological and personal support.

It is impossible to provide evidence that there is an analgesic effect from a sympathetic attitude of staff to patients. However it must make for greater patient and staff satisfaction.

In summary

• Mild to moderate pain should be treated with regular combination analgesia, using each technique to its maximum effect.
• There should be prophylaxis against expected side effects of treatment.
• Contra-indications to drugs must be respected.
• Opioids are the best drugs for severe pain. PCA is an effective form of administration.
• Epidural analgesia has major benefits in pain control and patient outcome. It also has risks.
• Local guidelines for standard care improve efficacy and safety.
• Non-drug analgesia should always be used as appropriate.

Key points

• Efficacy and safety are improved by use of local guidelines, staff and patient education, regular pain assessment and regular monitoring.
• Opioids are the gold standard of care for severe acute pain. NSAIDs are effective for moderate

pain, or as co-therapy for severe pain. Regional analgesia has important benefits but needs careful management.
• Regular combination therapy gives the best pain relief for the least side effects. The prescription should include a first and second-line analgesia plan, with prophylaxis against side effects of analgesia.
• The approach of staff to patients may have a profound effect on pain and suffering. Non-drug analgesia should be used whenever it is appropriate.
• Most post-operative pain can be controlled effectively by optimal use of common analgesic drugs and techniques.

Further reading

EBM Report: Acute pain management: scientific evidence 1999 Australian National Health and Medical Research Council. Full text on website www.health.gov.au/nhmrc/publications/

Harmer, M. & Davies, K.A. (1998). The effect of education, assessment and a standardised prescription on postoperative pain management. *Anaesthesia*, **53**: 424–430.

McQuay, H., Moore, A. & Justins, D. (1997). Treating acute pain in hospital. *Br. Med. J.*, **314**: 1531–1535.

Rowbotham & Macintyre (2003). *Clinical Pain Management: Acute Pain*. Arnold, London.

Rodgers, A., Walker, N., Schug, S., McKee, A., Kehlet, H., van Zundert, A., Sage, D., Futter, M., Saville, G., Clark, T. & MacMahon, S. (2000). Reduction of postoperative mortality and morbidity with epidural or spinal anaesthesia: results from overview of randomised trials. *Br. Med. J.*, **321**: 1493.

Web site: Oxford Pain Internet Site: www.jr2.ox.ac.uk/bandolier/booth/painpag/

M.G. Serpell

Introduction

In 1864 Silas Weir Mitchell and his associates published their monumental treatise on *Gunshot Wounds and Other Injuries of Nerves*. Their classic description was based on their experience of traumatic injuries during the American Civil War (Figure 25.1). Due to the fact that so very few nerve injuries were seen in civilian practice, little or no further mention was made of this syndrome until René Leriche published his observations following the German invasion of France in 1915 which left a trail of patients with nerve injuries.

Complex regional pain syndrome (CRPS) consists of a constellation of symptoms and signs in limbs, which usually follow traumatic injuries or events such as myocardial infarction or a stroke (Table 25.1). There are two types of syndrome:

• CRPS I – without nerve injury.
• CRPS II – with nerve injury.

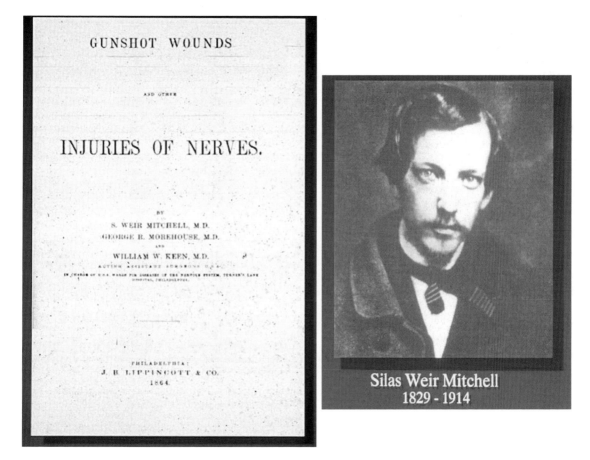

Figure 25.1 Silas Weir Mitchell.

Table 25.1	Examples of causes of CRPS	
Trauma	*Accidental*	Sprains, minor cuts, contusions, dislocations, fractures, crush injuries, traumatic amputation, burns
	Surgical	Tight plaster casts
		Tissue or nerve damage from any procedure
	Occupational	Repetitive strain injury such as pneumatic tool operators, typists etc.
Diseases	*Visceral*	Myocardial infarction
	Neurological	Cerebrovascular accident resulting in post-hemiplegic dystrophy
		Nerve damage by tumour invasion
	Vascular	Generalised angiopathies, frostbite, thrombosis

Both types can be further classified into those with (sympathetic mediated pain, SMP) or without (sympathetic independent pain, SIP) a sympathetic nervous system component to the pain (Jänig, 2002).

Severe degrees of pain or vasomotor changes may occur following seemingly insignificant injuries, which the patient may not even recall. CRPS predominantly affects the younger age group of the population and (if disabling) can have major potential economic implications. The natural history of CRPS is not known for certain due to the difficulties in diagnosis. However, it is considered by many experts to be mild and transient in nature, usually resolving spontaneously. Other cases stabilise into a mild disorder, while a small subset becomes chronic, severely disabling patients.

Diagnostic criteria

CRPS is difficult to diagnose, let alone treat. It was previously called 'reflex sympathetic dystrophy' (RSD) which reflected the consensus that these conditions involved abnormal reflex activity in the sympathetic nervous system. The term was revised in 1993 by a Special Consensus Workshop organised by the International Association for the Study of Pain (IASP) to that of CRPS (Harden *et al.*, 1999; Bruehl and Harden, 2002). The group felt that the term RSD had lost usefulness as a clinical designation because it had been used so indiscriminately that it was no longer clear what it meant.

In general, CRPS conditions (Figure 25.2) are manifested by a triad of:

* Pain.
* Vasomotor disturbances.
* Trophic changes.

The pain is usually constant and diffuse, but characteristically increases when the limb is dependent.

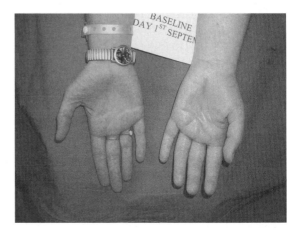

Figure 25.2 The patient has trophic changes of the left arm, which displays oedema of the hand and thin glossy skin. Reproduced from Varma, T.R.K. (2002). Neurosurgical techniques in the treatment of chronic pain. *Anaesth. Intens. Care Med.*, **3(1)** (by kind permission of The Medicine Publishing Company).

Unlike neuralgia, it does not have a segmental or peripheral nerve distribution, but is almost invariably associated with hyperaesthesia. While the initiating aetiological factors may be very different, the underlying mechanisms producing the symptoms are probably similar (if not identical) in all of these disorders. The common factor is local tissue damage initiating a reflex response, which in some way involves the sympathetic nervous system. Furthermore, the pain and the vasomotor disturbances are often improved or cured in the early stage of the condition by interruption of the involved sympathetic pathways.

A feature of the diagnostic criteria proposed by IASP (Table 25.2) is that they include a number of optional criteria, of which one must be present from each of the four categories. This results in the criteria lacking specificity and having a poor predictive value (about 40–60%).

Table 25.2 Diagnostic criteria for CRPS as proposed by IASP (Stanton-Hicks *et al.*, 1995)

A Initiating noxious event or cause of immobilisation
B Pain, allodynia or hyperalgesia, disproportionate to inciting event
C Evidence at some time of oedema, vasomotor or sudomotor activity in the painful region
D Diagnosis precluded by other conditions which could account for the symptoms

A new version of the diagnostic criteria has been formulated using principal component factor analysis (Harden *et al.*, 1999). This identifies clinical features of similar discriminating power and assigns them to clusters of different and independent discriminating power (Table 25.3). The inclusion of motor features enhances the diagnostic power and (when present) helps to distinguish CRPS from less complex or purely sensory neuropathies. Thus, if four of four categories of symptoms, in addition to two of four categories of signs, are required, the sensitivity and specificity have been calculated to be 0.7 and 0.94, respectively. This results in the greatest probability of accurate diagnosis of 80–90%. If the criteria are changed, so that only two of four categories of symptoms and two of four categories of signs are required, the sensitivity is high at 0.94 but the specificity falls to 0.36, resulting in a high proportion of false positive diagnosis (Bruehl and Harden, 2002).

Table 25.3 Proposed revision of diagnostic criteria for CRPS (Harden *et al.*, 1999)

1 Continuing pain disproportionate to inciting event
2 Must report at least *one symptom* in each of the *four* following *categories*:
   * Sensory: hyperaesthesia
   * Vasomotor: asymmetry in skin temperature and/or colour and/or skin colour changes
   * Sudomotor: oedema and/or sweating changes and/or sweating asymmetry
   * Motor/trophic: decreased range of motion and/or motor dysfunction and/or trophic changes
3 Must display at least *one sign* in at least *two* of the following *categories*:
   * Sensory: hyperalgesia and/or allodynia
   * Vasomotor: asymmetry in skin temperature and/or colour and/or skin colour changes
   * Sudomotor: oedema and/or sweating changes and/or sweating asymmetry
   * Motor/trophic: decreased range of movement and/or motor dysfunction and/or trophic changes

Diagnostic categories

Sensory

Sensory examination can be difficult if allodynia is severe. Assessment can be performed with bedside instruments (cotton wool, pin prick, joint position, hot and cold roller) or, more objectively, with quantitative sensory testing (mechanical and thermal detection and pain thresholds). Often there is hypoaesthesia or loss of sensation (occurring more commonly in CRPS II). Temperature and proprioception deficits are usually the first abnormalities to appear.

Vasomotor and sudomotor

Vasomotor and sudomotor changes can be spontaneous or induced. Skin colour changes vary between red, cyanosed, pale or mottled appearances. The limb may be hot or cold, possibly swollen and exhibiting hyperhydrosis or hypohydrosis.

Formal investigation of vasomotor function is done with:

* Skin blood flow doppler (measures blood flow into tissue).
* Infrared thermography (measures heat emission, an indirect corollary of blood flow).

Sudomotor function can be objectively measured by the 'gold standard' of qualitative sudomotor axon reflex test (QSART) (Sandroni *et al.*, 2003). This involves the activation of post-ganglionic sympathetic sudomotor nerve fibres by iontophoretic administration of acetylcholine into the skin. This initiates an action potential, which travels antidromically to the first branch and then orthodromically back to the skin to activate the corresponding second population of sweat glands, whose sweat output is measured. Other tests commonly performed prior to the availability of QSART include: sympathetic skin response (indirect measure of sweat production by the change in skin resistance following random electrical stimulation) and resting sweat output (measures baseline sweat production).

Previously, three phases of vasomotor/sudomotor abnormalities were accepted. In the early phase the limb was warm and pink with hypohydrosis (reduced sympathetic activity). This was followed by a phase of increased sympathetic activity (cold and pale with hyperhydrosis), culminating in a final dystrophic/atrophic phase. These three phases were artificial as there were too many exceptions to make it a clinically useful tool. Some individuals immediately develop the cold dystrophic phase, while others alternate intermittently between the various phases. Therefore, the new proposals for diagnostic criteria do not include any reference to the timing of the three phases.

Trophic

Trophic changes present as abnormal hair and nail growth, fibrosis, thin glossy skin and osteoporosis. The incidence varies between 13% and 60% and is more common with more prolonged symptoms. If a limb is cold at the onset, the condition is associated with increased trophic disabilities and warrants aggressive management.

Motor

The motor changes can be secondary to disuse atrophy or trophic changes to tendons and muscles. These result in a limb which is weak, restricted in range of movement and has impaired co-ordination. Fifty per cent of patients have postural or action tremor and 10% have myoclonus or dystonia. A 'neglect syndrome' has also been described.

Diagnosis and laboratory investigations

There is debate over whether the diagnosis of CRPS is enhanced by laboratory testing. Symptoms of CRPS are strongly correlated with positive laboratory results (Bogduk, 2001) but negative results are useful as they refute the diagnosis where clinical symptoms are weak. Thus, the numbers of false positive diagnoses of CRPS are reduced. If testing is performed, the relative approach (where measurements are compared to the normal side) is 20% more accurate than the absolute approach (comparing results to published normal values).

CRPS I and CRPS II

CRPS I

The incidence of CRPS I is uncertain, but it is more common than CRPS II. CRPS I is frequently misdiagnosed since symptoms and signs can appear unrelated to any precipitating cause (Jänig, 2002; Sandroni et al., 2003). The clinician may fail to recognise an organic basis and attribute them to psychogenic factors. Thus, patients are often mismanaged or neglected for long periods of time. This may allow the disease to progress from a potentially reversible to an irreversible state.

In CRPS I, the pain tends to be increased when the limb is dependent. It most commonly occurs in the younger age group, presumably because the young are more prone to trauma. There is also a female predominance (3 : 1), but no obvious explanation accounts for this. The incidence of CRPS I is about 1–2% following fracture of a limb (7–35% after Colles fracture) and 5% following myocardial infarction (resulting in shoulder/hand syndrome). After a stroke, the incidence is 12–55%, but the cause remains unknown in 10–25% of cases.

CRPS II

The diagnosis of CRPS II is usually an easier one to make. The initiating mechanism is related to obvious nerve injury and the resultant syndrome (particularly the burning pain) is characteristic.

The incidence of CRPS II is 1–5% following nerve injury. The median and sciatic nerves are most commonly affected, possibly related to a large sensory and sympathetic fibre component. Since nerve damage is involved in CRPS II, a greater degree of sensory deficits and involuntary movements of peripheral origin are observed.

Mechanism

Some investigators believe that CRPS is a psychiatric disorder and have labelled it a somatiform pseudoneurological illness. However, a consensus is emerging that it is predominantly a central nervous system (CNS) abnormality (Jänig, 2002). Although there are undoubtedly peripheral mechanisms, such as inflammation and neuropathic damage, both lead to central sensitisation and hyperexcitability.

Central mechanisms appear to be primarily responsible for the syndrome. Clinical findings supporting this include:

- Up to 50% of CRPS I patients develop hypoalgesia and hypoaesthesia in the ipsilateral quadrant or half of the body to the affected limb.
- The abnormal sympathetic activity is often not restricted to merely the damaged limb, but can occur in other limbs.
- The rapid onset of reduced sympathetic activity is similar to that which occurs after a stroke (and can occur on the 1st day). An acute stroke is not painful, suggesting that in CRPS the pain and sensory features are caused by parallel, but separate, mechanisms to the autonomic one.
- In normal conditions sympathetic activity varies in co-ordination with the respiratory cycle. In CRPS this reflex response of central origin is lost.

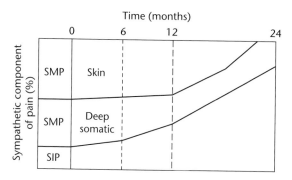

Figure 25.3 Graph displaying the different components of SMP and how these vary over time. Baron, R. (2002). *International Conference on Neuropathic Pain*, Bermuda, November; personal communication. SMP: sympathetically mediated pain; SIP: sympathetically independent pain.

Table 25.4 Treatment objectives of and therapeutic options for CRPS

Treatment objective	Therapeutic options
Pain	Neuropathic drugs
Sympathetic activity	Sympathetic blockade: upper limbs – Stellate ganglion block lower limbs – Lumbar sympathectomy either – intravenous regional sympathectomy using guanethidine, reserpine or bretylium
Motor dysfunction	Physiotherapy and occupational therapy
Inflammation and oedema	Steroids and anti-inflammatory drugs

The syndrome may or may not have a sympathetic component. Patients with SMP are diagnosed by either obtaining an analgesic effect from a sympathetic block or alternatively, the pain is exacerbated by sympathetic stimulation (e.g. total body cooling). Those patients with SMP also have a baseline pain, which is SIP. The proportion of SMP declines over time, which may explain why sympathetic nerve blocks are more effective in the early stages (Figure 25.3). Moreover, the proportion of SMP derived from the skin or deeper component is variable, with deep somatic hyperalgesia (pain on pressure of joints) present in 90% of cases (a finding unique to CRPS).

Treatment

Lack of understanding of the syndrome and lack of objective diagnostic criteria has resulted in a shortage of proper clinical trials (Sandroni *et al.*, 2003; Bogduk, 2001). However, the consensus is that the same general principles used in treating any chronic pain condition should apply. That is to say, treatment must be immediate and should comprise a comprehensive interdisciplinary setting, with emphasis on pain management and restoration of full function. This includes pharmacology and interventional procedures as well as physiotherapy and psychotherapy.

Preventative

The primary objective is to minimise further tissue trauma and provide optimal wound healing. Physiotherapy should be instituted early to prevent disuse atrophy and promote functional recovery. Two controlled studies have shown that stellate ganglion block (sympathetic blockade) or vitamin C (oxygen-free

radical antagonist) can prevent the onset of CRPS. Calcitonin may also confer some benefit (Bogduk, 2001).

Established CRPS

The treatment components of established CRPS should be directed at the predominant pathology (Table 25.4).

The most recent review of therapeutic strategies was performed by Kingery (1997):

- The only trial data to consistently demonstrate analgesic effectiveness was with oral corticosteroids.
- There is some evidence for:
  - Oxygen radical scavengers (e.g. topical dimethyl-sulphoxide and mannitol infusions).
  - Epidural clonidine.
  - Intravenous regional bretylium or ketanserin.
- There were conflicting results for intra-nasal calcitonin and intravenous phentolamine.

Treatments for which there was evidence of no benefit include:

- Intravenous regional guanethidine (IVRG) or reserpine. There is controversy over the usefulness of IVRG. It is still commonly used in many pain clinics because of anecdotal reports of benefit. The two reviews which concluded IVRG was not beneficial (Kingery (1997): eight studies and McQuay and Moore (1998): five studies) were based on studies, which had serious deficits in methodology. These deficits included poorly defined diagnostic criteria, small numbers of patients, differing doses and frequency of guanethidine administration and incomplete crossover.

- Droperidol.
- Atropine.
- Amputation of the limb – this resulted in pain relief in only two of 34 patients. Therefore, it should only be considered where there is uncontrolled infection or ischaemia.

Since Kingery's review, there has been further evidence of the benefits of the conventional neuropathic pain drugs, such as the tricyclic antidepressants, anticonvulsants, lidocaine infusions and opioids (Bogduk, 2001):

- Osteoporosis can be a feature of CRPS and one study using intravenous clodronate demonstrated significant benefits in analgesia.
- Intrathecal baclofen can reduce dystonias in the upper limbs (but inexplicably not those in the lower limbs).
- Sympathetic and somatic nerve blocks can be beneficial, particularly in the early phase of the syndrome.
- Spinal cord stimulation in combination with physical therapy has a significant but modest effect on pain at 6 months (but no effect on function or quality of life). The justification for such costly and invasive treatments must be questioned, when the benefits are so modest.

Key points

- Progress has been made in formulating diagnostic criteria for CRPS. Separate categories of cluster features of sensory, vasomotor, sudomotor and motor/trophic changes are used.
- Early sympathetic blocks and vitamin C may prevent the development of CRPS.

- Few studies of the therapeutic options are of sufficient standard or quality. The most helpful treatments appear to be steroids and bisphosphonates.
- The general consensus is that management should be aggressive, immediate and multidisciplinary, with the emphasis on pain management and restoration of full function.

References

Bogduk, N. (2001). Complex regional pain syndrome. *Curr. Opin. Anaesthesiol.*, **14**: 541–546.

Bruehl, S. & Harden, N.R. (2000). An empirical approach to modifting IASP diagnostic criteria for CRPS. In: Harden, N.R., Baron, R. & Jänig, W. (eds) *Complex Regional Pain Syndrome. Progress in Pain Research and Management*, Vol. 22. IASP Press, Seattle; pp. 303–313.

Harden, R.N., Bruehl, S., Galer, B. *et al.* (1999). Complex regional pain syndrome: are the IASP diagnostic criteria valid and sufficiently comprehensive? *Pain*, **83**: 211–219.

Jänig, W. (2002). CRPS-I and CRPS-II: a strategic view. In: Harden, N.R., Baron, R. & Jänig, W. (eds) *Complex Regional Pain Syndrome. Progress in Pain Research and Management*, Vol. 22. IASP Press, Seattle; pp. 3–13.

Kingery, W.S. (1997). A critical review of controlled clinical trials for peripheral neuropathic pain and complex regional pain syndrome. *Pain*, **73**: 123–139.

McQuay, H. & Moore, A. (1998). Intravenous regional sympathetic blockade (IRSB) for reflex sympathetic dystrophy. In: McQuay, H. & Moore, A. (eds) *An Evidence-Based Resource for Pain Relief.* Oxford University Press, Oxford; pp. 212–215.

Sandroni, P., Dotson, R. & Low, P.A. (2003). Complex regional pain syndromes. In: Jensen, T., Wilson, P. & Rice, A. (eds) *Clinical Pain Management – Chronic Pain.* Arnold, London; pp. 383–401.

Stanton-Hicks, M., Jänig, W., Hassenbusch, S. *et al.* (1995). Reflex sympathetic dystrophy: changing concepts and taxonomy. *Pain*, **63**: 127–133.

A.P. Baranowski

Some consultants in pain medicine are fortunate to have developed areas of 'specialised' interest and as such may regularly see a condition rarely seen by others. However, many pain consultants regularly see rare conditions as a one off. It is with this background that we need to consider the management of uncommon pain syndromes. This chapter aims to impart general principles. The general management techniques used for common conditions are applied to uncommon conditions.

Uncommon pain conditions include:

- *Connective tissue diseases*: For example, systemic lupus erythematosus (SLE), polymyalgia rheumatica and giant-cell arteritis. These are rare, but not without significant risks to sufferers. They often present initially with pain.
- *Metabolic diseases*: Although diabetes is very common, conditions such as porphyria and hyperparathyroidism are less frequent and can present with pain, but also life-threatening emergencies.
- *Nutritional deficiency*: This exists in many forms, as a result of dietary choice or co-incidental illness (e.g. Vitamin B1, B6 and B12 deficiencies).
- *Poisoning*: Lead, thallium, arsenic and mercury poisoning are all rare causes of non-acute pain.
- *Vascular*: Many pain conditions have a vascular component (e.g. thoracic outlet syndrome, steal-associated pain, Raynaud's and Paget's disease). Steal-associated pain may be surgically induced and very difficult to manage. Paget's disease is important in the differential diagnosis of back pain.
- *Urogenital pain syndromes*: These are increasingly being recognised but remain poorly understood. Interstitial cystitis, is a blanket term, often used inappropriately by both physicians and patients.
- *Headaches*: These are common, but many variants are rarely seen by the pain specialist (e.g. cluster headaches).

Connective tissue diseases

SLE

SLE has an incidence: 4.8–7.6 per 100,000 depending on country. The highest frequencies and severities are in women of Afro-Caribbean, Chinese, Asian and South American Indian ancestry. The aetiology is poorly understood, but the diagnosis is made when four of The American College of Rheumatology criteria are met. These include:

- Macular rash.
- Discoid rash.
- Photosensitivity.
- Oral ulcers.
- Arthritis.
- Serositis.
- Proteinuria.
- Neurological disorders.
- Haematological disorders.
- Immunological disorders with autoantibodies such as LE cells, anti-native DNA, anti-Sm.
- Presence of anti-nuclear antibody.

Patients' clinical features are listed in Table 26.1. They present two conflicting issues:

- Multiple pathologies may generate multiple mechanisms for pain; for example, an SLE patient presenting with lower limb ulceration may have a complex of pain due to: acute inflammation, ischaemia, infection and neuropathic (both peripheral and central) causes.
- Multiple pathologies may significantly effect treatment options.

While SLE patients may present with pain of many aetiologies, the commonest are musculoskeletal and related to:

a Primary pathology of the joints and muscles (e.g. arthritis and myositis).
b Secondary pathology in the muscles, due to chronic illness and disability (e.g. long periods of being bed bound and poor posture).

Table 26.1 Some of the common clinical features exhibited by lupus sufferers

System	Clinical features
Musculoskeletal	Arthritis, myositis, tendonitis
Cardiac	Pericarditis, endocarditis, myocarditis
Pulmonary	Pleurisy, atelectasis
Nervous	Peripheral neuropathy, spinal cord lesions, cerebritis, stroke, epilepsy
Urogenital	Cystitis, infertility
Renal	Nephritis
Vascular	Vasculitis, thrombosis
Haematology	Anaemia, thrombocytopaenia, lymphopaenia, leucopaenia, splenomegaly
Other	Uveitis, mucositis

c Muscle disease secondary to treatment (especially steroids).

Physiotherapy is a mainstay of treatment, but anti-inflammatory agents should be considered (e.g. non-steroidal anti-inflammatory drugs (NSAIDs) and steroids). These may be taken orally or injected locally, such as in the case of an enthasitis (inflammation of the tendon insertion into bone) or tendonitis. The injection must never be into the tendon itself, as rupture is a complicating factor. In certain cases of myositis generalised immunosupression may be indicated.

Neuropathic pain may manifest itself in various forms:

• Central nervous system (CNS) involvement (e.g. strokes and spinal cord infarction) may result in chronic debilitating central pain. In addition, the incidence of migraine and other types of headaches is increased.
• Peripheral nervous system (PNS) involvement includes: mononeuropathies, multiple mononeuropathies and polyneuropathies. These may be autoimmune, vasculitic or inflammatory in nature, or secondary to surgery or deformity.

General management of the primary cause is advocated, usually involving the use of steroids and (possibly) immunosupression. Specific neuropathic therapies (Chapter 20 & 42) may also be required and there may be a role for opioids (Chapter 40).

Vasculitic problems and Raynaud's phenomena may produce ischaemic pain, which can benefit from vasodilator treatment. In certain cases sympathetic blockade (e.g. lumbar phenol sympathectomy) or spinal cord stimulation are indicated. Ischaemic pains are often associated with the neuropathic changes of

central sensitisation. Consideration should be given to the use of neuropathic analgesics.

Visceral pain may occur from SLE affecting the internal organs. However, even if there is a visceral cause for the pain, treatment directed at the secondary referred hyperalgesia of the muscles should be considered. For instance, in patients with renal pain, there is often a referred hyperalgesia to the loin muscles, anterior abdominal wall, para-spinal muscles and the thoracic muscles. Treatment aimed at reducing muscle pain may limit the overall suffering.

In addition to the variety of pain presentations, multiple pathologies may affect treatment options. Therefore, patients must be fully evaluated by the pain team prior to instigating any treatment. Particular attention should be paid to the cardiovascular, respiratory, nervous and renal systems. Drug modifications may be necessary in the presence of dysfunction within these systems, and positioning for procedures may be compromised.

Caution is the key to invasive therapies. Patients with SLE are more likely to bleed as a result of thrombocytopaenia, the lupus anticoagulant and antiphospholipid syndrome. Moreover, because of the tendency to thrombosis in some patients, anticoagulant use is common. Injection-type treatments must be approached with caution and adequate preparation. In addition, certain drugs may interact with warfarin (e.g. carbamazepine), or increase the risk of bleeding (e.g. NSAIDs).

Non-invasive and non-pharmacological measures such as cognitive behavioural techniques can have a role in specific patients. However, their use may have to be modified to account for chronic illness and reduced life expectancy.

Polymyalgia rheumatica and giant-cell arteritis

The importance of these conditions is that the diagnosis may be missed when patients present to the pain clinic as a non-specific musculoskeletal pain. Polymyalgia is at one end of the disease spectrum, with giant-cell arteritis (and its life-threatening associations) at the other.

Polymyalgia rheumatica occurs predominantly in female patients (2:1) over the age of 60, though younger patients are seen and the diagnosis should not be excluded on the basis of age alone. Patients present with girdle pain and stiffness on waking, which may last for hours. This contrasts with non-specific musculoskeletal pain that often eases early on in the morning with mobilisation. General malaise, fatigue, depression, anorexia, weight loss and night sweats are frequently associated. Polyarthritis may also occur. The erythrocyte sedimentation rate (ESR) is usually raised with an average value about 40 mm/h. Liver function tests may show mild changes, but otherwise there is often little else to find. Corticosteroids in low doses are the mainstay of treatment, with response being both significant and rapid.

Giant-cell arteritis has an incidence of 18 per 100,000 in those aged 50 years or more. It may represent, in a more severe and specific form, the disease process that includes polymyalgia rheumatica. As with polymyalgia, the onset may be dramatic, with malaise, fever and anaemia. The main difference to polymyalgia is the presence of severe temporal features associated with the arteritis, namely: headache, scalp tenderness, skin ulceration, ischaemic pain of jaw and tongue, and nerve damage. Permanent blindness is a major risk. Arteritis may also affect the heart, aorta, peripheral vessels and nerves.

Polymyalgia and giant-cell arteritis require urgent management by a rheumatologist. For both the mainstay of treatment is corticosteroids.

Metabolic diseases

Acute intermittent porphyria

Presentation is usually at some point between puberty and the late 20s. It is an autosomal dominant condition, with variable clinical expression. Abnormalities of the porphobilinogen deaminase enzyme result in excess δ-aminolaevulinic acid (δ-ALA) and porphobilinogen.

Presenting pains may be:

- Severe abdominal pain: This is the most frequent presenting symptom, usually being central, colicky and intermittent in nature. The symptoms may resemble peritonitis, but bowel sounds are often normal and abdominal palpation may be benign. Changes in bowel habit, nausea and vomiting may further confuse the picture. The excess porphyrin excretion in the urine colours the urine a 'port wine' colour.
- Related to peripheral neuropathies, which have been known to result in fatal respiratory paralysis.
- Consequent upon central neuropathies: Autonomic dysfunction may be associated with hypertension, tachycardia, syncope and sweating. Psychosis is also common.

The treatment of the pain of acute intermittent porphyria may be difficult. It is first important to make the diagnosis and second not make matters worse by the use of inappropriate drugs. Opioids provide the foundation for the treatment of abdominal-type pains

and chronic visceral pain is often managed similarly. The main problem may then become one of drug addiction. The chronic use of opioids should be used with appropriate guidelines (Chapter 46).

If nerve blocks are required in a patient with acute porphyria then bupivacaine is regarded as safe, whereas lidocaine is probably unsafe. Corticosteroids have an equivocal record and may precipitate an acute episode. Sedation is best avoided unless absolutely necessary, since many of the drugs are contraindicated in porphyria.

Hyperparathyroidism

Approximately 80% of patients with hyperparathyroidism have a single parathyroid adenoma. Pain is common:

- Fifty percentage of patients present with renal colic. It is now well established that renal colic can cause CNS sensitisation that produces long-term muscle hyperalgesia and possibly visceral hyperalgesia. Chronic loin pain in patients that have passed a renal stone, but where there is no current evidence of a calculus, should be considered to demonstrate neuropathic and muscular pain components. Agents such as gabapentin and amitriptyline may have a role. Similarly, renal nerve blocks (reducing visceral input) and para-vertebral/epidural injections (attenuating muscle hyperalgesia) may be of help to the patient.
- Muscle weakness and pain affects over 50% of patients.
- Subchondral bone lesions with loss of integrity of the subchondral plate, gout and pseudogout may all contribute to joint pain. However, only a small proportion of patients (<2%) present with radiographic bone cystic lesions due to resorption.

Nutritional deficiency

Causes may be:

- Dietary.
- Following gastric or ileal surgery.
- Patients with small intestine lesions.
- Congenital deficiencies and abnormalities.
- Alcohol abuse.

Vitamin B$_1$ (thiamine)

Common symptoms and signs include:

- Painful paraesthesia in the feet.
- Proximal sensory symptoms.
- Distal motor weakness.

Vitamin B$_6$ (pyridoxine)

B$_6$ deficiency, may also produce a painful neuropathy; it is very rare and usually related to the use of medication such as the antihypertensive hydralazine or the anti-tuberculosis agent isoniazid.

Vitamin B$_{12}$ (hydroxycobalamin)

Vitamin B$_{12}$ absorption requires binding to intrinsic factor (which may be lacking). Anaemia is not a universal finding. Indeed deficiency may present with symmetrical lower limb neuropathy with associated:

- Paraesthesia.
- Ataxia.
- Hypoaesthesia.
- Muscle weakness.
- Faecal incontinence.
- Optic neuropathy.
- Psychiatric disturbances.

Correcting the deficiency (in all but the most severe states) usually corrects the sensory disturbance.

Poisoning

Poisoning by a variety of heavy metals is associated with a painful peripheral neuropathy.

Lead poisoning

Poisoning with lead is very rare in the UK. In the past the use of lead pipes and lead in paint were the main causes. Poisoning with lead produces a neuropathy that is predominantly motor. Chronic lead poisoning may produce chronic abdominal pain. Pain related to the resultant motor dysfunction and the pain of associated renal and haemopoitic pathologies may also be present. Diagnosis may be made clinically by detecting a black 'lead line' on the gingival margins, basophilic stippling of erythrocytes and elevated blood lead levels.

Thallium poisoning

This usually occurs following accidental ingestion of rodent poison. The early onset abdominal pain with diarrhoea is soon followed by the development of a mixed motor and painful sensory neuropathy. Central neurological symptoms, such as choreiform movements and optic neuropathy may occur. The acute poisoning may be treated with diethyldithiocarbamate that binds with the thallium.

Arsenical poisoning

Chronic arsenic poisoning is usually associated with gastrointestinal disturbances, anaemia and jaundice. The skin of the palms and soles thickens. White lines develop across the nails (Mees lines). Peripheral neuropathy affects the most distal parts first and spreads proximally, as a sensory neuropathy. Motor symptoms develop late in the illness. Treatment obviously involves removing the arsenic, but prognosis can be poor with persistent pain.

Mercury poisoning

Once again, a rare cause of a painful peripheral neuropathy. The pain starts in the periphery and moves centrally. Central symptoms associated with dementia, cortical blindness and ataxia may occur.

Treatment of the heavy metal poisoning is always the first concern. Often early treatment will result in less sensory dysfunction. Once the neuropathy is established management of the pain involves utilising the standard tools available to the pain specialist.

Rare vascular-associated pains

Pain associated with inadequate blood supply to tissues may be due to:

- Ischaemic stimulation of nociceptors.
- Peripheral sensitisation of nociceptors associated with inflammation.
- Infection.
- Tissue death and subsequent ulceration, including damage to nerve endings.
- Peripheral neuropathy.
- Central sensitisation.

Re-vascularisation alone will only acutely resolve the pain caused by ischaemia of the nerve endings. Time is then needed for the other processes to settle down and the patient may be left with long-term neuropathic pain.

Acute intermittent ischaemia is a less common event (e.g. Raynaud's syndrome, thoracic outlet compression, intermittent steal phenomenon and Paget's disease).

Thoracic outlet syndrome

The most common cause is a bony or fibrous band (i.e. cervical rib). If the band is fibrous it may be difficult to detect on X-ray. Ischaemic pain (from interruption of the brachial artery) may only be present when the arm is exercised, or raised above the head, when a unilateral pallor with hand pain is present. Venous occlusion may confuse the picture, producing oedema and a purple discolouration. Further confusion results from involvement of the brachial plexus, the lowest part of which is most commonly affected. Motor and sensory symptoms in the C8–T1 distribution may occur. In the first instance treatment is surgical removal of the rib.

Steal phenomena and pain

Ischaemic pain may occur when blood is diverted as a result of a 'steal phenomena'. Examples include:

- Arterio-venous fistulae, surgically induced to enable haemodialysis.
- Vascular tumours.

Management of the underlying cause normally resolves the pain.

Paget's disease

Around 5% of individuals over the age of 40 suffer with Paget's disease, but only approximately 1 in 20 of these will have symptoms. Commoner in men, this may represent a slow virus disease, though inheritance is also probably important.

Increased osteoclastic activity associated with increased vascularity may cause pain. However, the increased osteoblastic activity inappropriately producing new bone may also cause pain. Ectopic bone may distort a joint (producing an arthralgia), compress nerves (producing neuropathic pain) or irritate adjacent tissue (producing local inflammatory pain). The incidence of fractures is increased in Paget's disease.

The biphosphonates and calcitonins are the mainstay of specific drug treatments for Paget's disease. For pain management, simple analgesics should initially be utilised. NSAIDs have a role, as do tricyclic anti-depressants (TCAs), anti-epileptics and specific injections (e.g. intra-articular injections). Opioids may also be helpful in refractory cases.

Non-pharmacological treatments will include splints and physiotherapy (both conventional and chronic pain behavioural).

Urogenital pain

While this is not uncommon in the general population, it has historically been poorly recognised as a problem by the medical profession. Pain results from a large range of syndromes and pathologies. When assessing

these patients its essential to address: psychology, peripheral pathology (organ specific, muscular and neurological) and central processing.

Interstitial cystitis

Interstitial cystitis produces bladder pain and dysfunction. The specific criteria for definition are currently being revised, but are likely to include the guidelines of the National Institute of Arthritis, Diabetes, Digestive and Kidney Diseases Workshop (Gillenwater and Wein, 1988). Interstitial cystitis is primarily a diagnosis of exclusion and for this reason it is very important to effectively diagnose other pelvic pain syndromes.

Treatment of interstitial cystitis should be multidisciplinary (Table 26.2), but the evidence for efficacy is limited.

Table 26.2 Examples of treatment options for interstitial cystitis

Systemic medical treatment	NSAIDs Opioids Corticosteroids H1 and H2 antagonists (e.g. hydroxyzine, cimetidine) TCAs Sodium pentosanpolysulphate Antibiotics Prostaglandin (e.g. misoprostol) Immunosuppressants (e.g. azathioprine) Anticholinergics (e.g. oxybutynin) Anticonvulsants (e.g. carbamazepine, gabapentin)
Intravesicular treatment	Local anaesthetics Glycoproteins (e.g. pentosanpolysulphate) Heparin Hyaluronic acid Dimethyl sulphoxide Bacillus Calmette-Guerin (BCG) Vanilloids (e.g. capsaicin, resinferatoxin)
Interventional treatments	Bladder distension Transurethral resection, coagulation, laser therapy
Alternative	Bladder training Dietary restrictions Acupuncture Hypnosis
Surgical treatment	Supratrigonal cystectomy Subtrigonal cystectomy

Headaches

Headaches and facial pain have a high prevalence within the population causing a significant amount of distress and disturbance of daily activities. Individual conditions may be rare and difficult to diagnose. Management should be systematic with a stepwise approach to diagnosis and treatment being undertaken. Neurologists, dentists and maxillo-facial surgeons as appropriate must rule out serious pathology.

Cluster headaches

Cluster headaches are an example of a well-defined headache syndrome, which is rare and poorly understood, with management being empirical. They are more common in males than females (10 : 1) and manifest as severe attacks of unilateral pain in the ocular, frontal and temporal areas. Episodes of pain come in clusters, with each episode lasting from minutes to hours and with 1–10 attacks a day. The headaches are usually associated with ipsilateral autonomic dysfunction producing lacrimation, conjunctival injection, photophobia and nasal membrane hypersecretion and stuffiness. The aetiology of this distressing pain is unknown, though alcohol and vasodilators may precipitate attacks. Management tends to be empirical, with some benefit being gained in acute attacks from simple analgesics, sumatriptan and oxygen. Prophylactic use of calcium antagonists, ergotamine and methylsergide is known to be helpful. Remissions may occur, with attacks resuming every few years or so. As with any pain syndrome support from the pain team, especially the pain psychologist, is imperative.

Key points

- Rule out serious pathology and consider the rare.
- Involvement of all tissues (e.g. muscle, nerve, endocrine) must be considered.
- Best supported by a close working relationship with specialist colleagues.
- Inappropriate investigation and treatment can increase chronic pain behaviour.

Further reading

Bahra, A., May, A. & Goadsby, P.J. (2002). Cluster headache. A prospective study with diagnostic implications. *Neurology*, **58**: 354–361.

EAU Guidelines on Chronic Pelvic Pain. Fall, M., Baranowski, A., Fowler, C., Lepinard, V., Malone-Lee, J., Messelink, E.J., Oberpenning, F., Osborne, J.L. & Schumacher, S. (2004). *European Urology*, **46**: 681–689.

Gillenwater, J.Y. & Wein, A.J. (1988). Summary of the National Institute of Arthritis, Diabetes, Digestive and Kidney Diseases Workshop on Interstitial Cystitis, National Institutes of Health, Bethesda, Mayland, August 28–29, 1987. *J. Urology*, **140**: 203–206.

Pisetsky, D.S., Gilkeson, G. & St Clair, E.W. (1997). Systemic lupus erythematosus: diagnosis and treatment. *Med. Clin. North Am.*, **81**: 113–128.

Recommendations for the Appropriate Use of Opioids for Persistent Non-cancer Pain. A consensus statement prepared on behalf of the Pain Society; the Royal College of Anaesthetists, the Royal College of General Practitioners and the Royal College of Psychiatrists. March 2004. The Pain Society 2004.

27

R.F. Howard

Introduction

Childrens' pain has a history of misunderstanding and under-treatment. Despite enormous progress in recent years it still remains a significant clinical problem. It is important to recognize that all children, however immature, can experience painful events. This pain and its consequences must be anticipated, measured and safely managed to the best of our ability. Barriers to effective pain management are: insufficient core knowledge and the persistence of myths and misconceptions about pain in infants, children and adolescents (Table 27.1).

Table 27.1 Myths and misconceptions about childrens' pain

- A neonate cannot feel pain
- An active child is not in pain
- A sleeping child is not in pain
- Young children do not need strong painkillers
- Opioids are unsafe for infants and children
- Neonates and infants always get respiratory depression from opioids

---

The nature of pain in children

The measurement and treatment of childrens' pain are complicated by the enormous range in anatomical, physiological and psychological maturity which must be encompassed. From birth to adolescence tremendous maturational changes take place; many of which influence pain and its management. The nervous system continues to develop after birth and the processing of sensory information and motor responses are dependent on developmental age. Drug disposition is also age-dependent, potentially profoundly affecting both efficacy and toxicity of analgesics. While significant at all ages, this particularly complicates the management of infant pain. Moreover, because infancy is a time of enormous plasticity and adaptability, pain and its treatment may have consequences far and beyond the initial event. An understanding of the impact of developmental neurobiology and pharmacology is essential for safe and effective pain management in the neonate and infant.

Pain is a subjective experience and psychological factors greatly influence perceptions of the unpleasantness, quality and intensity of pain. Childrens' pain and related behaviour is modified by a complex interaction of emotional, situational, familial and developmental factors. Age appropriate treatment includes not only the selection of suitable analgesics at the correct dosage, but also non-pharmacological measures designed to reduce pain. These include:

- Close parental involvement.
- A suitable and sympathetic environment.
- Use of cognitive-behavioural and other psychology-based strategies. (Chapter 47)
- Allowing as much autonomy and sense of control as appropriate in individual settings.

General principles of pain management in children

Multi-modal or balanced analgesia

As the mechanisms of transmission of pain and maintenance of pain states are complex, it makes sense to treat pain with combinations of analgesics each having complementary modes of action on the different pathways and processes involved. The risk of adverse effects from treatment is often greater in children. A multi-modal approach theoretically allows maximum efficacy (by synergy) while limiting the dose of each agent, thereby improving the risk : benefit ratio. Local anaesthesia (LA) combined with paracetamol, non-steroidal anti-inflammatory drugs (NSAIDs) and opioids are the mainstay of analgesic pharmacotherapy. Newer agents, such as N-methyl-D-aspartate (NMDA) antagonists (e.g. ketamine) and $\alpha 2$ adrenergic agonists (e.g. clonidine) are becoming popular supplements in certain situations. As in adults, chronic pain states may be more responsive to alternative drugs and non-pharmacological techniques.

Pain assessment

Effective pain management depends on frequent measurements of pain, allowing assessment of the response to treatment and consequent adjustments to therapy (Table 27.2). Pain assessment in children can be a difficult and confusing matter; there is a profusion of instruments designed to measure pain. The decision to use a particular pain assessment tool may often be a pragmatic one. However, the most reliable tools will have been scientifically validated for the patient and setting for which they are designed (an example is shown in Figure 27.1).

Table 27.2 Pain assessment algorithm

Assess pain	Use a validated assessment tool
Plan	What intervention is required?
Implement	Appropriate analgesic intervention(s)
Evaluate	Reassess at frequent intervals

Monitoring and the treatment of side effects

Adverse effects can reduce the quality of pain control and lead to significant morbidity and even mortality. Fear of causing dangerous side effects (including respiratory depression, acute renal failure or increased intra-operative bleeding) is often cited as a reason to withhold analgesia. Less dangerous but bothersome effects are more common (e.g. nausea and vomiting, itching, drowsiness or constipation). Most adverse effects can be anticipated by suitable monitoring: they should be promptly detected and actively managed. Appropriate monitoring is determined by patient, treatment and setting – it should be audited for effectiveness and frequently reviewed. Education, well designed protocols, standing prescription orders and careful audit can all contribute to improvements in the quality of management.

Role of parents

The importance of parents and family in the management of childrens' pain must be recognized. The

(a) FLACC Score

Behavioural pain assessment

Categories	Scoring		
	0	1	2
Face	No particular expression or smile	Occasional grimace or frown, withdrawn, disinterested	Frequent to constant quivering chin, clenched jaw
Legs	Normal position or relaxed	Uneasy, restless, tense	Kicking, or legs drawn up
Activity	Lying quietly, normal position, moves easily	Squirming, shifting back and forth, tense	Arched, rigid or jerking
Cry	No cry (awake or asleep)	Moans or whimpers, occasional complaint	Crying steadily, screams or sobs, frequent complaints
Consolability	Content, relaxed	Reassured by occasional touching, hugging or being talked to, distractible	Difficult to console or comfort

(b) FACES Scale

Self-report pain assessment

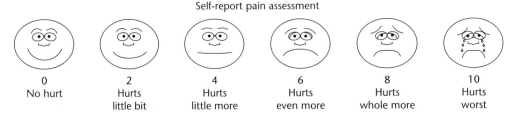

0	2	4	6	8	10
No hurt	Hurts little bit	Hurts little more	Hurts even more	Hurts whole more	Hurts worst

Figure 27.1 Behavioural and self-report pain measurement tools. (a) Behavioural pain assessment: The FLACC behavioural score for neonates up to age 7 years old (Merkel, S., et al. (1997). *Pediatric Nursing*, **23**: 293–27). Each of the five categories: **(F)** face; **(L)** legs; **(A)** activity; **(C)** cry; **(C)** consolability; is scored from 0 to 2 which results in a total score between 0 and 10. (b) Self-report pain assessment – FACES scale adapted from: Wong, D.L., Baker, C.M. (1988). *Okla Nursing*, **33**: 8. Suitable for children aged 3–4 years and above.

in-hospital care of children involves the establishment of a partnership between the parent and the primary nurse – a model of shared care facilitating good pain management. Parents can participate in pain management in hospital settings and will often be expected to continue treatment at home. They need education and support to allay anxieties, build confidence and be effective. In some circumstances, parental involvement may be limited to shared decision-making (e.g. during potent opioid analgesia in hospital). At other times parents may take complete control of analgesic management, including drug administration.

Pain management teams

Increasingly, pain control services specifically for children have been established, in order to improve management and facilitate good practice. Acute pain control teams dealing mostly with post-operative pain and led by an anaesthetist or specialist nurse, were the forerunners. Today, there is an increasing recognition that larger multi-disciplinary groups, with broadly based expertise and the ability to recognize and manage both acute and long-term pain, are more desirable.

The measurement of pain

Self-report

A personal and subjective assessment of pain intensity is generally considered to be the most accurate and desirable. This is perfectly possible for many adolescents and older children, who are able to understand and use a simple visual analogue scale (VAS) or other tool. However, it may not be suitable for young children, or the cognitively impaired. Children at the age of 3–4 years are usually able to report the degree of pain experienced. Therefore some form of self-report should be considered. A number of measurement tools, designed to help young children rate the intensity of pain have been developed (e.g. using images of faces showing increasing degrees of pain from which the child can choose the most appropriate – see Figure 27.1).

Behavioural

Observation for pain-related behaviour is an option for children who cannot self-report. It is important that behavioural tools are appropriate for age and setting, as behaviour is highly modified by developmental, affective and other factors. Facial expression and cry have been found to be the most reliable behaviours in the very young, followed by body posture and motor restlessness (Figure 27.1). Typically, an observer scores a number of such behaviours (sometimes with particular weightings) to achieve a final numerical assessment of pain. A large number of rating systems have been devised, utilizing an array of behaviours and validated for different ages and circumstances.

Physiological

Many physiological parameters have been used to assess pain, including: heart rate, blood pressure, sweating, plasma cortisol and catecholamines. The hope that a physiological measurement may accurately quantify pain has not been realized. Cardiovascular and humoral responses are characterized by a lack of specificity and sensitivity to pain. Physiological measures are also subject to homoeostatic mechanisms, which tend to reduce their value over time. Therefore they have generally been used to help assess the pain of brief stimuli rather than the ongoing pain.

Multi-dimensional

Pain assessment systems, combining several of the above measures have also been devised in attempts to improve accuracy. These tend to be rather complicated and time consuming, both to perform and interpret. Their place in routine practice is uncertain.

Pain in the neonate

Although development of the nervous system continues after birth, neonates as young as 26 weeks gestation have considerable maturation of nociceptive pathways and are able to mount both neurobehavioural and autonomic responses to a noxious stimulus. The hormonal stress response to surgery has been particularly well characterized and is clearly attenuated by anaesthesia and analgesia.

Sensory thresholds are lower in the neonate and reflex responses are more exaggerated. The receptive fields of sensory neurones are relatively larger and more overlapping, which may influence sensory discrimination and localization. Both the peripheral and central mechanisms of sensitization following injury or noxious stimulation appear to be developmentally regulated, as do many modulating influences, such as descending inhibitory controls (which develop later than afferent excitatory pathways). Nevertheless, sensitization after injury (causing pain and tenderness) has been demonstrated in both animal models and human neonates and is amenable to treatment with local anaesthetics and opioids. Due to the plasticity of the infant nervous system there is a concern that the response to pain, injury or analgesia at this age may initiate changes with important effects on subsequent development.

Body composition, metabolic rate and the function of hepatic and renal clearance mechanisms change with age and sex, affecting drug disposition and effect. In the neonate these lead to higher volumes of distribution, slower elimination, increased tendency to accumulation, higher plasma unbound or free fractions, with subsequent greater toxicity potential for many drugs. In addition, the immaturity of the respiratory system and of respiratory control mechanisms at birth predispose to acute respiratory failure in response to physiologically adverse or stressful circumstances for some time.

The need for adequate analgesia in the neonatal period has been heightened by studies showing that infants who undergo painful procedures without analgesia subsequently display relatively greater behavioural responses to pain than control subjects. Neonatal pain management depends on careful attention to analgesic doses and dose intervals, with sufficient monitoring for adverse effects in a monitored environment.

Analgesics

Local anaesthetics (LA)

LA techniques are versatile and have many advantages when used alone, or as part of a multi-modal technique. The efficacy and safety of LA has been empirically and experimentally established over many years. Bupivacaine in solutions of 0.25% or weaker is the most commonly used LA in children. The newer and less toxic agents, ropivacaine and L-bupivacaine, may be preferred on theoretical grounds but have not yet been fully investigated in paediatrics.

Topical LA

EMLA and amethocaine gel have revolutionized the management of procedural pain in children of all ages. They are effective for venepuncture, arterial puncture, lumbar puncture and other brief procedures. They also have been used to reduce pain of chest drain removal and for operative and post-operative pain of neonatal circumcision.

Infiltration LA

Wound infiltration, a simple and safe technique during surgery, has been shown to reduce post-operative analgesic requirements after many procedures including herniotomies, dental conservation and squint surgery.

Peripheral nerve blocks

A number of simple to learn and perform local blocks have been shown to be effective after surgery for all ages (Table 27.3).

Table 27.3 Efficacy of simple local anaesthetic blocks in children

Block	Procedure	Evidence level
Ilio-inguinal nerve	Inguinal hernia	**
	Orchidopexy	**
Penile dorsal nerve	Circumcision	**
Infra-orbital nerve	Cleft lip:	
	Child	**
	Infant	**
	Neonate	*
Axillary plexus	Hand surgery	*
Fascia Iliaca	Surgery to thigh/femur	*

*** Systematic review.

** One or more randomized controlled trials.

* Cohort study or non-randomized trials.

Central nerve blocks

Single dose and infusion epidural analgesia are frequently used in paediatrics for post-operative pain and other indications. Advantages are:

- There is little interference with other body systems (particularly cardiac and respiratory).
- Large regions of the body can be selectively blocked.
- It is possible to differentially block painful sensation by using low doses of LA.

Central nerve blocks are effective at all ages. Suitable equipment is readily available commercially for even the smallest infant. Recent experience of augmenting central local anaesthetic blocks with opioids, clonidine or ketamine has been encouraging, but their place is not fully established.

Paracetamol, NSAIDs and weak opioids

Paracetamol is a weak analgesic and anti-pyretic at all ages. NSAIDs are often used in combination with paracetamol and/or opioids (see Table 27.4). NSAIDs are avoided in neonates and in the presence of renal dysfunction. Aspirin-induced asthma is a contraindication. Codeine is popular but of low efficacy and may be unreliable in certain patients who cannot produce the active metabolite morphine. It should always be used in combination with paracetamol or NSAIDs.

Table 27.4 Analgesics suitable for mild and moderately severe pain, as part of a multi-modal strategy

Drug	Analgesic class	Routes admin	Doses
Paracetamol	Anti-pyretic–analgesic	Oral or rectal	90 mg/kg/day
			60 mg/kg/day term neonate
			45 mg/kg/day pre-term neonate
		Intravenous	90 mg/kg/day paracetamol
			180 mg/kg/day propacetamol
Ibuprofen	NSAID	Oral	20 mg/kg/day (5 mg/kg qds)
Diclofenac	NSAID	Oral	3 mg/kg/day (1 mg/kg tds)
		Rectal	3 mg/kg/day (1 mg/kg tds)
Ketorolac	NSAID	Oral	2 mg/kg/day (0.5 mg/kg qds)
		Intravenous	0.5 mg/kg qds
Codeine	Opioid	Oral	1 mg/kg qds
		Rectal	1 mg/kg qds
Tramadol	Opioid-like	Oral	1 mg/kg qds
		Intravenous	1 mg/kg qds

Table 27.5 Morphine – dosage/administration*

Route	Dose (mg/kg)	Schedule
Oral	0.2–0.4	4–6 times/day
Intravenous or sub-cutaneous	0.05–0.1	Initial/loading dose
Epidural	0.02–0.05	Initial/loading dose

*Note: Reduce doses for newborn. Respiration should *always* be monitored.

Table 27.6 Morphine infusion protocols

Intravenous	
Preparation	Morphine sulphate 1 mg/kg in 50 ml solution
Concentration	20 mcg/kg/ml
Initial dose	2.5–5.0 ml (50–100 mcg/kg)
Infusion	0.5–1.5 ml/h (10–30 mcg/kg/h)
Neonate	
Preparation	Morphine sulphate 1 mg/kg in 50 ml solution
Concentration	20 mcg/kg/ml
Initial dose	0.5–5.0 ml (10–100 mcg/kg)
Infusion	0.1–0.6 ml/h (2–12 mcg/kg/h)
Sub-cutaneous	
Preparation	Morphine sulphate 1 mg/kg in 20 ml solution
Concentration	50 mcg/kg/ml
Initial dose	1–2.0 ml (50–100 mcg/kg)
Infusion	0.2–0.4 ml/h (10–20 mcg/kg/h)

Opioids

Opioids are the most potent drugs available for severe pain. Morphine has been used most extensively in paediatric practice (Table 27.5). Dose intervals and infusion rates must be adjusted to compensate for slower elimination in the newborn (Table 27.6). The side effect profile of opioids is well recognized and respiration should be closely monitored during infusion therapy (Table 27.7). Respiratory depression is easily treated with naloxone.

Table 27.7 Monitoring for patients receiving opioids

Suggested monitoring for children receiving opioids	
Analgesia	Validated pain score: VAS > 3 requires intervention
Sedation	Sedation scale 0–4: >3 requires intervention
Respiration	Respiratory rate, pulse oximetry (in air): saturation <95% requires intervention in normal children
Cardiovascular	Heart rate/blood pressure: set age appropriate parameters
Nausea and vomiting	Nausea scale 0–3: >1 give anti-emetics

Nurse controlled analgesia

Nurse controlled analgesia (NCA) is a simple modification of continuous morphine infusion, using patient controlled analgesia (PCA) technology. It allows rapid and sensitive titration of analgesia within pre-defined limits. Protocols suitable for neonates are also available (Table 27.8).

Rectal formulations of these drugs are convenient and popular, although absorption is known to be slow and erratic requiring adjustments to both dosing and dosing interval.

Table 27.8 Morphine NCA and PCA infusion protocols

NCA

Preparation	Morphine sulphate 1 mg/kg in 50 ml solution
Concentration	20 mcg/kg/ml
Initial dose	0.5–5.0 ml (10–100 mcg/kg)

Programming

Background infusion	0.0–0.5 ml/h (0–10 mcg/kg/h)
NCA dose	0.5–1.0 ml (10–20 mcg/kg/h)
Lock-out interval	20 min

Neonatal NCA

Preparation	Morphine sulphate 1 mg/kg in 50 ml solution
Concentration	20 mcg/kg/ml
Initial dose	0.5–2.5 ml (10–50 mcg/kg)

Programming

Background infusion	0.0–0.5 ml/h (0–10 mcg/kg/h)
NCA dose	0.5–1.0 ml (10–20 mcg/kg)
Lock-out interval	20 min

PCA

Preparation	Morphine sulphate 1 mg/kg in 50 ml solution
Concentration	20 mcg/kg/ml
Initial dose	0.5–5.0 ml (10–100 mcg/kg)

Programming

Background infusion	0.0–0.2 ml/h (0–4 mcg/kg/h)
PCA dose	0.5–1.0 ml (10–20 mcg/kg)
Lock-out interval	5 min

Patient controlled analgesia

With adequate support children are able to understand and use PCA from around 5 years old. There is evidence that a small background infusion is beneficial, particularly at night and for younger age groups.

Novel analgesics (not in routine use)

Ketamine

Low doses (i.e. <1 mg/kg) of the NMDA antagonist ketamine have been found to be analgesic, administered systemically or epidurally. Single dose studies of 0.5 mg/kg have demonstrated a long lasting postoperative analgesia. Concerns about a direct neurotoxic effect of intrathecal ketamine and poor availability of suitable formulations have delayed further neuraxial evaluation.

Clonidine

The α2 adrenoceptor agonist clonidine has a wide spectrum of effects including: analgesia, sedation, hypotension and anti-sialogogue. It has been shown to be a useful analgesic orally and epidurally in the dose range 0.5–1.0 μg/kg, where it augments the effects of LA and other analgesics – improving both quality and duration. Excessive sedation and hypotension have been reported, but appear to be rare complications in children.

Chronic pain management

Estimates of the incidence of chronic pain in children are increasing as clinicians become more aware of the possibility of its existence. Neuropathic pain states do occur in children, as do musculoskeletal pain syndromes, chronic headache and abdominal pain. A number of medical conditions are also associated with chronic pain in children, notably:

- Sickle cell haemoglobinopathy.
- Rheumatic diseases (e.g. juvenile rheumatoid arthritis).
- Skin conditions (e.g. epidermolysis bullosa).
- Metabolic diseases (e.g. osteogenesis imperfecta).

Specialist services are often required for optimal management and suitable rehabilitative treatments and are increasingly becoming available.

Key points

- Infants and children of any age can feel pain.
- Developmental age profoundly influences pain assessment and treatment.
- Acute pain should be anticipated, treated and frequently assessed.
- Use a multi-modal analgesic strategy to treat pain.
- Chronic pain is also prevalent in children.
- The management of chronic pain requires a specialist team approach.

Further reading

Berde, C.B. & Sethna, N.F. (2003). Analgesics for the treatment of pain in children. *N. Eng. J. Med.*, **347**: 1094–1103.

Fitzgerald, M. & Howard, R.F. (2003). The neurobiologic basis of pediatric pain. In: Schecter, N.L., Berde, C.B. & Yaster, M. (eds) *Pain in Infants, Children and Adolescents*, 2nd edition. Lipincott Williams and Wilkins, Philadelphia.

Franck, L.S., Greenberg, C.S. & Stevens, B. (2000). Pain assessment in infants and children. *Paedtr. Clin. North. Am.*, **47**: 487–512.

Howard, R.F. (2002). Pain management in infants: systemic analgesics. *Br. J. Anaesth. CEPD Rev.*, **2**: 33–64.

Howard, R.F. (2003). Current Status of Pain management in Children. *JAMA.*, **290**: 2464–2469.

Pain in children (1998). In: Fields, H. (ed.) *Core Curriculum for Professional Education in Pain*. IASP Press, Seattle.

Peutrell, J.M. & Mather, S.J. (1997). *Regional Anaesthesia in Babies and Children*. Oxford University Press, Oxford, UK.

The Royal College of Nursing Institute (1999). *Clinical Guidelines for the Recognition and Assessment of Acute Pain in Children*. Royal College of Nursing Institute, London.

PAIN IN THE ELDERLY

28

A. Holdcroft, M. Platt & S.I. Jaggar

Demographics

The term 'elderly' refers to the oldest age group of the population. The age-range represented by this group has varied with the changing morbidity and mortality of both time and circumstances. Modern terminology also sometimes refers to the elderly, the aged and the extreme aged, relating to those over 65–70, 80 and 90, respectively. Key points on life expectancy at birth include:

- Early humans had an average lifespan of 20 years (reckoned from skeletal remains).
- At the beginning of the nineteenth century, in industrialized countries, life expectancy was 48 years. It has since improved by a reduction in deaths from infectious and parasitic diseases, poor nutrition and childbearing.
- More recently mortality from degenerative diseases, particularly heart disease and stroke, has fallen and deaths due to cancer have shown a modest reduction. Importantly, disability among the elderly has decreased (from 25% to 17% over the last 50 years in the USA) suggesting that longer life in old age is due to improved health, rather than merely prolonged survival with increasing disability.

Overall UK life expectancy at birth in 2002 was 75 years for males and 80 years for females. Reflecting these demographic changes, the term 'elderly' has changed from referring to those over 50 years in the early twentieth century, those over 65 years some 20 years ago, to those over 70 years currently.

Age brings degenerative disease, often associated with chronic pain, suggesting that pain plays a major part in the health of the elderly population. Recent US studies show that up to 26% of patients in long-term care admit to experiencing pain on a daily basis. However, when appropriate behavioural pain assessment scales are utilized, a 64% prevalence of pain has been documented in medical units.

Key physiological changes with ageing

- Ageing, or senescence, may be defined as the gradual reduction of organ and tissue function by reason of genetic (DNA and RNA) malfunction in cell metabolism, occurring over time.
- Age-related disease refers to chronic degenerative disease, such as atherosclerosis, hypertension and osteoarthritis. These aggravate the effects of ageing and may further shorten life expectancy.
- Ageing and age-related disease are both associated with reduced organ reserve that varies with genetic, disease, environmental, social and other factors.

Over the age of 80 years, individuals have a broader inter-individual variability, with a much wider spectrum of organ and tissue function. Thus, peers within a similar age group become increasingly distinctive, when compared to younger age groups. This means that health care professionals are less able to generalize or use rigid regimes of health care and individually designed treatment regimes may be of more benefit. The biologically 'old' patient often presents with a lifestyle that includes smoking, alcohol, drug abuse, 'unfit' lifestyle and poor nutrition (excess or lack of basic nutrients).

The effect of degenerative disease and ageing on 'vigour' (as defined by a measurable reduction in exercise capacity, mobility and physiological function) is of a gradual reduction, followed by a sudden falling off at the end of life. An increase in 'frailty' (the opposite of 'vigour') is often accompanied by a similar increase in pain-associated disease. However, the management of pain requires consideration of the physiological changes that occur with ageing, in regard to the ability of the body to handle and respond to drugs.

Physiological effects on pharmacokinetics and pharmacodynamics in the elderly

Ageing produces changes in body shape and composition (both tissues and organs). These result in alterations in both how the tissues handle drugs (pharmacokinetics) and how drugs affect the body tissues (pharmacodynamics). These changes show individual variation and there is little data to support specific values.

Pharmacokinetic changes

- Reduced total body water and extra-cellular fluid compartment. This may be due to:
  - Reduced renal function associated with ageing.
  - Reduced appetite and thirst.
  - Voluntary reduction in fluid intake (e.g. due to prostatism or depression).
  The effects of reduced total body water are to reduce the volume of distribution of water-soluble drugs, altering the activity levels. Important effects include the possibility of morphine overdose due to increase in free drug at the site of action.
- Reduced serum albumin and increased α_1-acid glycoprotein. This may be exacerbated by acute disease or malnutrition, altering serum levels of unbound drug. Important side effects may occur with agents usually bound to albumin (e.g. non-steroidal anti-inflammatory drugs, NSAIDs), while conversely, drugs bound to α_1-acid glycoprotein (e.g. alfentanil) may show less efficacy.
- Decreased tissue perfusion and blood flow consequent upon reductions in:
  - Cardiac output (secondary to reduced heart rate and ejection fraction).
  - Circulation (secondary to arterial disease).
  - Autoregulation.
  This will influence the rate of drug uptake and rate of rise of target organ concentration.
- Increased fat, with reduction in lean body mass, resulting in an increased volume of distribution for fat-soluble drugs, prolonging their elimination and half-life. Thus, side effects of lipid-soluble agents (e.g. diamorphine) may be problematic.
- Hepatic function changes:
  - Reduced hepatic mass and blood flow, decreasing elimination rates of drugs with high clearance (e.g. intravenous (i.v.) lidocaine).
  - Reduced oxidative metabolism of many drugs by cytochrome P450 enzymes. Clearance typically decreases 30–40% in those drugs affected, including opioids (e.g. morphine, pethidine, dextro-propoxyphene) and NSAIDs (e.g. ibuprofen and naproxen). However, since the rate of drug metabolism can vary greatly from person to person, individual titration is important.
  - Drugs requiring complex multi-stage metabolism (e.g. amitriptyline) are particularly likely to demonstrate altered pharmacokinetics in the elderly. Simple metabolic pathways, such as conjugation, are less affected.
- Renal function changes:
  - Significant reductions in kidney mass and blood flow in the renal cortex, with concomitant reductions in glomerular filtration rates.
  - Once creatinine clearance falls below 30 l/min, renal excretion is significantly affected. This is of particular importance where drugs or their metabolites (e.g. nor-pethidine) are toxic. Nor-pethidine neurotoxicity (presenting as coma or convulsions) is increased in the elderly.

Pharmacodynamics

With ageing there are changes in:

- Receptors – numbers and activity decrease.
- The autonomic nervous system, in particular:
  - Increased circulating catecholamines.
  - Increased parasympathetic tone.
  - Downregulation of peripheral adrenergic receptor function.
  - Reduced vasomotor responsiveness.
  Together, these effects contribute to an age-related impairment of reflex baroreceptor function. This may be exacerbated by drugs that cause vasodilatation (e.g. morphine), resulting in postural hypotension, especially when used concurrently with diuretics or adrenergic blocking drugs.
- Neuronal activity, including loss of neuronal cells and 'chemical drive' (i.e. transmitter production and release). This results in reduced, slower nervous system integration and co-ordination, which may be exacerbated by neuroactive agents.

Interestingly, despite all the pharmacokinetic and pharmacodynamic changes outlined above, experimental human volunteer research suggests that pain sensation alters little with age, but may be altered by psychomotor dysfunction.

Assessment of pain in the elderly patient

There are often difficulties in pain assessment of an elderly patient, which may contribute to under-treatment of pain. Sometimes a hospital environment is contributory. These problems relate to:

Communication

- *Hearing difficulties*: Deafness is commoner in the elderly and may not always be obvious (especially if it is not acceptable to the patient).

- *Visual problems*: Using visual analogue scales is only appropriate if the patient can see (and understands how to use) them.
- *Intellectual alteration*: The patient not understanding what is being said by the health care professional (or indeed, vice versa) may bring significant communication problems (especially if the patient's native language is foreign).
- *Cultural changes with time*: Age differences between health care professionals and patients frequently result in generational communication problems. Many elderly patients have a different approach to pain, often having had to put up with pain for much of their lives. They may not recognize their 'normal' background pain as anything significant. This stoical ethos may be seen especially in those who have survived war and trauma in the past. A past history of violence and torture also significantly affects the patient's view and understanding of pain. Lastly, they may under-state their pain so as 'not to upset the doctor'.

The presence of multiple pains

There may be several different pains caused by different disease entities, or several different causative complicating factors. Pain may be:

- Consequent upon inter-current diseases which may:
  - Themselves cause pain.
  - Exacerbate other pain syndromes.
- Secondary to treatment modalities (e.g. scarring from radiotherapy).
- Reflective of general illness or debility (e.g. bedsores).
- Nociceptive, visceral and neuropathic pain – often occur in combinations especially in the pain of cancer.

Pain assessment (see also chapters 10,11,12)

- As elderly patients often react more slowly, clinicians should allow ample time to perform any pain assessment.
- Cognitively impaired patients require simple pain scales and more frequent assessments.

Different tools may be required because behaviour differs with cognitive impairment. Instead of complaining about pain, cognitively impaired patients may become quiet or more noisy, demonstrating the importance of observing changes in behaviour that may signal pain. The 'Doloplus' behavioural scale has been developed by a team of French and Swiss geriatricians to assess pain among elderly, non-verbally communicating patients, or patients with cognitive impairment.

The scale uses somatic, psychomotor and psychosocial reactions of the patient to diagnose pain severity.

International recommendations for pain management in the elderly

- Assessment should focus on:
  - Recording events leading up to the present pain complaint.
  - Establishing a diagnosis, a plan of care and a likely prognosis.
- The risks and benefits of various assessment and treatment options should be discussed with patients and family, with consideration for patient and family preferences in the design of any assessment or treatment strategy.
- Patients with persistent pain should be reassessed regularly for improvement, deterioration or complications.

Surgery and pain

Research shows that the under-treatment of pain can have many serious consequences, including:

- Physiological complications (e.g. muscle breakdown and weakness).
- Psychosocial impairments (e.g. anxiety and depression).
- An overall decrease in quality of life.

It seems wiser to avoid these hazards, especially in the elderly. Consequently, it is prudent to ensure that iatrogenic pain (e.g. postoperative) is appropriately and adequately controlled, to minimize stress to the patient and optimize recovery.

Management (see also Chapter 50)

Basic management

- Oral intake (food, fluids and medication).
- Output (bowels and bladder function).
- Social support (e.g. to encourage mobilization, cerebration).

Individualize pain management protocols taking into account

- Co-morbidity (e.g. arthritis) may prevent operation of patient-controlled analgesia (PCA), necessitating alternative analgesic regimes.

- Polypharmacy:
  - Check all drug prescriptions for potential interactions.
  - Compliance may be reduced due to communication and cognitive difficulties.
- Central nervous system (CNS) function – drugs should be titrated against effect.
- Renal and hepatic function needs regular monitoring.

Institute guidelines for appropriate management

- Regional techniques to reduce systemic effects (e.g. respiratory depression and vomiting from opioids).
- Regular pain and nausea assessment.
- Regular prescriptions for analgesic drugs.
- Maintain bowel motility (laxatives).

Day case surgery (see also Chapter 18)

The majority of ambulatory procedures in the elderly are operations to remove cataracts, when local anaesthetic nerve blocks can be used with the patient staying awake. In the past decade guidelines (recommending avoidance of day case surgery in patients over 65 years) have been relaxed. This resulted from an increasing awareness of the wide inter-individual variability observed in this age group.

The conditions for discharge for the elderly are the same as for younger patients (i.e. when stable with adequate pain relief and accompanied). However, it is particularly important that the social circumstances and support needed by this group are appropriately assessed, if the practice is to be undertaken safely.

Key points

- The elderly population is large, expanding and has more biological variability than younger groups.
- The ageing population is getting fitter and healthier. Pain from chronic inflammatory disease (e.g. arthritis) is increasing.
- Improved understanding of the effects of ageing on pharmacokinetics and pharmacodynamics should improve pain control.
- Maintenance of mobility and basic functions is a priority through choice of adjuvant medications.

Further reading

Fries, J.F. (2003). Measuring and monitoring success in compressing morbidity. *Ann. Intern. Med.*, **139**: 455–459.

Moller, J.T., Cluitmans, P., Rasmussen, L.S., Houx, P., *et al.* (1998). Long-term postoperative cognitive dysfunction in the elderly ISPOCD1 study. ISPOCD investigators. International study of post-operative cognitive dysfunction. *Lancet*, **351**: 857–861.

The Management of Persistent Pain in Older Persons (2002). AGS Panel on Persistent Pain in Older Persons. *J. Am. Geriatr. Soc.*, **50(suppl. 6)**: 205–224.

Won, A., Lapane, K., Gambassi, G., Bernabei, R., Mor, V. & Lipsitz, L. (1999). Correlates and management of non-malignant pain in the nursing home. SAGE Study Group: Systematic Assessment of Geriatric drug use via Epidemiology. *J. Am. Geriatr. Soc.*, **47**: 936–942.

29

A. Baranowski & A. Holdcroft

Society has long been aware of the multiple differences between men and women, including the variable responses to pain. This chapter will address the evidence relating to:

- Why pain experiences might differ between the sexes.
- Pain syndromes specific to men and women.
- How the response to treatment might differ between the sexes.

Definitions

Sex is the classification of living things, generally as male or female according to their reproductive organs and functions assigned by the chromosome complement.

Gender is a person's self-representation as male or female, or how that person is responded to by social institutions on the basis of the individual's gender presentation.

Sex dependent is the differences that are dependent on physical attributes (e.g. body fat content) (Table 29.1).

Classical experimental studies of normal individuals demonstrate that in comparison to men, women report:

- Lower pain thresholds.
- Higher pain intensities.
- Less pain tolerance.

The pain history of a man may not be as detailed as a woman, because he prefers not to expand on lack of control over pain. Physicians must be aware that men self-report less than women, actively eliciting the necessary history and encouraging disclosure. Study results can vary depending on the:

- Type of stimulus.
- Site of the stimulus.
- End point (e.g. the experiment ends at either patients' maximum tolerance, or after a fixed amount of time).
- Environment.
- Food intake.
- Anxiety.
- Cognitive differences.

Electrical stimuli produce larger sex differences than thermal stimuli. Furthermore, when these are applied in somatic areas that have interaction with viscera from the reproductive tract, further sex differences can be measured. Disease states can also alter sex differences in experimental pain. For example, women with dysmenorrhoea may have less tolerance to noxious muscle stimulation than men or those women without dysmenorrhoea.

Effects of sex steroid hormones

From fetal life to senescence, sex steroid hormones influence all the major body systems. Their

---

Table 29.1 Effects dependent on body composition

	Males	Females	Comments
Fat	↓	↑	Drug Vd increased in women if lipid soluble
Water	↑	↓	Drug Vd increased in men if water soluble
Other components (e.g. protein binding of drug to α_1 acid glycoprotein)	↑	↓	Effect depends on type of molecule. Drug toxicity increased if more free drug available (e.g. lidocaine)

Vd: volume of distribution.

non-genomic activity (externally on cell membranes) is more acute than their genomic effects that have multiple interactions, for example, in neurotransmitter and enzyme synthesis. In the foetus their effects can be described as 'organising' and are responsible for actions such as the phenotypic structure of hepatic enzyme systems responsible for drug metabolism.

Growth is dependent on the effects of sex steroid hormones during childhood and adolescence, as are physical characteristics for drug distribution. In the immune system and hypothalamopituitary axis these hormones mediate the interactions between inflammation, stress, pain and the cardiovascular system. Specific hormones such as, progesterone can alter nociception during reproductive cycles. Epidemiological studies reveal that it is during this time that pain disorders start to exhibit sex differences. But, it is important to remember that psychosocial events are occurring concomitantly, for example, schooling, games and risk-taking behaviours (which may involve trauma).

It is during the childbearing years that regular menstruation in women can be associated with cyclical uterine and pelvic pain that has a muscular component, so-called muscle hyperalgesia. At this time trauma-induced pain is more common in men. Later in life, the sex hormone cycles in women are terminated during the menopause, often resulting in a loss of sex differences in epidemiological studies (Table 29.2).

Table 29.2 Life events and potential changes in the body

Event	Change
Fetal	Organisation
Childhood	Growth
Adolescence	Social expectations
	Reproductive function
Senescence	Deterioration of systems

Sex differences in central nervous system organisation and function

When the brain is imaged during a painful sensation, regional activation is widespread and outside the traditional centres for pain transmission. These results vary between subjects, but also between sexes. Within the genetic female during the menstrual cycle, painful thermal stimulation can result in different patterns of activation depending on the time of the cycle, despite similar pain intensity ratings.

Sex steroid effects on non-genomic cellular functions are diverse. Neuroactive chemicals (and their receptors) such as gamma amino butyric acid (GABA), N-methyl-D-aspartate (NMDA), glutamate and neurokinin A can co-localise and/or be modulated by sex steroid hormones, thus providing mechanisms for sex differences within the nervous system.

Specific sex-related disorders

Chronic pelvic pain affects both sexes. In many cases there are overlapping mechanisms, even if the presentations are slightly different due to different sex characteristics. Specific end organ diseases (e.g. chronic infective orchitis, painful dysmenorrhoea and balanitis) relate to reproductive tract structures. Thus, in females they may present to obstetric and gynaecology departments. Less specific pains result from nerve damage and muscle dysfunction (particularly of the pelvic floor) of these organs.

Pain disorders in men

Penile pain

It is unusual for a patient to present with chronic pain primarily in the penis. The penis is a somatic organ and as such is subject to pain associated with:

- Trauma.
- Infection.
- Inflammation.
- Ischaemia.

However, pain may be referred to the penis; classically its tip, from:

- Base of the bladder (e.g. associated with interstitial cystitis).
- Prostate (e.g. chronic inflammatory prostatitis).
- Pelvic floor muscle dysfunction.
- Consequent upon nerve damage (secondary to arachnoiditis, sacral trauma and pelvic tumours).

Such conditions are usually associated with other localising symptoms, such as urinary frequency/urgency, areas of numbness or hyperaesthesia. Intermittent chronic pain may be associated with Peyronie's disease, where the penis is distorted on erection, with fibrous bands within the tunica albiginea making penetrative sex painful.

The primary function of the penis is reproduction. As a result, chronic painful conditions of the penis will have psychosexual consequences (including impotence and anxiety related to sex). Thus, chronic penile pain may negatively affect relationships, resulting in

Table 29.3 Possible causes of testicular pain

Causes arising in testis, epididymis and scrotum	Causes arising in alternate sites
Trauma – Surgical – for example, – vasectomy/herniorraphy – Non-surgical	Groin problems (e.g. muscle tears, enthesitis, scar tissue and muscle dysfunction)
Tumour	Aortic or femoral aneurysms (remember testicular blood supply is intra-abdominal)
Infection – Bacterial – Viral	Entrapment neuropathy (e.g. ilioinguinal, iliohypogastric or genitofemoral)
Physical – Torsion – Varicocoele – Hydrocoele – Spermatocoele	Referred pain from: – Pelvis (e.g. prostate disease) – Spine (e.g. osteoarthritis) – Nervous system (thoracic disc)

enthasitis = inflammation of the attachment of a tendon to a bone

extreme distress. Although uncommon, psychological distress (particularly related to sexual life events) may also manifest as penile pain. As with all chronic pain, both the physical and the psychological aspects of penile pain need to be managed.

Testicular pain

The testis is a visceral organ subject to the usual characteristics of visceral pain (see Chapter 21). It is the only easily accessible true visceral organ. Therefore, much of the early work on visceral pain was based on testicular research.

Both acute and chronic pain conditions affecting the testis are well described in urological textbooks (Table 29.3). However, referred pain from the spine, local muscles and tendons may also present with testicular pain, as does neuropathic pain (lower thoracic and upper lumbar spine (T10–L2), sacral roots (S1–S3), intra-abdominal and pelvic nerve plexi, genitofemoral, ilioinguinal and pudendal nerves). Appropriate examination and scans (magnetic resonance imaging (MRI) spine and pelvis, possibly with stir images or gadolinium enhancement) will be necessary. However, there still remain a significant number of patients with testicular pain (probably >25% of presentations) where the cause is not identifiable and the result of treatment is poor. Scrotal pain syndrome is the accepted terminology for idiopathic testicular pain when the pain is not localised to either the body of the testis (testicular pain syndrome) or the epididymis (epididymal pain syndrome).

Patients with identifiable lesions amenable to surgery, may show a 50% reduction in pain. The higher success rates are observed when there is evidence of hydrocoele, spermatocoele or varicocoele. In the absence of these the results of epididymectomy and orchidectomy are poor (20% and 60% success rates, respectively), although microsurgical testicular denervation has produced favourable results in expert hands.

However, surgery should not be attempted without good cause, as it is itself a cause of pain. Approximately 33% of patients will still complain of pain 1 year post vasectomy with 5% seeking further medical advice. Surgery is probably indicated in less than 1%, with asymptomatic epididymal cyst being frequent and symptomatic sperm granulomas benefiting from epididymectomy.

Patients without an identifiable cause should be treated conservatively following a trial of antibiotics. Transcutaneous electrical nerve stimulation (TENS), simple analgesics, neuropathic analgesics (amitriptyline is said to be particularly helpful) and nerve blocks may provide benefit in some patients. The complex nature of the innervation of the testis suggests that nerve blocks at multiple levels may be required. Some specialists in this area find L1 lumbar sympathectomies to be helpful, but the supporting evidence base is weak. Spinal cord stimulation has been tried but it is still early days.

Prostate pain syndrome

The term prostate pain syndrome was introduced by the International Continence Society to describe a constellation of symptoms and signs comprising:

• The occurrence of persistent or recurrent episodic pain, felt primarily in the region of the prostate.

- Associated with symptoms suggestive of urinary tract and/or sexual dysfunction.
- No proven infection or other obvious pathology, in particular no inflammatory cells or infection within the urine/prostate secretions are present.

The European Association of Urology has accepted that it should replace terms such as prostadynia and chronic non-bacterial prostatitis. They account for 90% of prostate pain.

By definition the aetiology and pathophysiology of the prostate pain syndrome remains a mystery. Possible causes that may be relevant to individual patients are found in Table 29.4.

Table 29.4 Possible causes of prostate pain syndrome

Obstructive voiding	• Bladder neck dysfunction • Detrusor-sphincter dysfunction • Dysfunctional voiding • Urethral stricture
Pelvic floor muscle dysfunction	• Incoordinate muscle relaxation • High resting tone
Unrecognised prostate pathology	• Chronic loculated infection • Autoimmune pathology • Intra-prostatic ductal reflux of urine • Chronic infection with urinary tract commensals assumed harmless
Neuropathic	• Complex regional pain syndrome • Pudendal nerve irritation

Investigation should involve quality of life questionnaires, urodynamics, and pelvic ultrasound examination. Examination of expressed prostatic secretions is being replaced by simple urine analysis in many centres as the more invasive approach does not appear to be any more sensitive and false negatives may also occur due to the trauma of the massage. Pelvic floor muscle electromyogram (EMG) assessment is available in some centres to diagnose peripheral nerve problems.

All patients should be treated with at least one course of antibiotics under the guidance of a urologist. Following this, treatment options include:

- Tricyclic agents (level 1b evidence).
- α2 adrenergic blockers (level 1b evidence).
- Simple analgesics should be considered.
- Diazepam and baclofen may help if there is evidence of sphincter dysfunction or pelvic floor muscle spasm.
- Training of the pelvic floor muscles with biofeedback surface EMG may also help pelvic floor muscle spasm.

- Stretching the pelvic floor muscles (by an osteopath or chiropractor) has also been found to be useful in certain cases.
- Some urologists will milk the prostate by a *per rectum* massage while others will recommend regular ejaculation. However, there is little research evidenced for this.
- TENS.
- Acupuncture.
- Transrectal hyperthermia is used in some centres, but there is little published supporting data.
- Radical prostate surgery probably does not have a role.
- Transurethral resection and bladder neck incisions may have a role if obstructive voiding has been demonstrated.

The wide range of treatments attempted reflects the difficulties of current management. However, the role of a pain management psychologist with an interest in chronic urogenital pain is invaluable in a specialist pain clinic.

Pain disorders in women

Endometriosis

Endometriosis is associated with the presence of endometrial tissue outside the uterus. It mainly presents as infertility in young women. The diagnosis is commonly made at 25–28 years following laparoscopy. Clinical complaints include:

- Pelvic pain (70%).
- Menstrual pain (dysmenorrhoea in 71–76%).
- Dyspareunia (vaginal hyperalgesia in 44%).
- Severe pain (a mean of 3.2 on a scale of 1–4).
- Positive family history (26–33%).
- No symptoms (6–8%).
- Only 13–17% use pain medications.

One of the recognised associations is of urinary tract symptoms. The involvement of other viscera with the potential for viscero-visceral and or viscero-somatic interactions should be considered (Chapter 21). Hormonal therapies such as gonadotrophic releasing hormone agonists are presently the main medical treatment. They may be used with or without surgery (laser, cauterisation, resection, hysterectomy).

Vulvar pain syndromes

Women commonly report vulval discomfort.

- The localised vulvar pain syndrome (also known as vulvodynia or vulvar vestibulitis) occurs in young women. They describe pain localised to the introitus, provoked by local stimulation (e.g. vaginal penetration). It is clinically elicited by cotton bud sensitivity in the vestibular area (usually posterior).

- The diffuse vulvar pain syndrome (also known as dysaesthetic vulvodynia or essential vulvodynia) exhibits neuropathic features in the distribution of the pudendal nerve. It usually presents in the older woman who reports poorly localised pain that burns, stings or is sharp like a knife. In some cases an allodynia type of response may be available, although in others examination is normal.

The mechanisms for these conditions are poorly understood. Co-existing disease such as candidiasis should be excluded, as should pudendal nerve damage. Low dose tricyclic antidepressants may be helpful at night and other neuropathic analgesics should be considered.

Sex differences and therapies

Drug effects can be divided pharmacologically into pharmacokinetic and pharmacodynamic. Physical differences between the sexes can alter drug distribution (Table 29.1). In contrast to men, women have:

- Larger percentage of fat.
- Smaller muscle mass.
- Lower blood pressure.
- Biological rhythms relating to reproduction.

Variation in drug pharmacokinetic profiles reflect these.

Opioids

In a meta-analysis of postoperative morphine use (with patient controlled analgesia, PCA), men consumed almost two and a half times more morphine than females. This may reflect underlying differences in:

- Pathways mediating pain sensation.
- Pain tolerance.
- Psychological factors (e.g. anxiety and previous pain).
- Frequency of side effects.

Sex differences in response of dental pain to the kappa opioid receptor (KOP) agonists nalbuphine, buprenorphine and pentazocine have been demonstrated to be time and dose related. Specifically, women seem to achieve statistically significantly more analgesia with kappa agonists than do men. This altered responsiveness to kappa opioid drugs may be clinically utilised if women do not respond to mu opioid receptor agonists (MOP).

Both gender and age influence MOP binding in the brain as measured by positron emission tomography (using ^{11}C carfentanil as the marker). Women have higher opioid binding during their reproductive years supporting the prediction that women are more sensitive to opioid analgesics during their reproductive years. Anatomically the brain regions demonstrating MOP binding are also different, particularly the thalamus and the amygdala.

One of the main reasons for differences between the results of animal and human experiments using morphine analgesia is in its metabolism. Rodents convert morphine solely to morphine-3-glucuronide (M3G). This metabolite is a functional morphine (M) antagonist, with a M3G:M ratio of 6.6:1 in females and 0.7:1 in male rats. Thus, male rodents exhibit greater analgesic responses to morphine than females. In contrast, human glucuronidation of morphine is into two compounds, M3G and morphine-6-glucuronide (M6G). M6G is a more potent analgesic agent than morphine (and indeed is about to enter phase 3 trials as an analgesic agent in its own right). Women exhibit greater opioid analgesia than men and differences in metabolism may be a significant factor.

Non-steroidal anti-inflammatory analgesics

Tolerance to experimentally induced electrical pain after the administration of ibuprofen shows a similar profile in men and women. However, the effect on pain tolerance is both greater in magnitude and more long lasting in men. Despite these experimental findings, no time-related sex differences have been observed in clinical postoperative dental pain.

Drug effects on sexual performance

Many drugs used for the management of non-acute pain may affect male sexual performance. This may critically affect compliance with therapy and should be specifically considered (Table 29.5).

Table 29.5 Drugs prescribed in pain clinics and their effect on male sexual performance	
Antidepressants	• Reduce orgasmic sensation • Delay or inhibit ejaculation

Carbamazepine	• May block testosterone production with subsequent:
	   – Testicular atrophy
	   – Gynaecomastia
	   – Galactorrhoea
	 • May inhibit ejaculation

Opioids including tramadol	• Reduce libido and potency

Key points

- Women report pain more frequently and of higher intensity than do men.
- A pain history should be sensitive to sex or gender-related events.
- The response to pain may be affected by sex and gender.
- Analgesic efficacy may be altered by sex and gender.
- Side effects may differ between the sexes.
- The classification of specific sex disorders is under scrutiny.

Further reading

Baker, L. & Ratka, A. (2002). Sex-specific differences in levels of morphine, morphine-3-glucuronide, and morphine antinociception in rats. *Pain*, **95**: 65–74.

Chia, Y.Y., Chow, L.H., Hung, C.C., Liu, K., Ger, L.P. & Wang, P.N. (2002). Gender and pain upon movement are associated with the requirements for postoperative patient-controlled iv analgesia: a prospective survey of 2,298 Chinese patients. *Can. J. Anaesth.*, **49**: 249–255.

Kest, B., Sarton, E. & Dahan, A. (2000). Gender differences in opioid-mediated analgesia: animal and human studies. *Anesthesiology*, **93**: 539–547.

Wizemann T.M. & Pardue M-L. (eds) (2001). *Understanding the Biology of Sex and Gender Differences*, Institute of Medicine of the National Academy of Sciences.

Zubieta, J.K., Dannals, R.F. & Frost, J.J. (1999). Gender and age influences on human brain mu-opioid receptor binding measured by PET. *Am. J. Psychiat.*, **156**: 842–848.

THE ROLE OF EVIDENCE IN PAIN MANAGEMENT

PART

4

CLINICAL TRIALS FOR THE EVALUATION OF ANALGESIC EFFICACY 30

L.A Skoglund

During the past two decades our understanding of mechanisms involved in pain transmission or modulation has progressed. Such progress is habitually followed by novel analgesic treatments introduced into the clinic. The initial euphoria created by the introduction of new treatments often recedes as the new treatment is tested in the clinical environment.

Clinical trials are the definitive umpire of the usefulness or otherwise of analgesic treatments developed following basic science discoveries. This fact is quite often overlooked in the scientific community, where research discoveries almost instantly attain religious status, with clinical research receiving less status and priority. However, many health providers now realise that analgesic treatments require justification by documented clinical effectiveness. Consequently increasing efforts are attempting to improve the quality of analgesic trials. This chapter addresses some of the major practical problems that can determine the outcome of a clinical analgesic trial.

Types of clinical analgesic trials

Clinical trials are basically done for three reasons:

1 The pharmaceutical industry conducts small- and large-scale trials as part of their investigational new drug (IND) programmes (see Table 30.1). IND programmes are based on commercial contracts between the industry and clinics. Large-scale trials are usually undertaken by contractual research organisations (CROs) consisting of collaborating clinics.
2 Clinical trials are routinely conducted at academic institutions as part of academic training programmes.
3 Many clinical trials also arise from a genuine problem-solving interest in specific clinical problems. The aim is to identify the optimum analgesic treatments for specific painful conditions.

Several well-founded combinations exist between these three reasons for a trial.

Table 30.1 Development programme of a new drug following pre-clinical testing

Investigational new drug (IND) application

Phase 1 trials
The new drug is tested in small groups of volunteers ($n < 100$) for the first time. This evaluates safety and dose range in addition to identifying unexpected or adverse effects.

Phase 2 trials
The drug is given to a larger group of patients (<500). This assesses efficacy and further evaluates safety.

Phase 3 trials
The study drug is given to large groups of patients (up to several thousand). This allows confirmation of effectiveness, monitors side effects and compares it to commonly used treatments. Such information aims to ensure that the drug or treatment may be used safely.

New drug application (NDA)
Phase 4 trials
Post-marketing studies delineate additional information including: the risks, benefits and optimal use of the novel treatment. This is required by regulatory authorities to ensure identification of potential new adverse effect profiles.

Clinical trials may be of a variety of types. An explanatory trial aims to elucidate a biological principle, assuming that a chosen pain model will yield test results that are generally applicable to other pain conditions. In contrast, a pragmatic trial attempts to find the better analgesic treatment in a particular pain condition (Max and Laska, 1991). A practical approach to clinical trials is to distinguish between comparative and exploratory trials. Comparative trials are those in which the effects of differing treatments are compared. Exploratory trials are trials where new analgesic techniques/technologies, the pain insult itself, or analgesic treatments for new or unproven indications are investigated. The distinction between an explanatory/pragmatic and comparative/exploratory trial is not always clear.

Trials may be conducted in several ways depending on the purpose:

1 In open trials the investigator and the participant know the treatment.
2 In single-blind trials the investigator knows the treatment while the participant does not. If the purpose of the trial demands it, the opposite is also possible.
3 In double-blind trials neither the investigator nor the participants know the treatment.

Blinding of the data analysis is often overlooked when doing single-blind and double-blind trials.

Controlled clinical trials may encompass both explanatory and pragmatic trials. A controlled clinical trial aims to make the patient's experience a clinical setting where everything is as similar as possible, with the exception of the variable to be tested. The gold standard in clinical trial methodology is the double-blind, randomised, controlled clinical trial (RCCT). Both complete blindness, and randomisation, is essential to minimise the possibility of introducing bias into the trial results compromising their interpretation.

Trials to good clinical practice standards

Some of the best-designed trials are the industry-sponsored trials undertaken as part of IND programmes. The drug companies dedicate the generous financial resources necessary to complete the programme within the shortest possible time. Basic Phase 2 and 3 trials (Table 30.1) are outsourced to clinics *via* CROs. If supplemental Phase 3 trials are requested by the authorities for additional documentation of a problem (analgesic efficacy or safety), companies, pressed for time, often approach clinics outside the CRO to do additional trials. Approached by a pressed drug company, it is not easy for clinics to withstand the temptation of unexpected funding, but rapid completion will be required and the logistics of this may be difficult to organise.

Many drug companies will (depending on cost and industry priorities) also help clinicians undertaking clinical trials. However, potential marketing advantages arising from your idea will be important. There is often a reverse correlation between the enthusiasm for sponsoring your idea of a clinical trial and the time elapsed since the drug reached the market. Naïve and ill-founded approaches to drug companies are usually not rewarded with success.

Table 30.2 Practical problems that should be addressed prior to commencing a clinical trial

- Does my clinic have any experience with the trial methodology needed for this trial?
- What logistical support do I need for the trial?
- Do I have the clinical setting required for the trial?
- Do I have the finances necessary to undertake the trial?
- Do I have the time necessary to conduct and satisfactorily monitor the trial?
- Do my superiors fully support the trial?
- Do my subordinates fully support the trial?
- Do my colleagues accept the premise of the trial?

Practical problems concerning a clinical trial

The most unpleasant task prior to commencing a clinical trial is consideration of the potential problems associated with its instigation. If these problems are not satisfactorily dealt with before the trial, the trial will either fail or be very difficult to complete (Table 30.2). Never underestimate the resources needed to complete a trial. A successful trial depends upon everyone involved in the trial organisation understanding the benefits that will accrue from a well-run trial. It is not wise to believe that a trial can be planned and then delegated to hospital staff as an add-on to their daily routines. In large hospitals, with staff working in shifts, a delegated trial will never rate as high as the exercise of the daily duties. Thus, it will never receive the attention it needs for effective completion.

Even highly motivated people lose their motivation over time when a trial drags out due to 'unexpected' problems consequent upon bad planning. Seasonal lack of patient recruitment (because nobody checked expected recruitment rates by comparison with historical data) is a frequently encountered example of poor planning in large-scale trials. A well-conducted clinical trial is best done by a trained team, dedicated to the task of trial completion, closely monitored by a project leader (or a single dedicated clinician). The last option can be extremely time consuming and expensive.

Designing a clinical trial

The answers to several important questions (Table 30.3) will determine the logistical requirements a trial will demand. Existing literature regarding the question you want your study to answer must be critically reviewed. By doing so you will establish the precise aims of the study.

Table 30.3 Questions needing answers before designing a clinical trial

- Which specific question(s) do I want to answer with the trial?
- Which pain insult is best suited for the trial?
- How many patients reach my clinic with this pain insult every week/month/year?
- Which pain measurement method will I utilise?
- How large is the variance of baseline pain in the patients after the chosen pain insult?
- Which outcome measure will I use?
- Can I make an assessment of the outcome difference? This is relevant so that a reasonable estimate of sample size can be made.
- Do I need a pilot study before the actual clinical trial?
- Is it possible to make a special operating procedure (SOP), which all parties involved in the trial will adhere to?

Table 30.4 Options to be considered for clinical trials

- Comparative or exploratory trial?
- Double blind or single blind?
- Controlled or non-controlled?
- Is randomisation necessary?
- Parallel groups or crossover?
- Outpatient or in-patient setting?
- Single-dose or multiple-dose protocols?
- Total number of participants needed?
- Are race considerations important?
- Are gender considerations important?

There are many options to consider depending on the purpose of your trial (Table 30.4). An exploratory trial is best suited as an addition to the daily routines at the clinic. It is very useful as a pilot study to see if an analgesic method is effective. Exploratory trials do not necessarily require blinding of treatment. Such trials are also necessary to obtain information about pain insults. They form part of the validation process, to see if a particular pain model is useful.

Comparative drug trials are always the most logistically demanding. They require stringent procedures. In simplistic terms, comparative trials usually compare one analgesic drug or treatment with another, to assess which is the better. An optimal comparative drug trial contains a minimum of three arms (drug treatments). The arms are: the experimental drug, a standard active drug and a placebo. The purpose of the standard and the placebo is twofold. It is necessary for a trial to show sufficient down- and upside sensitivity.

Sensivity of a trial

The concept of downside sensitivity implies that the model is sensitive enough to separate the analgesic efficacy of a standard drug from that of the placebo. The concept of upside sensitivity implies that the model can separate the experimental drug from the standard drug (Cooper, 1991). The ideal standard is the best available standard analgesic drug. It is not uncommon to choose as standard a non-optimal drug or a non-optimal dose of the standard. This practice may be understandable since upside sensitivity may be difficult to achieve. However, such trials should be discouraged since they limit the interpretation of the drugs' efficacy.

Placebo medication has traditionally been one of the basic requirements for a trial to be judged a 'high-quality trial'. However, ethical considerations in association with the Declaration of Helsinki have seriously questioned the use of placebo medication in clinical trials. In particular, the use of placebos may be difficult to justify where it is not possible to adequately consent a patient. There is always a balance between the need for an inherent quality-control (by the use of placebo) and ethical considerations. One way to avoid the use of placebo in a trial is to include two doses of the standard drug. Two doses, one in each end of the known dose – response profile of the standard drug can be used. The downside sensitivity is valid if your model is able to discriminate between the two doses of the standard control drug.

Factors which might introduce bias in your trial

One major cause for concern in analgesic clinical trials is the possibility of imbalance of baseline pain (Roberts and Torgerson, 1999). Key factors that might influence baseline pain involve issues, such as gender, age, race, the pain insult (such as the choice of surgical pain insult) and pre- and peri-operative medication (including choice of anaesthetic). The question of possible influence of gender and race on pain is currently very topical (Keefe et al., 2002). Distinct racial differences in analgesic requirements have been reported (Houghton et al., 1992), as has the effect of gender on susceptibility to opioids (Sarton et al., 2000).

With the racial homogeneity of the European/North American population changing towards a more heterogenous population, the aspect of possible racial influences on a clinical pain trial needs consideration. For pragmatic studies, or studies with low patient numbers, it is wise to use homogenous patient populations (similar race, age and gender). Studies with large patient samples allow for a more flexible view as regards variance of age, although it may be best to avoid extremes. As the influence of gender and race are still disputed balancing the treatment groups with respect to gender and racial composition is advocated, even in trials with large patient numbers.

It can be dangerous to pool several different surgical techniques causing pain insults unless you have categorised the pain intensity and duration associated with each type. Changing anaesthetic techniques or medications during a trial can also cause problems with baseline pain, unless you have characterised the pain resulting from the different techniques used. Different pain assessors may cause within-group bias due to different verbal or non-verbal patient instructions. As a rule do not underestimate the possibility of bias introduction. Check your model frequently and never deviate from an established SOP – which describes in detail how the trial shall be conducted and the structured case report form (CRF).

It is necessary to estimate a clinically meaningful treatment difference based on your chosen pain measure. This estimate is the basis for the calculation of the number of patients (sample size) within each treatment group needed to identify a real treatment difference. Statistical textbooks offer traditional methods to perform sample-size calculations. Furthermore, several online Internet services and computer programs are available. A common error when undertaking sample-size calculations is failure to add a specified percentage (e.g. 10–20% based on experience) to the calculated number of participants to compensate for dropouts.

Choice of primary outcome variable

Pain is an individual and subjective experience resulting from complex central nervous signal processing of inputs from memory, emotional status and nociceptive transmission. The aim of clinical trials in pain is to measure a difference in either:

- Intensity of this subjective experience (i.e. pain intensity).
- Magnitude of subjective reduction in pain intensity (i.e. pain relief) as a consequence of different analgesic treatments.

A decision is required as to which of these two should be the primary measure.

Outcome measures in analgesic trials should preferably contain the following requirements:

a   Ease in use by the participants of the trial.
b   Sensitivity sufficient to detect difference among treatments.
c   Clarity for the clinicians who will use the treatments (Max and Laska, 1991).

Indirect measurements (such as the use of analgesic tablet counts or reduction of concomitant medication) are not good measures of analgesic efficacy. Use outcome measures that have a proven record of efficacy and validity (e.g. visual analogue scale (VAS) or numerical rating scale (NRS) (Max and Laska, 1991)). Such scales allow comparisons with other studies using the same scores (Moore *et al.*, 1997).

The primary variable of efficacy, outcome, is the principal measure of the variable to be tested and has a major impact factor when interpreting the results. A summed measure of VAS or NRS is usually used as the primary outcome variable. Secondary variables are allowed. Remember that sample-size calculations for the primary and the secondary variables are not necessarily the same.

The protocol and presentation of data

Some clinical investigators believe that designing the study (developing the protocol) and the subsequent task of presenting the data are two separate issues. They should not be considered as such. Poor reporting of a high-quality trial will not change practice. Moreover, inclusion in a meta-analysis will be precluded, further decreasing the appropriate dissemination of important data. The Consolidated Standards of Reporting of Trials (CONSORT) statement defined absolute transparency with respect to reporting of details of the design, conduct, analysis and interpretation of trials data (Table 30.5). This emphasis on the quality of papers, primarily reporting the results of RCCT's also has an important secondary purpose. It forces clinical investigators to consider the items contained in the CONSORT statement while at the planning stage of a clinical trial. The investment in time and resources used when designing a trial is repaid when the time comes to presenting the results of the trial. A well-designed trial, with a well-defined outcome variable, yields results that are much easier to publish. Such a trial will have a greater chance of being accepted in high-impact journals and included in meta-analyses (Deveraux *et al.*, 2002). One of the ultimate aims for a clinical investigator should be to see their papers included in the foundation of knowledge upon which health providers base their clinical decisions.

Table 30.5 How to write a paper from a trial using CONSORT standards (checklist of items to be included when reporting a randomised trial)

Item	Report description
Paper section and topic	*Descriptor*
Title and abstract	How participants were allocated to intervention (e.g. 'random allocation', 'randomised' or 'randomly assigned'
Introduction	
Background	Scientific background and explanation of rationale
Methods	
Participants	Eligibility criteria for participants and the settings and location where the data were collected
Interventions	Precise details of the interventions intended for each group and how and where they were actually administered
Objectives	Specific objectives and hypotheses
Outcomes	Clearly defined primary and secondary outcome measures, and, when applicable, any methods used to enhance the quality of measurements (e.g. multiple observations, training of assessors)
Sample size	How sample size was determined and, when applicable, explanation of any interim analyses and stopping rules
Randomisation	
Sequence generation	Method used to generate the random allocation sequence, including details of any restriction (e.g. blocking, stratification)
Allocation concealment	Method used to implement the random allocation sequence (e.g. numbered containers or central telephone), clarifying whether the sequence was concealed until interventions were assigned
Implementation	Who generated the allocation sequence, who enrolled participants, and who assigned participants to their groups
Blinding	
Participant flow	Flow of participants through each stage (a diagram is strongly recommended). Specifically, for each group report the numbers of participants. Randomly assigned, receiving intended treatment, completing the study protocol, and analysed for the primary outcome. Describe protocol deviations from study as planned, together with reasons
Recruitment	Dates defining the periods of recruitment and followup
Baseline data	Baseline demographic and clinical characteristics of each group.
Numbers analysed	Number of participants (denominator) in each group included in each analysis and whether the analysis was by 'intention-to-treat'. State the results in absolute numbers when feasible (e.g. 10 of 20, not 50%)
Outcomes and estimation	For each primary and secondary outcome. A summary of results for each group and the estimated effect size and its precision (e.g. 95% confidence intervals)
Anciliary analyses	Address multiplicity by reporting any other analyses performed, including subgroup analyses and adjusted analyses, indicating those pre-specified and those exploratory
Adverse effects	All important adverse effects in each intervention group
Discussion	
Interpretation	Interpretation of the results, taking into account study hypotheses, source of potential bias or imprecision, and the dangers associated with multiplicity of analyses and outcomes
Generalisability	Generalisability (external validity) of the trial findings
Overall evidence	General interpretation of the results in the context of current evidence

Adapted from Moher *et al.*, 2001.

References

Cooper, S.A. (1991). Commentary. Single dose-analgesic studies: the upside and downside of assay sensitivity. In: Max, M.B., Portenoy, R.K. & Laska, E.M. (eds) *The Design of Analgesic Clinical Trials. Advances in Pain Research and Therapy*, Vol. 18. Raven Press, New York; pp. 117–124.

Deveraux, P.J., Manns, B.J., Ghali, W.A., Quan, H. & Guyatt, G.H. (2002). The reporting of methodological factors in randomized controlled trials and the association with a journal policy to promote adherence to the consolidated standards of reporting trials. *Control Clin. Trial.*, **23**: 380–388.

Houghton, I.T., Aun, C.S., Gin, T. & Lau, J.T. (1992). Interethnic differences in postoperative pethidine requirements. *Anaesth. Intens. Care*, **20**: 52–55.

Keefe, F.J., Lumley, M.A., Buffington, A.L.H., Carson, J.W., Studts, J.L., Edwards, C.L., Macklem, D.J., Aspnes, A.K., Fox, L. & Steffey, D. (2002). Changing face of pain: evolution of pain research in psychosomatic medicine. *Psychosom. Med.*, **64**: 921–938.

Max, M.B. & Laska, E.M. (1991). Single-dose analgesic comparisons. In: Max, M.B., Portenoy, R.K. & Laska, E.M. (eds) *The Design of Analgesic Clinical Trials. Advances in Pain Research and Therapy*, Vol. 18. Raven Press, New York; pp. 55–95.

Moher, D., Schulz, K.F. & Altman, D.G. (2001). The CONSORT statement: revised recommendations for improving the quality of reports of parallel-group randomization trials. *Ann. Intern. Med.*, **134**: 657–662.

Moore, A., Moore, O., McQuay, H. & Gavaghan, D. (1997). Deriving dichotomous outcome measures from continuous data in randomised controlled trials of analgesics: use of pain intensity and visual analogue scales. *Pain*, **69**: 311–315.

Roberts, C. & Torgerson, D.J. (1999). Baseline imbalance in randomised controlled trials. *Br. Med. J.*, **319**: 185.

Sarton, E., Olofsen, E., Romberg, R., den Hartigh, J., Kest, B., Nieuwenhuijs, D., Burm, A., Teppema, L. & Dahan, A. (2000). Sex differences in morphine analgesia. *Anesthesiology*, **93**: 1245–1254.

Further reading

Coggon, D. (2003). *Statistics in Clinical Practice*, 2nd edition. BMJ Books, London.

Duley, L. & Farrell, B. (eds) (2002). *Clinical Trials*. BMJ Books, London.

Jadad, A.R. (1998). *Randomised Controlled Trials*. BMJ Publishing Group, London.

Max, M.B., Portenoy, R.K. & Laska, E.M. (eds) (1991). The design of analgesic clinical trials. *Advances in Pain Research and Therapy*, Vol. 18. Raven Press, New York.

Tramer, M.R. (ed.) (2000). *Evidence Based Resource in Anaesthesia and Analgesia*. BMJ Books, London.

Web sites for further information

FDA Office for Good Clinical Practice (http:\\www.fda.gov/oc/gcp/default.htm)

The International Conference for Harmonisation (ICH) (http:\\www.ich.org)

European Medicines Agency (EMEA) (http:\\www.emea.eu.int)

Bandolier Home Page – Evidence based health care (www.jr2.ox.ac.uk/bandolier)

CONSORT statement (http:\\www.consort-statement.org)

H.J. McQuay

What constitutes evidence?

Finding and using the best available evidence should be part of our professional lives.

There are several interlinked strands:

- Finding the evidence.
- Appraising the evidence.
- Making the evidence (doing trials or systematic reviews (SRs)).
- Using the evidence.

SRs and large randomised trials constitute the most reliable sources of evidence we can muster (Table 31.1). Put simply, they are the best chance we have to determine what is true.

Where do you get the evidence?

The randomised controlled trial (RCT) is the most reliable way to estimate the effect of an intervention.

Table 31.1 Type and strength of efficacy evidence (Oxford centre for evidence-based medicine levels of evidence, May 2001)

Level	Therapy/prevention, aetiology/harm
1a	SR (with homogeneity) of RCTs
1b	Individual RCT (with narrow confidence interval)
1c	All or none*
2a	SR (with homogeneity) of cohort studies
2b	Individual cohort study (including low quality RCT, for example <80% follow-up)
2c	'Outcomes' research; ecological studies**
3a	SR (with homogeneity) of case–control studies
3b	Individual case–control study
4	Case-series (and poor quality cohort and case–control studies)
5	Expert opinion without explicit critical appraisal, or based on physiology, bench research or 'first principles'

http://www.cebm.net/levels_of_evidence.asp
* i.e all cured or none cured
** relating to a type of study design

The simple principle of randomisation is that each patient has the same probability of receiving any of the interventions being compared. Randomisation abolishes selection bias because it prevents investigators influencing who has which intervention. Randomisation also helps to ensure that other factors, such as age or sex distribution, are equivalent for the different treatment groups. Inadequate randomisation, or inadequate concealment of randomisation, lead to exaggeration of therapeutic effect (Schulz *et al.*, 1995).

This is elegantly demonstrated in an SR of transcutaneous electrical nerve stimulation (TENS) in postoperative pain. Seventeen reports on 786 patients were randomised studies in acute post-operative pain. Of these, 15 demonstrated no benefit of TENS over placebo. Nineteen other reports had pain outcomes, but were not RCTs. In 17 of these 19, TENS was said by the authors to be analgesic (Moore *et al.*, 2003).

To produce valid reviews of evidence a systematic search is necessary. To be qualitative or quantitative, they need to include all relevant RCTs. How many eligible RCTs exist? Commonly the total is unknown. Usually reviewers are only sure that they have found all the RCTs for newer interventions. In practice, constrained by time and cost, reviewers have to compromise hoping that what they have found is a representative sample of the unknown total population of trials. The more comprehensive the searching, the more trials will be found and any conclusions will then be stronger.

Retrieval bias is the failure to identify reports that could have affected the results of an SR or meta-analysis. This failure may be because trials are still ongoing, or completed but unpublished (publication bias) or because although published the search did not find them. Trying to identify unpublished trials by asking researchers has a very low yield and is not cheap. Registers of ongoing and completed trials are another way to find unpublished data, but such registers are rare.

The importance of basing SRs on the highest quality evidence (randomised trials) is obvious. The process is laborious, but the Cochrane Library has listed citations of RCTs, easing the process. For topics that are not mainstream the hand-searching process will still have to be done.

While databases can tell us how well the patient or the health care professional thought the intervention worked any conclusions about treatment efficacy are subject to the selection and observer bias which RCTs are designed to minimise. Estimates of treatment efficacy from database data are therefore likely to be overestimates. Other influences, such as the medical condition itself and other drugs, may confound the issue.

Trials: quality and validity issues

Once you have found all the reports of the trials relevant to your question you need to confirm that these reports meet certain *quality standards* and ensure the trial is *valid*.

Imagine a situation where you found 40 relevant trial reports. You then discover that 20 say that the intervention is terrific, while 20 conclude that it should never be used. Delving deeper you find the 20 'negative' reports score highly on your quality standards scale, but the 20 'positive' reports score poorly. What then will you conclude? Without a quality scale you would vote for the intervention. With the quality scale you would vote against.

The quality scale should include measures of bias. Bias is the simplest explanation why poor quality reports give more positive conclusions than high quality reports. The quality standards that you require cannot be absolute, because for some clinical questions there may not be any RCTs. Setting RCTs as a minimum absolute standard would therefore be inappropriate for all the questions we might want to answer. In the pain world however, there are two reasons for setting this high standard and requiring trials to be randomised. The first is that we do have, particularly for drug interventions, quite a number of RCTs. The second is that it is even more important to stress minimum quality standards of randomisation and double blinding when the outcome measures are subjective.

Developing and validating a quality scale

What makes a trial worthy of the label 'high quality'? In this context, quality indicates the likelihood that the study design reduced bias. Only by avoiding bias is it possible to estimate the effect of a given intervention with any confidence. The simple scale as shown in Table 31.2 was designed to assess this.

Table 31.2 Scale (3 point) to measure the likelihood of bias

1 Was the study described as randomised (including the use of words such as randomly, random and randomisation)?
2 Was the study described as double blind?
3 Was there a description of withdrawals and dropouts?

Give a score of 1 point for each 'yes' and 0 points for each 'no'. There are no in-between marks

Give 1 additional point if:	On question 1, the method of randomisation was described **and** it was **appropriate** (table of random numbers, computer generated, coin tossing, etc.)
and/or:	If on question 2 the method of double blinding was described **and** it was **appropriate** (identical placebo, active placebo, dummy, etc.)
Deduct 1 point if:	On question 1, the method of randomisation was described **and** it was **inappropriate** (patients were allocated alternatively, or according to date of birth, hospital number, etc.)
and/or:	On question 2 the study was described as double blind but the method of blinding was **inappropriate** (e.g. comparison of tablet versus injection with no double dummy)

Validity of trials

A study may of course be both randomised and double blind, and describe withdrawals and dropouts in copious detail (scoring well on this quality scale) and yet be invalid. Examples include:

- The injection of morphine into the knee joint to reduce pain after arthroscopy. In some trials this was made after the operation without knowledge of whether the patients had enough pain for the intervention to make a difference. If they had mild pain it is possible that the success ascribed to the intervention was due to an initial absence of pain.

- A review proclaimed fewer patients would die after major surgery if they had regional plus general anaesthesia. The statistical significance leading to this important conclusion came from a number of small trials with 30% mortality rates; the rates are so high that one questions the validity of the trials. A subsequent big RCT showed that the conclusion was wrong – there was no difference (Rigg *et al.*, 2002).

SRs: quality, utility and output

Judging quality of SRs

SRs of inadequate quality may be worse than none, because faulty decisions may be made with unjustified confidence. Quality control in the SR process, from literature searching onwards, is vital. Judging the quality of an SR is encapsulated below (Oxman and Cook, 1994):

- Were the question(s) and methods stated clearly?
- Were comprehensive search methods used?
- Did explicit methods determine articles to include?
- Was methodological quality of the primary studies assessed?
- Were selection and assessment of the primary studies reproducible and unbiased?
- Were differences in individual study results explained adequately?
- Were results of the primary studies combined appropriately?
- Were reviewers' conclusions supported by the data cited?

Outcome measures chosen for data extraction should also be sensible. Usually this is not a problem, with reviewers using all that is available. Problems may be due to inadequate outcome measures in the original trials, but this will determine the clinical utility of the review.

The questions an SR should answer for us are:

- How well does an intervention work (compared with placebo, no treatment or other current interventions)?
- Is it safe?
- Will it work safely for the patients in our practice?

Not all data can be combined in a meta-analysis: qualitative SRs

It is often not possible or sensible to pool data, resulting in a qualitative rather than a quantitative SR. Combining data may not be sensible if trials:

- Were of poor quality.
- Contained no quantitative data.
- Used different outcomes (e.g. continuous and dichotomous data).
- Had different follow-up periods.

Making decisions from qualitative SRs

Making decisions about whether or not a therapy works from a qualitative SR may look easy. In the

example of TENS in acute pain, 15 of the 17 RCTs showed no benefit compared with control. The thinking clinician will realise that TENS in acute pain is not an effective analgesic. The problem with this simple vote counting is that it may mislead. It ignores the sample size of the constituent studies, the magnitude of the effect in the studies and the validity of their design even though they were randomised (Moore *et al.*, 2003).

Evaluating efficacy

Combining data: quantitative SRs

There are also two parts to the 'does it work?' question:

- How does it compare with placebo?
- How does it compare with other therapies?

Whichever comparison is being considered, three stages of examining a review should follow:

- L'Abbé plot (L'Abbé *et al.*, 1987).
- Statistical testing (odds ratio or relative risk).
- Clinical significance measure (e.g. number-needed-to-treat (NNT)).

L'Abbé plots

This simple scatter plot yields a surprisingly comprehensive qualitative view of data. Even if the review does not present data in this way, it can be produced from information on individual trials presented in the review tables. Figure 31.1 contains data from an

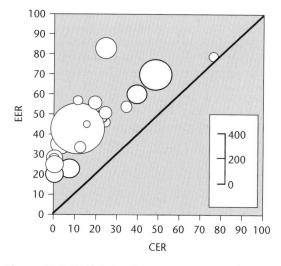

Figure 31.1 L'Abbé plot of Experimental Event Rate (EER; % >50% relief on treatment) against Control Event Rate (CER; % >50% relief on placebo) for RCTs of paracetamol 1000 mg.

updated SR of single dose paracetamol in acute pain. Each point on the graph is the result of a single trial (with the size of each point being proportional to the size of each trial). What happens with paracetamol (experimental event rate (EER)) is plotted against the event rate with placebo (control event rate (CER)).

Trials where experimental treatment proves better than control (EER > CER) lie in the upper left of the plot. Paracetamol was better than placebo in all the trials. If experimental drug is no better than control/placebo then points fall on the line of equality (EER = CER). If control/placebo is better than experimental then points lie in the lower right of the plot (EER < CER).

Visual inspection gives a quick and easy indication of the level of agreement among trials. Heterogeneity is often assumed to be due to variation in the EER – the effect of the intervention. Figure 31.1 shows that CER can also be a source of heterogeneity; even though the controls were all matched in relatively homogeneous acute pain conditions. They explain the need for placebo controls if ethical issues about future trials arise.

Variation in control (placebo) response rates   The overwhelming reason for large variations in placebo rates in pain studies (and probably in other clinical conditions) is the relatively small group sizes in trials. Group sizes are chosen to produce statistical significance through power calculations – for pain studies the usual size is 30–40 patients for a 30% difference between placebo and active analgesic. An individual patient can have 0–100% pain relief. Random selection of patients can therefore produce groups with a range of placebo responses. Mathematical modelling shows that while group sizes of up to 50 patients show a statistical difference 80–90% of the time, as many as 500 patients per group are needed to approximate clinical impact.

Thus, small trials should be treated with circumspection, understanding that variation is probably artefactual.

- *Heterogeneity*: Clinicians making decisions on the basis of SRs need to be confident that like are being compared with like. The crucial issues are whether the trials are clinically homogeneous and sufficiently large.
- *Indirect versus direct comparisons*: What clinicians really need are the results of direct comparisons of the different interventions, so-called head-to-head comparisons. These are rarely available, and what we have to work with are comparisons of each of the interventions with placebo. The methods illustrated here tell us how fast each competitor runs

against the clock, rather than who crosses the line first in a head-to-head challenge.

Statistical significance

When it is legitimate and feasible to combine data, the odds ratio and relative risk (or benefit) are the accepted statistical tests to show that the intervention works significantly better than the comparator.

Odds ratios   The ratio of the odds of having the target outcome in the experimental group, relative to the odds in favour of having the target outcome in the control group.

Where CERs are high (certainly when >50%), odds ratios should be interpreted with caution, since they may overestimate benefit.

Relative risk   The proportional increase in rates of an outcome between experimental and control patients in a trial, calculated as:

$$\frac{(EER - CER)}{CER}$$

where EER and CER are the experimental and CERs, respectively.

With event rates above 10% relative risk produces more conservative figures.

How well does the intervention work?

Clinical significance

While odds ratios and relative risks can show that an intervention works compared with control, they are of limited help in telling clinicians how well the intervention works – the size of the effect or its clinical significance. NNT may be more useful on an individual patient level, where the choice of analgesic (for both professional and patient) will be made on the balance between efficacy and risks.

Effect size

Effect size estimates the amount of treatment benefit using the standardised mean difference between treatment groups. The method can use continuous scale data, rather than the dichotomous data needed for the NNT. The output of the effect size estimation, the z-score, is in standard deviation units, and is therefore scale-free. The method was used widely in early psychology meta-analyses. Many clinicians find it difficult to understand or use.

NNT

The NNT is the number of people who have to be treated for 1 to achieve the specified level of benefit.

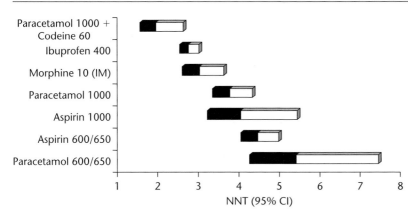

Figure 31.2 NNT for 50% pain relief in post-operative pain (single dose drug treatments). The NNT point estimate is at the junction of the black and white bar segments. Black bar segment is the lower 95% confidence interval (CI), white is the upper.

This concept is proving to be a very effective alternative as the measure of clinical significance. It has the crucial advantage of applicability to clinical practice demonstrating the effort required to achieve a particular therapeutic target.

The NNT is the reciprocal of the absolute risk reduction given by the equation:

$$NNT = \frac{1}{(IMP_{act} / TOT_{act}) - (IMP_{con} / TOT_{con})},$$

where:
IMP_{act} = number of patients given active treatment achieving the target.
TOT_{act} = total number of patients given the active treatment.
IMP_{con} = number of patients given a control treatment achieving the target.
TOT_{con} = total number of patients given the control treatment.

Advantages
The advantage of the NNT is that it is clinically intuitive, it is treatment specific and describes the difference between active treatment and control/placebo. The level of benefit used to calculate NNT can be varied, but NNT is likely to be relatively unchanged, since changing threshold changes results for both active and control. The threshold used for the single dose analgesic data (see Figure 31.2) was 50% pain relief. This is a difficult target for analgesics. Furthermore, in cancer pain, patients feel a treatment is beneficial if it produces 30% relief. What is judged worthwhile relief may vary with the clinical context.

An NNT of 1 describes an event that occurs in every patient given the treatment, but in no patient in a comparator group. This could be described as the 'perfect' result. There are few circumstances in which a treatment is close to 100% effective and the control/placebo completely ineffective. Therefore, NNTs of 2 or 3 often indicate an effective intervention. For unwanted effects, NNT becomes the number-needed-to-harm (NNH), which should be as large as possible. Whether the NNH is acceptable depends on the context as well as the value. If 1 in 10 patients vomit after your new anaesthetic this might be acceptable (NNH 10 compared with the old anaesthetic), 1 in 2 might not (NNH 2).

It is important to remember that NNT is always relative to the comparator and applies to a particular clinical outcome. The duration of treatment necessary to achieve the target should be specified.

Confidence intervals
The confidence intervals of the NNT are an indication that 19 times out of 20 the 'true' value will be in the specified range. If there is inadequate or conflicting data then the NNT may not have finite confidence intervals, and the statistical tests (odds ratio or relative risk) will not be statistically significant. An NNT with an infinite confidence interval may still have clinical value as a benchmark, but should be treated cautiously until further data permits finite confidence intervals.

Disadvantages
The disadvantages of the NNT approach are apparent from the formula:

- It needs dichotomous data (i.e. 'yes' or 'no'). Continuous data can be converted to dichotomous for acute pain studies (so that NNTs may be calculated) by deriving a relationship between the two from individual patient data.

- It will be sensitive to trials with high CERs. As CER rises, the potential for treatment specific improvement decreases: higher (and apparently less effective) NNTs result. So, NNT needs to be treated with caution, with comparisons only being made confidently if the pooled trials do not show major variation in their CERs.

Evaluating safety

Estimating the risk of harm is a critical part of clinical decisions. SRs should report adverse events as well as efficacy (including rare but important adverse events). Large RCTs apart, most trials study limited patient numbers. New medicines may be launched after trials on 1500 patients (Moore, 1995), missing such rare but important adverse events.

The absence of information on adverse effects in SRs reduces their usefulness.

Rules of evidence

The gold standard of evidence for harm – as for efficacy – is the RCT. The problem is that in the relatively small number of patients studied in RCTs rare serious harm may not be spotted. Rare and serious events (including death) cannot and should not be dismissed just because they are reported in case reports rather than RCTs.

NNH

For adverse effects reported in RCTs, NNH may be calculated in the same way as NNT. When there is low incidence it is likely that point estimates alone will emerge (infinite confidence intervals). Major harm may be defined in a set of RCTs as intervention-related study withdrawal. Precise estimates of major harm will require much wider literature searches to trawl for case reports or series. Minor harm may similarly be defined in a set of RCTs as reported adverse effects.

Key points

- High quality evidence requires high quality trials.
- In the ideal world you will have three numbers for each intervention, an NNT for benefit and NNHs for minor and major harm.
- These methods can be used to show the effectiveness or otherwise of a range of interventions.
- If effective the NNT may act as a benchmark of just how effective a particular intervention is. This becomes the yardstick against which alternative interventions should be judged.
- Clinical decisions on whether or not to use the intervention for an individual patient can utilise such figures. Figure 31.2 ranks the analgesics by their efficacy estimate. In particular situations a safer, although marginally less effective drug, may be preferred.
- Safety estimates usually result from lower quality studies.

References

L'Abbé, K.A., Detsky, A.S., O'Rourke, K. (1987). Meta-analysis in clinical research. *Ann. Int. Med.*, **107**: 224–233.

Moore, T.J. (1995). *Deadly Medicine.* Simon & Schuster, New York.

Moore, A., Edwards, J., Barden, J. & McQuay, H. (2003). *Bandolier's Little Book of Pain.* Oxford University Press, Oxford.

Oxman, A.D., Cook, D.J. Guyatt, G.H. (1994). Users' guides to the medical literature. VI. How to use an overview. *J. Am. Med. Assoc.*, **272**: 1367–1371.

Rigg, J.R.A., Jamrozik, K., Myles, P.S. *et al.* (2002). Epidural anaesthesia and analgesia and outcome of major surgery: a randomised trial. *Lancet*, **359**: 1276–1282.

Schulz, K.F., Chalmers, I., Hayes, R.J. & Altman, D.G. (1995). Empirical evidence of bias: dimensions of methodological quality associated with estimates of treatment effects in controlled trials. *J. Am. Med. Assoc.*, **273**: 408–412.

TREATMENT OF PAIN

GENERAL PRINCIPLES

SECTION

5a

C. Pither

Patients go to doctors not because a disease process starts or reaches a certain level; but rather to get help with problems that they perceive to have a medical solution. This is important as it underpins the reason that only approximately 15% of patients visiting their general practitioners (GPs) have identifiable pathology, and the observation that some people visit their doctor weekly, while others virtually never attend.

The way that physicians tackle the challenge of helping the person in front of them varies substantially between hospital medicine and primary care. In hospitals the above point, while perhaps not forgotten, becomes irrelevant in the reductionist pursuit of the cause of the problem that drives investigation and treatment. In primary care on the other hand, a much more problem-focused approach is adopted. The model is broader and acknowledges that the needs of the whole person must be addressed.

Patients with chronic pain attending hospital pain clinics fall somewhere between these two polarities. Pain clinicians rightly consider themselves to have a sophisticated scientific understanding of pain and practice evidence-based medicine. However, they also advocate a biopsychosocial model, where issues beyond the purely biological are taken into account. At least half of pain clinic patients will not have a clearly identifiable pathology to account for their pain; ultimately pain is always a subjective experience known only to the sufferer. Thus, not only the pain, but also the outcome of interventions, will always be reliant on the patients' subjective account. This is not the case in many other areas of medicine (e.g. the success of a hernia repair or alterations to peak flow in asthma treatment). Therefore the patients' subjective report of benefit replaces the objective evidence that might guide treatment (e.g. of raised blood pressure).

Chronic pain can seldom be cured. This is a fact, perhaps accepted more by the seasoned clinician than the Young Turk. This is not the same as saying it cannot be helped. It can, often very considerably, but total relief usually remains an elusive Utopian end point. If cure is an unrealistic goal in the majority of patients, what then replaces it?

Relief of pain is a valid therapeutic goal in its own right. Indeed it can be seen as one of the fundamental tenets of medicine. But what relief is enough? If relief can only be judged by the sufferer, should it rightly be left for the patient to determine the end point of treatment? Is relief of pain without change in function acceptable? The mother who administers her child paracetamol to ease frequent headaches is acting in accord with ethical and common sense principles, as is the nurse delivering optimal opioid analgesia to a patient recovering from surgery. Why then might we feel uneasy about a GP giving nightly pethidine injections to his wife troubled by insomnia due to neck pain, or the 30-year-old factory worker unable to work due to back pain because he claims lying recumbent is the only position in which he is pain free?

It will be clear from the above brief discussion that the goals and aims of chronic pain treatment require analysis and reflection. It behoves the potential specialist in the field to be aware of some of the issues involved. This chapter is not the place for a full analysis of these, but will instead suggest some general principles which should be born in mind by all those prescribing treatment for chronic pain.

Belief not blame

When patients tell doctors how they feel (worried, sad, frustrated, happy, etc.) the doctor seldom doubts the reality of the experience. Why then do doctors doubt patients' reports of pain? When a doctor cannot readily explain a pain, or when the descriptions of pain are out of proportion to what they believe to be appropriate, doctors sometimes give the impression that they doubt the sufferers' experience. Phrases such as 'I'm not sure how much pain he/she is really having' or 'there is a lot of overlay' are still too often heard in the hospital setting.

When faced with a person telling us they have pain with little evidence of tissue pathology we are seemingly faced with a dilemma. The reverence that is bestowed upon the scientific method within medical training directs us to believe the science. Simple humanity compels us to hear the voice of suffering. How can the two be reconciled? In practice there is no dichotomy: it is my view that to disbelieve a patient in this way amounts to medical negligence. Not only does such a standpoint irretrievably damage the therapeutic relationship and prevent the delivery of effective therapy, but it also promotes exaggeration and abnormal pain behaviour. This can lead to confirmation (in the eyes of the physician) that the person's problems are not 'real' or as severe as they claim. Unfortunately, pain specialists inherit many patients who have been damaged in this way by their passage through the medical system. Disbelief never paves the way to successful therapy.

Pain specialists see those unfortunate patients who are most troubled and most disabled by their pain. It is now clear that the development of distress and disability is predicated by psychosocial variables not physical pathology. Epidemiological data clearly show that by definition, this patient group are disadvantaged in terms of education, social support, income, housing, etc. It is therefore possible to subtly imply that the patients are responsible for their own predicament. Patients are very adroit at detecting this blaming, which once again poisons the therapeutic relationship. I believe that this is akin to blaming a person for receiving a poor education.

Patients are often more logical in their thinking and behaviour than we give them credit for. A person with pain acts and behaves in a manner predicated by their perception of their illness. If this perception is wrong and they are exhibiting unhelpful pain behaviours (e.g. resting excessively or taking too many tablets) it is inappropriate to blame them before enquiring why they are acting as they are. Frequently it will be the messages given to them by doctors and therapists that have informed their beliefs and underpin their actions.

The message is simple: never doubt the patients' subjective experience, nor blame them for their disability.

Communication

Pain patients are often heard to say that their visit to the pain clinic was the first time they were listened to and believed. Good communication between doctor and patient is vital. This may require specialist training. Anaesthetists who take the time to go on communication skills training courses may do more for their patients than attending 10 years worth of scientific meetings.

Realism and honesty are the mainstays of effective communication. It is often surprising what patients will cope with if they are given clear messages. The false hope of cure, implied by blind reassurance that all will be fine, may only serve to delay the adaptation required for successful acceptance of a chronic illness.

Patients do require adequate explanations of their symptoms, which can be a challenge when so much uncertainty surrounds the causes of pain. In spite of this, one must beware over-simplistic explanations, such as 'trapped nerve' or 'bulging disc'. Rather, it is necessary to explain how complex chronic pain states are, and how many mechanisms are involved, while moving on from the truism that the fundamental abnormality may not be identifiable. It is important that the sufferer sees chronic pain as a disorder of neural and musculoskeletal function, rather than structural damage.

Map the treatment plan

Given that the treatment offered is unlikely to cure, it is crucial to help the patient understand the aims and objectives of the proposed therapy. The programme will probably commence with pain relieving interventions and drugs. Later, rehabilitation techniques, directed at reducing distress, improving function and abetting coping, are instituted if the pain cannot be relieved.

Patients arrive in pain clinics often polarised in their attitudes. Some expect a cure, while others despair after being told that they cannot he helped. A positive treatment outcome is much more likely if:

a The patient can be engaged in treatment in a collaborative fashion.
b Their part in the therapeutic relationship is made clear at the outset.

It is important that they understand that they will not be abandoned, even if the pain relieving techniques are unsuccessful. The valued physician is the one who can help the person who cannot be helped by drugs or interventions.

Focus on function not pain

In the context of chronic pain, changes to pain intensity mean little if there is no change in function. The patient will not understand this, being unable to see further than the need for pain relief. A treatment that improves pain levels but does not allow an improvement in functional level is of little value and the benefit soon palls. Even low-intensity pain can cause secondary distress and depression: it is not the pain level that irks – it is its presence. Patients need to understand from both the specialist and clinic staff that:

- Therapy will focus on function as well as pain.
- Improvements in activity level and functional capacity are valid end points in their own right.
- Any improvement takes time to occur. Remember that if the development of distress and dysfunction has taken 2 years, it may take a similar time to regain health.

With many spinal and musculoskeletal conditions improvements in strength, range of movement, posture and fitness, will result in reductions in pain. However, the pain relief comes later after the change in function. This needs to be explained to the patient as a rationale for engaging in rehabilitation.

Similarly, anxiety, negative thinking patterns, poor stress management, a tendency to catastrophise and fear that pain equates to damage, can all be thought of as psychological dysfunctions which, if improved can enhance quality of life, irrespective of pain intensity.

Do no harm

Chronic pain is never simply a problem within the tissues. It always encompasses neural mechanisms involving spinal and cortical processing influenced by the meaning of the pain, low mood, fear, etc. There is no pain that cannot be made worse by an inappropriate intervention. This may occur secondary to tissue damage (due to error or mishap), but also through psychological mechanisms (secondary to: inappropriate or overly aggressive interventions, inadequate explanation, or erroneous messages given during the procedure), which can cause much hurt and harm in the longer term.

Happily the age of widespread use of neuro–destructive techniques has passed, largely due to recognition of their limitations. It still behoves the aspiring pain specialist to be extremely cautious about performing destructive techniques in benign pain states.

Rules of prescribing

For many specialists prescribing remains the mainstay of treatment, with the expectation that appropriate medications can reduce the level of pain by up to 50%. However, is must not be forgotten that as many patients find drugs are not the answer to their problem and cease taking medications, as end up taking multiple drugs in more than the recommended dose. It has never been the case that a certain level of pathology requires a certain dose of drug. Most patients who

reduce or stop their analgesics do not notice an increase in pain in the longer term, indicating uncertainty about the exact mechanisms of action in chronic administration. Furthermore, physicians tend to prescribe stronger painkillers on the basis of patient distress, rather than tissue pathology. This is illogical as analgesics are not effective anxiolytics.

Various recommendations can be made:

1 Drugs alone seldom improve function in chronic pain states.
2 Give clear explanations of effects and side effects. Is the drug intended to reduce pain alone? (or at all?), or does it have other actions? (e.g. aiding sleep?). Patients may cease taking a potentially useful drug if it causes side effects that they were not warned about.
3 Let patients titrate the dose within limits set by the physician.
4 If a drug is unhelpful stop it.
5 Avoid two drugs from the same class, or compound analgesics with additional doses of one component.
6 Be prepared to go up a step in strength if large doses of a lower strength drug are not effective.
7 Avoid polypharmacy.
8 Try not to give strong drugs on the basis of distress alone. Analgesics do not solve sad lives.
9 Set dose limits from the outset.
10 Communicate with patients' primary care physicians, to agree a prescribing strategy.
11 Allow patients to stop drugs if they wish.

Key points

- All medical treatment requires detailed knowledge of evidence of efficacy for the proposed treatment, and its appropriateness within that individual. In addition, pain clinic treatment requires practitioners to formulate treatment approaches that take into account the patients psychosocial status, along side the biology of the disease.
- Relief of pain is a valid end point, but is seldom achievable to the extent that it enables functional improvement and reduction of distress in its own right. Half a pain is still a pain. Those who find pain distressing frequently find it is just as problematic at a lower intensity.
- Effective treatment starts with good communication and ends with the patient taking responsibility for their own condition. The role of the pain specialist as healer–director in the sad theatre of 'the pain clinic' is not for everyone. However, it can provide sufficient rewards for those with oceans of empathy, a phlegmatic attitude and the hide of a rhinoceros.

A. Howarth

Pain has been viewed in the past as many things, ranging from a philosophical concept to a religious manifestation of wrong doing. It is now recognized as a complex phenomenon with biological, psychological, social and spiritual issues needing to be considered. Pain chronicity potentially impacts greatly on an individual's well being, requiring management, rather than treatment aimed at a cure. Medical management may in many cases reinforce the characteristics exhibited by patients with chronic pain. It may raise their hopes and expectations of a cure and total pain relief, which is not realistic – chronic pain is unlikely to go away. Therefore, patients should be encouraged to get on and live with their condition, by taking control and managing their illness and health, rather than being controlled by it.

Self-management of health by patients with any chronic illness is well established. The aim is to provide the person with the knowledge and skills to enable them to become the active participant in their day-to-day management. In doing so the emphasis and responsibility of a patient's health shifts from the doctor in the health care environment, to the patient in their home environment. Self-management of health, implemented through a multidisciplinary team (MDT) offers a comprehensive approach to this.

The core elements of an MDT

Multidisciplinary pain centres were established in the 1950s and are recommended by International Association for the Study of Pain (IASP) as the desirable way to manage chronic pain (Bond *et al.*, 1991). Many things including a person's psychological or psychiatric state, cultural differences, and past experiences and beliefs of pain, affect the experience and perception of pain and reduce quality of life. The aim of multidisciplinary pain management is not only to relieve pain, but also to restore activities of daily living and normal patterns of behaviour, while helping patients develop coping strategies.

The core elements of an MDT are doctors, nurses, psychologists and psychiatrists, in addition to physiotherapists and occupational therapists.

Doctors

Anaesthetists with skills in regional anaesthesia have been the forerunners in the development of multidisciplinary pain clinics. Moving on from the administration of nerve blocks, they are increasingly utilizing a biopsychosocial approach. The relationship between the doctor and patient is changing from a paternalistic relationship to one where patient autonomy is promoted. Doctors are in a prime position to promote and provide liaison between the MDT and other professionals, for example neurologists.

Nurses

The role of the nurse in the MDT is that of patient care, education, research and co-ordination. Nurse specialists trained in pain management deliver expert care. Their role in co-ordinating services involves liasing between the MDT and other disciplines including social workers, counsellors, training and enterprise councils, disablement resettlement officers and housing associations. This liaison develops social support, often vital for patients with chronic pain.

Psychologists and psychiatrists

Patients often expect a doctor to offer a cure. However, chronic pain is rarely cured, causing patients to experience helplessness, hopelessness, depression and social withdrawal. Cognitive behavioural approaches, utilized by psychologists and psychiatrists, help patients achieve the best level of physical and emotional functioning possible. This involves coping strategies including relaxation, pacing and addressing issues, such as control, anxiety and depression.

The role of the psychiatrist in the management of chronic pain is to detect pathological states, such as severe depression and suicidal thoughts. Input from a psychiatrist involves diagnosis and treatments, including psychotropic medication, psychotherapy, biofeedback and distraction methods.

Physiotherapists and occupational therapists

Physical therapy involves the restoration of function through graded fitness programmes and education.

Thus the physiotherapist can reduce disability and pain, increasing patient stamina and improving confidence. The cognitive behavioural approach aims to improve patient fitness, mobility and posture and counteract the effects of disuse.

Occupational therapists work closely with physiotherapists in:

- Goal setting.
- Activity planning.
- Pacing.
- Assessing domestic circumstances.
- Advising on activities of daily living and aids.

Multidisciplinary treatment

A MDT is only as good and useful as its ability to communicate between the disciplines. It requires regular meetings with transference of information between disciplines sharing a common philosophy and goal, in order to achieve effect.

The patient journey in a multidisciplinary pain clinic is one of change. Often one treatment will support and make possible another, for example analgesia and physical therapy. Hence the necessity for individualized treatment regimes and regular review of patient progress. Clinics vary considerably in what they offer patients, depending upon the skills of their team members and the resources available. One may make an initial assessment, another recommend a plan of care and someone else support pain management on an on-going basis. Team members have to be consistent in their explanations, helping the patient to accept the chronicity of their problems and encouraging self-management.

Some hospitals have pain management programmes (PMPs) where groups of patients interact with the MDT. This improves insight, explains why they are experiencing pain and what it means, in addition to offering help and advice. The aim of such programmes is not to remove the pain. Rather they help patients to change their behaviour and improve their functioning and quality of life, while experiencing on-going pain. This biopsychosocial approach is used often in conjunction with treatments based in cognitive behavioural therapy. Programmes are usually for outpatients on a weekly or bi-weekly basis. Inpatient programmes are costly and are usually reserved for those who need more intensive intervention and rehabilitation.

The efficacy of multidisciplinary pain clinics

Clinical effectiveness is the extent to which specific clinical interventions, when deployed in the field, for a particular patient, do what they intend to do. Evidence for clinical effectiveness of specific pain management treatments has been produced. When combined with evidence of cost effectiveness this may enable funding support for MDT. One issue in studies is that of long-term follow-up. Current studies often limit follow-up to 6 or 12 months, making it difficult to establish the long-term efficacy of study interventions.

Many reports regarding the efficacy of MDTs focus on the input of certain disciplines, such as nursing, physiotherapy, psychology and doctors, while patients are attending a programme or receiving treatment from the entire MDT. The results from systematic reviews (conducted through the Cochrane database) investigating the effectiveness of the multidisciplinary approach to pain management suggest that high quality trials are needed in this area. One randomized controlled study by Keller *et al.* (1997) evaluated the effect of multidisciplinary pain management for outpatients with chronic low back pain. Improvement was found in areas of pain measurement, functional capacity, disability, muscular strength, self-efficacy, depression, well being and posture immediately post-intervention. Improvement in pain measurement, posture, self-efficacy and well being was maintained at 6 months post-intervention.

An extensive and complex review of outpatient services for the treatment of chronic pain was undertaken by McQuay *et al.* (1997). This systematic review aimed at reviewing studies and papers to establish the effectiveness of interventions on a number needed to treat (NNT) basis, for example for ibuprofen (Chapter 31). However, only individual interventions were considered, providing controversial results. The report proposed that there was little evidence to support the efficacy of transcutaneous nerve stimulation (TENS), relaxation, guanethidine blocks, epidural steroids, intra-articular steroids for shoulder pain and spinal cord stimulation. Others have provided systematic review support for epidural steroids in sciatic pain, TENS for osteoarthritis of the knee, intra-articular steroids and one randomized, controlled study supporting relaxation therapy. Many of these interventions are commonplace in multidisciplinary pain clinics and are classed by both clinicians and patients as being clinically effective and beneficial.

When considering McQuay's review, two points in particular illustrate the problems of studying the MDT. Firstly, interventions were examined in isolation (i.e. a unimodal approach). In reality multidisciplinary management does not occur like this and interventions may complement each other. Secondly, some of the interventions were found to be ineffective.

However it is possible that the scoring systems establishing the efficacy of one type of intervention may not apply to a different type of intervention.

Key points

The multidisciplinary approach aims to:

- Reduce pain levels.
- Restore ability to carry out activities of daily living.
- Help people develop strategies to cope with their pain.

Further reading

Bond, M.R., Charlton, J.E. & Woolfe, C.J. (eds) (1991). Desirable characteristics for pain treatment facilities: report of the IASP taskforce. *Proceedings of the VI World Congress on Pain*. Amsterdam, Elsevier.

Keller, S., Ehrhardt-Schmelzer, S., Herda, C., Schmid, S. & Basler, H.D. (1997). Multidisciplinary rehabilitation for chronic back pain in an outpatient setting: a controlled randomised trial. *Eur. J. Pain*, 1: 279–292.

McQuay, H.J., Moore, R.A., Eccleston, C., Morley, S. de C. & Williams, A.C. (1997). Systematic review of outpatient services for chronic pain control. *Health Technol. Assess. Prog.*, 1(6).

Pain Society Desirable Criteria for Pain Management Programmes. A report of a working party of the pain society, London 1996.

PHYSICAL TREATMENTS

M. Thacker & L. Gifford

Physiotherapy, due to its knowledge of science and rehabilitation offers the potential to revolutionise the management of the pain and alleviate much suffering.

Patrick Wall

Introduction

Physiotherapy is a movement and rehabilitation based profession. It is impossible to define a generic role for physiotherapists as they are engaged in all major areas of medical practice. Physiotherapists/physical therapists from all backgrounds have frequent contact with patients in pain; it is estimated that over 90% of all patients seen by physical therapists have pain at presentation.

The original aim of the profession was to return people to function. However, during the period from the 1970s to the early 1990s musculoskeletal therapists shifted from rehabilitation to tissue-specific, modality-focused approaches that were heavily dependent on passive interventions. This trend has recently reversed and resulted in the profession receiving growing attention as a valuable tool in the management of pain.

The various modalities used to treat and manage pain can be broadly divided into passive and active therapies. The evidence base for specific modalities remains weak. The problem in the clinic is that therapists tailor concurrent therapeutic inputs and interventions/exercises to the individual, making it difficult to evaluate the efficacy of the intervention and/or a given dosage/regimen. Thus, randomised controlled trials have been difficult to apply to the assessment of specific interventions. However, recent literature suggests that physiotherapy is starting to develop an evidence base.

Models of care

Traditional physiotherapy approaches have linked to a biomedical model with an emphasis on detection and treatment/alleviation of a specific pathology. Recently this association has been superseded by a broadening acceptance of a biopsychosocial (bio-behavioural) model. As a result there has been a shift away from modality-specific treatments to broader based interventions including many components utilised by cognitive behavioural therapy (CBT). Core principles emphasise the prevention of chronicity (as opposed to narrowly focusing on the alleviation of symptoms) and involve self-management and rehabilitation strategies.

Referral patterns to physical therapy facilities and their organisation are starting to reflect the key role of rehabilitation. Thus, this therapy should not be regarded as a tertiary service after 'medical treatment' is complete or has failed. In order to provide these facilities, a major reorganisation of services has to be planned, with a shift of resources. One example is the management of low-back pain, which has led to increasing support for the physical management of other conditions/areas of the body (e.g. for the management of whiplash and work-related upper limb disorders).

Clinical reasoning

Historically, findings from history taking and physical examination were used in a selective way that promoted individual bias and a trial-and-error approach to management. Jones advocated the acceptance of a clear reasoning framework for physiotherapists (see Figure 34.1) that leads to rational and evidence based interventions involved in the management of pain. His suggestion for the use of 'hypothesis categories' has now gained widespread acceptance among many therapists. The concept was based on the hypothetical deductive reasoning models validated in other spheres of medicine.

An integrated strategy

We propose that the best way to integrate a broad based reasoning model into clinical practice is via a 'shopping basket approach'. This model integrates

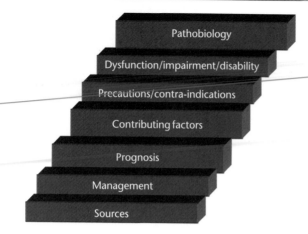

Pathobiology

Dysfunction/impairment/disability

Precautions/contra-indications

Contributing factors

Prognosis

Management

Sources

Figure 34.1 Categories of the clinical reasoning hypothesis that should be addressed when managing patients (adapted from Jones, 1992).

new developments in patient management with existing therapies and approaches. The emphasis is biased towards patient self-management, responsibility and involvement, rather than being over-dominated by passive and pain-focused treatments. It contains six interrelating compartments that can be assessed with the potential for treatment or management:

- Biomedical factors.
- Psychosocial barriers to recovery.
- Activity and participation capabilities and restrictions.
- Physical impairments.
- Physical fitness.
- Pain.

The paradigm presents a system viewing problems from a multidimensional perspective, therefore encouraging the management of all aspects and components of presenting problems. Although a degree of prioritisation is still required it attempts to place equal emphasis on both physical and non-physical components, treating and managing them together.

Biomedical factors

Paramount to the safety and success of this multifaceted approach is the ability of therapists to triage patients based on medical referral and individual assessment. They must recognise/detect serious pathology/injury and/or the presence of conditions that require referral for further medical investigation and management, in addition to other potentially important biomedical factors experienced by the patient (e.g. involvement of the nervous system, healing and strength of damaged tissues, type/mechanism/category of pain).

Questions that can be used to establish the biomedical aspects of the patient's condition include:

1 *Is the condition serious, requiring further investigation or appropriate medical management and intervention?* For example central nervous system (CNS) or other serious pathology (tumour, fracture, biomechanical instability, inflammation).

2 *Is there nervous system dysfunction?* Pain conditions with frank impairment of nerve function are not uncommon. A competent neurological examination that reveals normal function provides reassurance for both therapist and patient. Thus, it is recommended that clinicians report modest deficits of nerve function (e.g. decreased or absent calf reflex in a nerve root neuralgia like sciatica) to patients, before attempting to normalise these disorders. This physician reinforcement of signs and symptoms can support cognitive approaches to pain management.

3 *Are the tissues that hurt (or that may be responsible for the hurt) stable or strong enough to be progressively loaded in order to maintain and restore function?* Since early mobilisation is a primary goal, clinicians and patients must feel confident that repairing/healing structures are capable of being loaded. Progressive/graded loading and reactivation require an atmosphere of confidence. To create this, clinicians should consider issues including:
   - Time since onset.
   - Details of injuring mechanisms and forces involved.
   - Mechanical stability of the tissues.
   - Healing time/stage.
   - General health, age and well being of the patient.

Waddell's 'physiologic view of health' is a useful guide. It applies a powerful (and often under-rated and misunderstood) rationale for the inclusion of movement as part of an overall patient management programme:
   - Continued use is essential to maintaining health: 'use it or lose it'.
   - Function stimulates and maintains structure.
   - Use improves functional capacity, fitness and performance.
   - Movement promotes healing.

Additionally, movement and normal goal orientated activity, when performed in the right atmosphere and context, are very potent painkillers.

A consideration of whether the underlying processes are adaptive or maladaptive may be relevant. Inflammation associated with normal early healing is adaptive. This suggests that the logical clinical option is to avoid interventions that dampen inflammatory mechanisms and focus on appropriately paced rehabilitation. Graded mobilisation of activity, paying respect to early vulnerability of healing tissues, in combination with adequate pain control and management is currently recommended. However, if inflammation continues it may be maladaptive/undesirable. Management options include physiotherapy modalities, possibly in association with non-steroidal anti-inflammatory drugs (NSAIDs) or other inflammation modifying drugs. Maintenance, modification or restoration of function remain vital considerations and have been shown to have positive long-term benefit.

4 *What pain mechanisms are operating and can they be considered adaptive/helpful or maladaptive/unhelpful?* Pain mechanism determination may be a hypothetical exercise, but can be useful in providing prognostic and management clues (e.g. long standing pain out of proportion to any tissue abnormality is likely to be difficult to ameliorate via standard treatments). Existing guidelines suggest that the presence of a neurogenic component lengthens the required treatment programme.

5 *Are there any other interventions available that can help in the management or treatment of the presentation?* It is desirable to combine physiotherapy, psychological and medical interventions alongside a central reactivation process. Patient outcome is vastly improved where a central interdisciplinary unity integrates diagnosis, the management plan and goals. Work on interdisciplinary clinical pathways for chronic regional pain syndrome by the International Association for the Study of Pain (IASP) seems particularly encouraging. We would probably do far better to adopt such tactics for all pain conditions.

6 *Is the presentation a common syndrome?* The identification and categorisation of presentations into common syndromes can be of value. Many have established natural histories that patients should understand, accept and adjust to. A great deal more research into the natural history of common conditions is urgently required.

Psychosocial barriers to recovery

Many physiotherapists actively screen for, identify and appropriately manage relevant psychosocial components. It is important to emphasise that this is not about seeking to label a patient's problem as psychologically mediated, but an attempt to identify and manage some of the barriers to recovery that might be present. The aim is to improve outcomes.

The 'flagging system' for spotting patients with the potential to develop chronicity (see Chapter 22) has now been adopted in physiotherapy to provide:

- Methods for screening for psychosocial factors.
- A systematic approach to assessing psychosocial factors.
- Strategies for improving management.

Thus a number of key psychological factors have been identified:

- A belief that back pain is harmful or severely disabling.
- Fear-avoidance behaviour patterns, with reduced activity levels.
- Tendency to low mood and withdrawal from social interaction.
- Expectation that passive treatments rather than active participation will help.

These psychosocial factors relate to:

1 Patient characteristics:
   - Misunderstanding causation (a belief that hurt = harm).
   - High levels of distress at the onset of an acute pain problem.
   - Catastrophising (fearing the worst).
   - External locus of control (expecting others to cure the problem).
   - Doctor and treatment shopping.
   - Substantial anger (at initiating cause, pain itself and medical profession).
   - Fear/avoidance of pain and activity.
2 Outside influences:
   - Work/benefits.
   - Compensation/litigation.
   - Family reinforcement of illness.
3 Doctor/therapist dependent factors:
   - Unclear diagnosis or mixed messages from different professionals.
   - Unclear explanations of pain.
   - Inadequate assessment.
   - Unrealistically optimistic promises regarding outcome.
   - Reinforcing passivity of patient.
   - Reliance only on medication or rapid referral.

Main and Watson have described a 'rule of thumb' for assessment of psychosocial factors:

A: Attitudes and beliefs about the pain.
B: Behaviours.
C: Economic and compensation issues.
D: Diagnosis and treatment issues.
E: Emotion.

F: Family.
W: Work.

Questioning around these factors might include:

A: 'Attitudes' and beliefs about pain may reveal beliefs that bones are 'crumbling' and joints "worn out" and that activity may lead to further damage.

B: 'Behaviour' may reveal a passive attitude to recovery with patients avoiding activity, resting a great deal, using medication excessively and coming to depend on various supports and walking aids.

Clearly a primary focus of physiotherapy is to help the patient re-evaluate their situation, understand the consequences of passivity and to gain agreement for (and start) a graded and goal orientated programme of reactivation and normal activity.

Activity and participation capabilities and restrictions

There is now compelling evidence to support paced approaches focusing on the maintenance of and/or the early return of function/activity/work in acute and chronic management. Benefits include:

- *Distraction*: Being occupied diverts attention away from pain.
- *Activity*: Reverses the negative effects of deconditioning.
- *Circulation*: Movement promotes exchange of metabolites and healing. Injured tissues heal in proportion to the demands put on them.
- *Safety*: Supported patients can find that they are able to start to move normally and without severe pain. This is a unique skill provided by physiotherapy. Patients begin with exercises and activity quotas they feel confident with and build from there. Starting levels are easy to determine during the patient interview or physical assessment.

Unfortunately, physiotherapy still carries the stigma of bullying, due to outdated treatment paradigms and lack of understanding of the wider issues in pain. Adequate and appropriate functional goals must be negotiated, while accepting the continued need for pain control. Pacing of rest and activity is a key to building confidence. Initial modest activity should build via progressive increments to more regular participation for longer periods. The principle is similar to that used in fitness training and in the rehabilitation of sports injuries.

Physical impairments

The management of physical impairments is the area in which physiotherapists excel. A tendency to over-indulge in this area at the expense of the others is not surprising, since physiotherapists have long specialised in the examination and correction of 'physical abnormalities'. Dragging a physiotherapist away from an impairment-dominated intervention may be as difficult as persuading a surgeon to put away his or her scalpel. Both have their place and can be highly appropriate, but more generalised approaches may be far more beneficial.

Techniques and approaches that are commonly used for the management of impairments and associated pain include:

- Passive mobilisation, manipulation and massage.
- Active exercise – aimed at improving:
  - Muscle imbalance and stabilisation.
  - Proprioceptive neuromuscular facilitation (PNF) – an advanced form of flexibility training involving both contraction and stretching of muscles.
  - Other specific exercises (e.g. various forms of stretching and strengthening).
  - General exercise techniques.
- Movement retraining.
- Desensitisation programmes – as with allergy treatment exposing the individual to gradually increasing amounts of the problem stimulus, in a supportive framework.

Physical fitness

The detrimental effects of inactivity, immobilisation, disuse and deconditioning, and the beneficial effects of attending to and reversing these effects are now promoted for the management and treatment of musculoskeletal pain. It is therefore essential that any reasoned management programme for pain include a structured fitness regimen. The ability to prescribe, dose and support patients along this process are essential skills for physiotherapists involved in pain management.

Pain

The proposed mechanisms by which most physiotherapy modalities have their effects on pain have been reviewed in detail (see Further reading). Most authors report paradigms that are dominated by tissue based mechanisms, although there is growing attention on CNS mechanisms that may be involved. Acknowledgement of psychophysiological effects of interventions are important and may be mediated via:

- Belief and enthusiasm (patient and therapist mediated).
- Learning and conditioning.

- Expectation.
- The therapeutic alliance.
- Changes in attention and stress.

These are still inadequately voiced, but it is clear that:

- Providing support, safety and treatment, often involving touch, care and passive treatment for those who are in acute pain and vulnerable is a natural and possibly highly evolved behaviour that is likely to be linked to positive, recovery-enhancing, physiological mechanisms.
- Passive pain relieving modalities alone appear to be inadequate. They should not be seen to form the main thrust of a given treatment plan. Graded withdrawal of passive pain relieving modalities and the quick inclusion of patient directed pain management, graded reactivation and self-management in the acute and sub-acute phases are recommended.

Many therapies and approaches that physiotherapists use, in particular the 'complementary therapies' (but also many of the various manual therapies) can be associated with what Evans (2003) calls 'crackpot theories'. He suggests that these theories promote a continuing schism between orthodox and complementary approaches. Unfortunately, doing away with the crackpot theories that provide alternative therapies with some of their appeal might actually rob them of their effectiveness, by destroying the vital belief that enables them to mobilise the placebo response.

- Passive modalities may help individual patients through pain flare-ups. Provided patients remain employed and active or quickly return to normal daily routines their use is warranted. But, the patient must always have a role to play, with care employed to prevent unnecessary dependence on therapy. When used strategically, selective treatment (active or passive) of identified physical impairments can provide direction to specific self-management exercises.

Modalities and strategies commonly used by physiotherapists for pain relief

Sole use of any of the modalities listed below is to be avoided. They should be seen as an adjunct and used in combination with appropriate education and functional retraining/reactivation. With this approach they may increase the ease of movement and patient confidence, key factors for effective self-management.

- Passive/hands on:
  - Passive movement, mobilisation and manipulation.
  - Various forms of massage and touch (e.g. friction massage, connective tissue massage).
- Active:
  - Stretching.
  - Large through range movements – 'pendular' exercises.
  - Repeated movements.
  - Clenching/isometric contractions.
  - Self-massage, mobilisation, frictioning, etc.
  - Relaxation and resting techniques.
  - Motor control and awareness of movement retraining.
  - Exercise classes.
  - Functional restoration programmes.
  - Being occupied – work, socialising, home.
- Electrotherapies:
  - TENS (see Chapter 36).
  - Short wave diathermy ($\pm$pulsed), where the electrical current produced is said to heat the tissues and provide analgesia.
  - Interferential therapy, another form of electrical stimulation, using low-frequency currents. The physiological basis of any analgesia is unclear.
  - Laser.
- Ultrasound:
  - The massaging effect provided by these devices is comforting. In addition blood circulation is thought to improve.
- Thermal modalities:
  - Heat.
  - Cold.
- Acupuncture (see Chapter 37).

We introduced this chapter with acknowledgement of how physiotherapists are struggling with proof of efficacy. The common criticism is that modalities are 'merely' a placebo or are totally ineffective. This position is highly understandable since most clinical trials and meta-analyses of research into the effectiveness of physiotherapy modalities are inconclusive, or show little valuable effect. However, we feel that the important conclusion to draw from this situation is that the trials *show lack of evidence rather than evidence of lack of effect*. Issues to acknowledge and problems to overcome include:

- Individuals will demonstrate unique responses both to different therapies and therapists. Therapists, just as patients, tend to gravitate towards techniques and modalities they feel comfortable with and perceive as effective. Future research needs to strategically draw from both the quantitative and qualitative/interpretive research paradigms for the full scope of biopsychosocial influences and the effects of more holistic management to be revealed.

- The label "placebo" is not at all helpful, but a better understanding of the placebo certainly is. We consider the following quote:

  The failure to demonstrate superiority over placebo need not imply lack of efficacy; it may imply similarity of mechanism. Comparison of a treatment with a placebo is therefore not a comparison of two mechanisms, only a comparison of their ability to activate the same mechanism ...

  Lawes (2002)

Key points

- *Self-management*: Interventions are geared towards patient control, rather than adhering to any prescriptive and rigid therapist determined plan of action. Hence therapist input requires the provision of information, guidance and negotiated agreement of any tasks or goals.
- *Information*: Reassuring explanations and clear advice – is very useful and should in part be driven by an understanding of the patient's beliefs and attributions regarding their pain and the nature of their problem.
- *Goal setting*: These should always be attainable, personally relevant, interesting and measurable. They should be set in three domains:
  - *Physical*: relating to exercise programmes.
  - *Functional tasks*: relating to everyday activities.
  - *Social*: relating to pleasurable social activities.
- *Graded exposure*: Tackling activities and physical tasks that are feared and/or avoided because of pain, or the belief that they will cause further pain and damage. Thus, physical confidence is restored via agreed graded progressions and pathways. As confidence and skills are improved the later stages may include increased loading, more functional tasks as well as performing the tasks faster.
- *Pacing*: This strategy enables patients to control exacerbations of pain by regulating activity and rest more efficiently. A major aim is to prevent the common 'over-activity-pain-rest' cycle that so often leads to failure, reinforcement of the pain sensitive system and a gradual reduction of performance.
- *Reinforcement skills*: This includes encouraging patients with:
  - Their own efforts.
  - Recognising their improvements and achievements.
  - Attributing them to their own efforts.
- *Acquisition of problem solving skills*: Helping patients work through and find ways of overcoming problems they encounter in their physical reactivation programmes and then to be able to generalise the skill to day-to-day life problems.

Further reading

Evans, D. (2003). *Placebo. The Belief Effect*. Harper Collins, London.

Hurley, M.V. (2003). Muscle dysfunction and effective rehabilitation of knee osteoarthritis: what we know and what we need to find out. *Arthritis Rheum.*, 49: 444–452.

Jones, M.A. (1992). Clinical reasoning. *Phys. Ther.* 72: 875–884.

Klaber-Moffett, J.A. (2002). Back pain: encouraging a self-management approach. *Physiotherap. Theor. Pract.*, 18: 205–212.

Main, C.J. & Watson, P.J. (2002). The distressed and angry low back pain patient. In: Gifford, L.S. (ed.) *Topical Issues in Pain 3. Sympathetic Nervous System and Pain Management: Clinical Effectiveness*. CNS Press, Falmouth.

Thacker, M.A. & Gifford, L.S. (2002). A review of the physiotherapy management of complex regional pain syndrome. In: Gifford, L.S. (ed.) *Topical Issues in Pain 3. Sympathetic Nervous System and Pain Management: Clinical Effectiveness*. CNS Press, Falmouth.

Watson, P.J. (1999). Psychosocial assessment. The emergence of a new fashion, or a new tool in physiotherapy for musculoskeletal pain? *Physiotherapy*, 85: 530–535.

A. Hartle & S.I. Jaggar

The conduction of action potentials along nerve fibres may be blocked by physical and pharmacological methods. The susceptibility of nerve fibres to such block is affected by their state of firing, their size and whether myelinated or not (e.g. Aδ fibres are myelinated and C-fibres are not). Nerve conduction may be blocked anywhere along the pain pathways, from nerve ending to the central nervous system.

Physical means of neural blockade include:

- Cold.
- Heat.
- Pressure.

Larrey described refrigeration anaesthesia during the French retreat from Moscow (1812), but in modern anaesthetic practice, the use of cold to achieve conduction block is largely limited to transient, topical anaesthesia (e.g. ethyl chloride spray). The application of heat may be used to produce permanent nerve block (e.g. radio–frequency lesions of the trigeminal ganglion in the treatment of trigeminal neuralgia). Pressure neural blockade is usually inadvertent (poor positioning on the operating table), but remarkably effective. It provides a portion of the analgesia observed with the use of intravenous regional anaesthesia (Bier's block).

Pharmacologic nerve block may be temporary (using local anaesthetics or other agents, e.g. pethidine) or permanent (using neurolytic chemicals).

Temporary/reversible pharmacological nerve blockade in the acute setting (e.g. surgery)

History of local anaesthetics

The introduction of cocaine (a naturally occurring alkaloid ester) by Koller and Freud for topical eye anaesthesia (1884), led to enthusiastic experimentation with the agent. Halsted and Hall performed head, face and limb nerve blocks on each other, and Bier described the use of cocaine in the subarachnoid and epidural spaces. Cocaine's usefulness was unfortunately limited by both its toxicity and its capacity for addiction (as discovered by many of the early experimenters). Less toxic ester agents were then introduced, including procaine (1904) and chloroprocaine (1952). Although improvements on cocaine, these esters were associated with frequent allergic reactions (possibly due to their common metabolite, *para*-aminobenzoate).

The first local anaesthetic amide, lidocaine, was introduced in 1947. Subsequently, more amides have been commercially released, including bupivacaine, ropivacaine, prilocaine, etidocaine and mepivacaine.

Action

Local anaesthetics are weak bases that bind to sodium channels from within the axon. They have a membrane-stabilising effect, preventing sodium entry during depolarisation. Thus, the threshold potential is not reached and propagation of the action potential is prevented.

Since their site of action is intra-cellular, local anaesthetics must diffuse across the cell membrane (best achieved by the unionised form and enhanced by nerve activity). Alkalinisation of local anaesthetic solutions increases the pH and the proportion of unionised agent, speeding passage through the membrane and hence onset. Vasoconstriction maintains the concentration of local anaesthetic at the site of injection. Therefore, the use of 'quick mix' solutions (e.g. 20 ml 2% lidocaine, 1 ml of 1 : 10,000 epinephrine and 1 ml 8.4% sodium bicarbonate solution) for rapidly supplementing and enhancing epidurals has been suggested. There is evidence that this does achieve anaesthesia with a faster onset than local anaesthetic alone. However, the need to mix solutions is time consuming and significantly increases the risk of drug errors; thus the clinical significance of this approach remains to be proven.

The addition of opioids or alpha 2 agonists (e.g. clonidine) has not been shown to have any clinical benefit except in neuraxial blocks (see Chapter 43).

Use

Local anaesthetic nerve blocks can be used to provide:

- Analgesia (e.g. single shot as a supplement to general anaesthesia or long-term infusion for post-operative pain relief).
- The sole anaesthetic technique.

The latter requires meticulous attention to technique and the use of the appropriate agents in the correct doses (i.e. the right dose of the right drug in exactly the right place).

It is a misconception (often firmly believed by surgeons) that some patients are so sick that surgery may only be performed under local anaesthesia. While this may be true for some, patients with severe cardiac or respiratory disease may do better with the degree of physiological control afforded by general anaesthesia. Indeed, they may be less able to cope with some of the physiological effects of nerve blocks (e.g. the phrenic nerve paralysis that inevitably accompanies interscalene nerve block or lumbar sympathectomy following lumbar plexus block).

If this subgroup of high-risk patients is to benefit from regional anaesthesia, it is important that nerve blocks are performed by properly trained and competent regional anaesthetists, not occasional practitioners. Where appropriate, techniques to locate the nerves to be blocked should be used to improve accuracy and reduce complications.

On any occasion when a local anaesthetic technique is planned, there must be appropriate preparation for the management of:

- Complications.
- Block failures (total or partial).

The use of significant sedation ('anaesthesia without airway control' or 'almosthaesia') can produce a lethal combination.

Advantages

- When a nerve block (or blocks) is used alone as the sole form of anaesthesia, then many of the side effects and complications of general anaesthesia are avoided. These include a potential reduction in the incidence of atelectasis and thromboembolism.
- Well-performed nerve blocks may provide intra-operative and post-operative analgesia, reducing the need for other analgesics with problematic side effects (e.g. those of opioids – see Chapter 40).
- There is evidence for earlier, more effective mobil-isation and rehabilitation of patients under-going major orthopaedic surgery under regional anaesthesia.

Disadvantages

- Performing any nerve block requires special equipment and experience, and inevitably takes time.
- Certain blocks may be technically very challenging (inevitably in the patients in whom general anaesthesia is best avoided, e.g. the obese).
- Nerve blocks have their own particular complications and may fail.
- Patients may find lying on an operating table for more than a short period of time uncomfortable.

Contraindications

As for any procedure, absolute contraindications include:

- Patient refusal.
- Practitioner unfamiliarity with technique.
- Known hypersensitivity to the agents to be used.

Relative contraindications relate to specific patients and techniques. Local infection, coagulation disorders and anatomical variation are examples. In some patients, rare specific complications might have an exaggerated effect on their future life (e.g. brachial plexus injury in a concert pianist).

General principles

With the possible exception of minor local infiltration, the same requirements apply to nerve blocks as to general anaesthesia: pre-block assessment, informed consent, adequate monitoring, trained assistance and facilities for resuscitation must be available. The risk–benefit profile of the technique planned (particular to the patient and procedure) must be considered, if avoiding general anaesthesia is surgically preferable.

Nerve blockade in the setting of chronic pain

In the setting of chronic pain, neural blockade may be used:

- To facilitate diagnosis.
- As a prognostic indicator of the effectiveness of permanent neurolytic techniques.
- As a therapeutic option.

To demonstrate validity, inserted nerve blocks must be accurately located.

Blockade of the 'pain pathway' may be undertaken at a variety of levels:

- Trigger points, for example in the management of fibromyalgia.

- Intra-articular, for example sacro-iliac blocks administered for sacro–iliac pain.
- Specific nerves, for example facet joint blocks administered for back pain. In the past, these were considered to be intra-articular in nature, but it is now thought that conduction in specific facet joint nerves is blocked either within or without the joint.
- Ganglion blockade, for example trigeminal ganglion.
- Plexus blockade, for example coeliac plexus blockade – a systematic review suggests that this is useful in pain arising from abdominal malignancies. The retroperitoneal plexus that surrounds the abdominal aorta and arteries supplying the upper gastrointestinal tract may be reached from anterior or posterior approaches. Both sympathetic and parasympathetic nerves will be blocked. Large case series suggest that there is a major complication rate of ~0.07% in experienced hands.
- Sympathetic blockade, for example stellate ganglion block. This is commonly utilised for upper limb complex regional pain syndrome (CRPS), but no level 1 or 2 evidence supports its use.
- Neuraxial blockade:
  – Spinal blocks, for example saddle block administered for pelvic pain from disseminated cervical cancer. Although some power in the legs may be retained (if cephalad spread is avoided), abnormalities in the function of both urinary and anal sphincters commonly result.
  – Epidural block, for example lumbar epidural steroids for chronic back pain. Systematic reviews have demonstrated their efficacy in both short-term (up to 3 months, with a number needed to treat (NNT) of 7.3) and long-term (3 months – 1 year, with an NNT of 13) outcomes.

Different durations of blockade may be produced by a variety of agents.

Short-term pharmacological agents:

- *Local anaesthetics*: usually used for diagnostic and prognostic blocks.
- *Steroids*: considered to act by reducing inflammation. The American Society of Anesthesiologists supports their use for local injection (following neurological evaluation), but cautions that general health must be kept under review because of the potential systemic effects of steroids. If administered via the epidural route, caution must be taken to avoid inadvertent subarachnoid injection, which is associated with arachnoiditis.

Long-term permanent pharmacological agents

Long-term permanent pharmacological agents producing neurolytic effects:

- *Alcohol*: first used in 1933. This is a hypobaric solution, which thus rises to the highest point if inserted into cerebro-spinal fluid (CSF). Nerves blocked will depend upon final location of the solution. Alcohol destroys the relationship between an axon and its covering myelin sheath, and further damages the neuron after binding to cell surface proteins. It is associated with an initial severe burning pain (which may be ameliorated by mixing it with a local anaesthetic), replaced by a warm, numb sensation. The analgesic effects cannot be assessed for 12–24 h.
- *Phenol*: a hyperbaric agent in use since 1936 which is provided in a variety of concentrations (6–10%). In comparison with alcohol, it is more sparing of motor function and is associated with an immediate local anaesthetic effect. Prolonged analgesic efficacy cannot be assessed until 3–7 days after injection.
- *Botulinum toxin (type A)*: initially used to treat muscle spasm, but it appears to have some utility in the prophylaxis and treatment of headache, although level 1 evidence is still lacking. Its duration of action appears to be 3–6 months.

Physical methods

- *Heat (radio-frequency ablation)*: Localised radio waves produce heat, thereby destroying nerves. Since 'rewiring' may occur over the space of several months, it is important (as when other techniques are used) to ensure that appropriate physiotherapy is undertaken in the pain-free period.
- *Cold (cryotherapy)*: Used to destroy nerves. Initially considered not to be associated with neuritis, but this is now known to occur.

Risk/benefit assessment

All neural blockade techniques are associated with a range of risks and benefits. Where long-acting agents are given, the importance of potential risks is increased – since these too might be expected to last for a prolonged period of time. Under such circumstances, it is particularly important to ensure that the risks have been clearly discussed with the patient (and important relatives and care-givers). In general, the risks of neurolytic agents will include:

- *Tissue necrosis*: consequent to damaged vascular supply.

- *Painful neuritis*: considered consequent to neural rewiring, which takes several months to develop. However, if the patient is unlikely to survive this long, this may not be of great importance.
- *Motor paralysis*.
- *Autonomic paralysis*: which may importantly include control of urinary, intestinal and sexual function.

It is clear that while these are major risks of neurolytic techniques, their importance to the individual patient will depend upon a variety of factors. These will include not only current pain, but also the response to other treatment modalities, functional ability, life expectancy, and social circumstances and support. However, with the advent of reliable, transportable and robust infusion pumps, the requirement for long-acting agents might be expected to decrease.

Technique

Nerve blocks may be performed:

- Based solely on anatomical principles (e.g. ring blocks, inguinal field blocks):
  - *Acute setting*: usually performed with anatomical knowledge.
  - *Chronic pain setting*: guidance using fluoroscopic or computed tomographic (CT) control is standard practice.
- By accurate location of the nerve to be blocked:
  - Traditionally performed by seeking paraesthesia within the distribution of the nerve targeted – this requires a conscious patient for whom the experience may be unpleasant.
  - Recent technological improvements have allowed precise localisation of nerves by seeking motor responses with a nerve stimulator. These allow blocks to be performed in sedated or anaesthetised patients (without neuromuscular block), but are not without their limitations (see below).

Each technique has its proponents and there is little evidence that either technique is preferable from the safety point of view.

Awake or asleep?

Although patients may prefer to be asleep for a nerve block, there is a body of opinion that recommends for safety reasons the patient stay awake. In particular, the awake patient is able to complain of:

- Pain during injection of local anaesthetic, which may be associated with intra-neural injection.
- Early symptoms of inadvertent intravascular injection (including circumoral tingling, anxiety or light headedness) that usually precede convulsions or cardiovascular collapse.

We recommend that nerve blocks should be performed in an anaesthetised patient only in rare circumstances. These would include:

- Children.
- Major acute trauma.
- Where the patient has refused to have the technique performed awake (and been counselled appropriately).

Equipment

Needle design

Traditionally, *short-bevelled* needles have been used for nerve blocks outside the neuraxis. The short bevel is thought to allow the anaesthetist to 'feel' the passage of the needle through tissue planes, and hence reduce the risk of nerve damage.

There is some evidence that while this is true, if damage is caused, it may be more severe than when a long-bevelled 'hypodermic' needle is used. Recently 'pencil-point' needles (now well established in spinal anaesthesia) of varying designs, have been introduced for peripheral nerve blocks. As yet there is little evidence of any clinical superiority of any one design.

The '*isolated*' needle technique described by Winnie is undoubtedly much easier and more accurate than using a syringe directly connected to a needle, because the weight of the syringe and its contents is removed, permitting precise, controlled needle placement. There is also much less likelihood of movement of the needle during aspiration, injection of the local anaesthetic or changes of syringe (if needed).

Insulated needles (where electrical current is only transmitted at the bevel) allow much more accurate needle placement, with greater success, when a nerve stimulator is used.

Nerve stimulators

These devices allow precise localisation of nerves, with enhanced block performance. They range in complexity and ease of use:

- *Current flow*: Passage of up to 5 mA through the needle tip is often possible. However, starting currents greater than 2.0 mA should rarely be necessary. In practice, one should either reduce the current or manoeuvre the needle – not both at the same time – this is a recipe for frustration! If the nerve block is to be used alone for anaesthesia, an appropriate motor response should be obtained at a current of less than 0.5 mA (usually indicating the needle tip is within 1 mm of the nerve).

It is wise to record a 'motor threshold' (i.e. the lowest current at which a response can be elicited). A motor threshold of less than 0.2 mA suggests that the tip of the needle lies within the nerve and it should therefore be repositioned (to avoid intraneural injection).

- *Stimulus duration*: If it is possible to vary this, it is important to select a duration less than 0.4 ms, at least in awake patients. Short duration stimuli produce a primarily motor fibre response, with little pain (since pain fibres require a longer stimulus).
- *Stimulation frequency*: This is more a matter of personal taste; we find with more than 2 Hz motor stimulation is uncomfortable for the patient, and may make it more difficult to appreciate small changes in needle placement.

A description of all nerve blocks that are possible to use in the acute/chronic setting is obviously beyond the remit of this chapter. However, we hope the following will illustrate some of the advantages of the variety of blocks available, using the upper limb as a basis.

- *Central neuraxial blockade*: Provide bilateral motor, sympathetic and sensory block. Inevitable sympathetic blockade may cause hypotension. Risks include causing damage to the spinal cord and also post-dural puncture headache. Rarely used for the upper limb, although recent work has described the use of stimulating epidural catheters introduced at the lumbar level and directed cephalad.
- *Major plexus blockade*: Brachial plexus blocks are categorised by their approach (interscalene, supraclavicular, infraclavicular, etc.). Every year new approaches are described, but it is probably more useful to think of what Paola Grossi described as the 'line of anaesthesia'. Unlike the leg, a single brachial plexus injection can provide anaesthesia for the whole upper limb. In principle, more proximal approaches are appropriate for more proximal operations (e.g. interscalene approach for shoulder surgery). The neck is full of vital structures. Unfortunately, all of these have at some stage had large volumes of local anaesthetic injected into them (the cervical spinal cord, vertebral artery and even the cuff of a laryngeal mask airway!). The axillary approach has far fewer serious complications and is eminently suitable for surgery to the hand, although tourniquet pain can be difficult to manage. Recent work suggests that a technique of seeking each of the four terminal branches of the plexus confers

high success, but loses the advantage of a single injection, although with only one skin entry site.
- *Individual nerve blocks*: The terminal branches of the plexus may be blocked by individual injections at the elbow and wrist. At these points the courses of the nerves are subject to more anatomical variability and require different entry sites for each block. They may be useful to supplement deficiencies in plexus blocks (e.g. ulnar nerve may frequently be 'missed' in interscalene blocks).
- *End branch blocks*: Digital nerve blocks may be performed for minor distal surgery, either at the base of the digit, or at the mid-carpal level. This latter has the advantage of avoiding the potential risk compromising the blood supply to the digit.

Similar deliberation should be undertaken when applying blocks to lower limbs or other regions. In all cases the particular advantages and disadvantages should be considered.

Key points

- Regional blocks may provide analgesia in the absence of systemic side effects.
- Side effects of blocks may relate to:
  - Traumatic effects of needle insertion.
  - Side effects of pharmacological agents – local or general.
  - Effects of blockade of nerves or plexuses themselves.
- Nerve blockade requires an accurate anatomical knowledge and specific training.
- In acute pain after surgery nerve blockade is not the 'panacea' for the seriously ill patient – better physiological control will often be provided by well-performed general anaesthesia than poorly performed regional anaesthesia.
- Reversible/selective nerve block can assist mobilisation and improve function in chronic pain patients.

Further reading

Stanton-Hicks, M. (2001). Nerve blocks in chronic pain therapy – are there any indications left? *Acta Anaesth. Scand.*, **45**: 1100–1107.

Rigg, J. & Jamrozik, K. (1998). Outcome after general or regional anaesthesia in high-risk patients. *Curr. Opin. Anesthesiol.*, **11**: 327–331.

Horlocker, T.T. & Caplan, R.A. (2001). Should regional blockade be performed on anesthetized patient? *ASA Newslett.*, **65**.

A. Howarth

Principles of transcutaneous electrical nerve stimulation

Transcutaneous electrical nerve stimulation (TENS) is the electrical stimulation of peripheral nerves for temporary analgesic effects.

Historically the description of using electricity in pain medicine is not new:

- 2500 BC Egyptian Fifth Dynasty – stone carvings depict the use of electrical fish to treat pain.
- 400 BC Hippocrates – electrical fish used for treatment of headaches and arthritis.
- 46 AD Scribonius Largus – electrical ray fish used for gout.
- 1756 Richard Lovett – first English textbook on medical electricity.

Theories of pain modulation using TENS

Spinal pre-synaptic inhibition (traditional TENS)

The gate control theory suggests that stimulation of large diameter, fast conducting afferent sensory (Aβ) fibres produces pre-synaptic inhibition within the dorsal horn (DH) of the spinal cord. This may effectively block further transmission in smaller, slower conducting (nociceptive) afferent C-fibres, which may be carrying noxious information.

TENS exploits this part of Melzack and Wall's theory. Persistent TENS stimulation can produce pre-synaptic inhibition of noxious information in the afferent C-fibres. Similar effects can be produced by vibration and rubbing, but these modes cannot be used for prolonged periods, thus negating analgesic efficacy.

Supra-spinal endogenous opioid peptide production (acupuncture-like mode of TENS)

Peripheral electrical stimulation may also excite higher centres causing the release of endogenous opioids.

These opioids have a descending inhibitory effect at the DH, binding to receptors on nociceptive afferent neurones, so inhibiting the release of substance P (SP).

Placebo

Responses to placebo are not only psychological, but also physiological. Exploiting the placebo effect can be regarded as a form of endogenous analgesia. Knowledge of the placebo response should improve potential effectiveness clinically and its use can only enhance rational therapy.

Patients may benefit from the placebo effect after receiving any form of treatment or contact with a health care professional. This, in addition to any actual benefit consequent upon any electrical stimulation they feel during treatment, can only be helpful.

Direct mechanical inhibition of damaged nerves

A peripheral effect has been hypothesized but evidence is weak.

Modes of application (Figure 36.1)

Pulse frequency (rate)

The pulse frequency (some times called pulse rate) is the number of pulses per second, or Hertz (Hz) of current delivered. The frequency range typically available in TENS units is 0–250 Hz (1 Hz = 1 cycle per second).

Pulse duration (width)

The pulse duration or width is the length of time each pulse lasts, usually in microseconds (μs). The common clinically useful range of adjustment is 100–200 μs.

Electrodes

Each channel on a TENS unit has an anode and a cathode. The anode is usually black, it is positively charged and is sometimes represented by a + sign. The cathode is usually red and is negatively charged;

(a)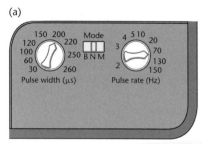

(b)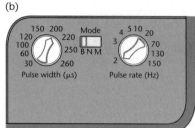

Figure 36.1 *TENS settings.* (a) High frequency in conventional TENS and (b) low frequency, used in acupuncture + burst TENS mode.

Table 36.1 Modes of TENS stimulation

	Conventional/traditional	Acupuncture, with burst mode	Modulated
Electrode site	Cathode placed: • Over/just proximal to painful site • Segmentally • Both	• Initially place anode proximally over the associated myotome with the cathode placed distally • If the effect is limited reverse polarity	• Not well defined in the literature – often down to trial and error
Frequency	High (80–100 Hz)	Low (2 Hz)	• 20–40 Hz for extended periods • 80–100 Hz for short periods
Pulse duration (width)	200 μs	200 μs	200 μs
Intensity	Low (start at ~2× sensory threshold)	High (start ~3× sensory threshold)	Not defined in literature ~2× sensory threshold seems sensible starting point
Mechanism of action	'Gate control'	Endogenous endorphin stimulation	Postulated to ↑ blood flow and rhythmic muscle contraction, ↓ing inflammatory exudates. At high frequency may also modulate pain gate
Sensation	Local, non-painful, tingling, paraesthesia	Tingling, with visible muscular contraction in the associated myotome	Strong, non-painful sensation at the peak of modulation cycle perceived as a massaging effect
Efficacy	• Rapid onset • Short duration	• Slower onset • Potentially longer lasting	• Variable
Assessment	Minimum 20 min	20 min	20 min
Treatment duration	At least 60 min	Maximum 45 min	Several hours at low frequency
Treatment frequency	Unlimited	4–5× per day ideal. No upper limit	Unlimited

it is sometimes represented by a − sign. The electrical current travels from the anode to the cathode, so the sensation is usually stronger under the cathode.

Modes

Table 36.1 describes more about modes.

Clinical application of TENS

Assessment

Initially the cause of pain should be established. Undiagnosed pain is a contraindication to treatment.

Stimulation sites

The sites used for stimulation are thought to be one of the primary factors in the efficacy of TENS (Figure 36.2). However, there is little conclusive evidence regarding the correct placement of electrodes. It may, therefore, be necessary to operate a degree of trial and error when initially treating patients.

There are four areas to which electrode placement in TENS can be applied:

1 The painful area.
2 Peripheral nerves.
3 Spinal nerve roots.
4 Motor, trigger and acupuncture points.

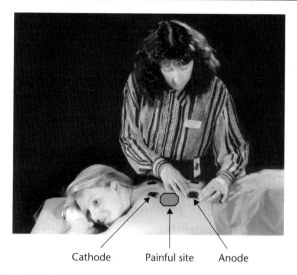

Cathode   Painful site   Anode

Figure 36.2 Application of a TENS machine.

Painful area

This is the most commonly used site. With conventional TENS the aim is to achieve stimulation around the painful area. Good effect is usually achieved by placing the cathode over the most painful site, producing stimulation and paraesthesia over the site of the pain. Initial assessment to ensure that the patient has full sensation before applying the pads should avoid skin irritation.

If the patient finds the application of TENS to the painful area too uncomfortable (e.g. with peripheral nerve injuries) then alternate electrode sites must be found. An area with normal sensation proximal to an area of hypersensitivity may be appropriate. Alternatively, contra-lateral limb application may be appropriate for phantom limb pain.

Peripheral nerves

Electrodes can be applied over peripheral nerves with cutaneous distribution in the painful area (e.g. median or sciatic nerves). Anatomical knowledge is required to ensure that electrodes are applied where peripheral nerves are most superficial and susceptible to stimulation.

Spinal nerve roots

Electrodes can be applied parallel to the vertebral column. This stimulates the nerve roots emerging from the spinal cord and supplying the affected dermatome or myotome. Acupuncture TENS is often used in this

manner to produce a muscle twitch. Again anatomical knowledge is necessary to identify appropriate sites. The use of dermatome and myotome charts (demonstrating skin and muscles innervated by particular nerve roots) is useful. Pad size is important and most standard electrodes are around 5-cm wide. This usually allows two adjacent nerve roots to be stimulated simultaneously. Bilateral application may be useful in degenerative low back pain, while unilateral pads will be more appropriate for shoulder pain.

Motor, trigger or acupuncture points

Motor points are the point of entry of a motor nerve into a muscle. Stimulation of these points are used for acupuncture TENS when muscle contraction is required. Trigger and acupuncture points can be used for stimulation. Trigger points are areas of tenderness, whereas acupuncture points reflect specific points used in traditional Chinese medicine. However, the two sites often overlap.

Good electrode positioning requires accurate assessment of the cause and location of the pain, in addition to knowledge of the type of TENS to be used. Conventional TENS requires paraesthesia and is, therefore, not suitable for use over bony prominences. Acupuncture TENS, which requires a muscle twitch, needs the electrodes to be placed over a muscle related to the area of pain.

TENS pads

Traditionally gel, black carbon rubber pads and tape have been used. However, this is messy, difficult for the patient to manage at home and leaves the patient susceptible to skin irritation and allergies to the tape. If this is the only option then hypoallergenic tape such as micropore should be used along with electro-conductive gel manufactured for the purpose – *not* KY Jelly. However, the use of self-adhesive reusable electrodes promotes patient use and compliance.

The distance between the electrodes is important. If they are too close together then the current will 'short' and bypass the patient, yet if they are too far away from each other then stimulation may be lost. Ideally pads should be at least a 'pads width' apart.

Sensory thresholds

The level of intensity where any sensation of electrical stimulation is felt can be regarded as the sensory threshold of stimulation. Although it is unique to individuals, most will lie within a normal range – which becomes familiar with clinical practice.

Conventional mode TENS stimulation should be at about twice the sensory threshold, but never painful. Using acupuncture (burst) type TENS, stimulation should be at about three times the sensory threshold, or where a muscle contraction is observed.

Duration and frequency of stimulation

The duration and frequency of stimulation required will depend upon the pain problem, the mode being used and the circumstances of the patient.

Recommendations from the literature and the instructions that accompany machines vary dramatically. The following is a combination of evidence and clinical experience.

On continuous mode the machine should be used for at least 1 h at a time. Contrary to popular belief, it can be used virtually constantly. Problems encountered if this is necessary are usually related to skin irritation and tolerance. These can be avoided by treatment breaks, or by rotating stimulation sites.

With acupuncture TENS the muscle twitch can cause muscle fatigue. It is, therefore, recommended that stimulation last no longer than 30–45 min at a time. However, this can be repeated four to six times a day.

The patient's pain problem may mean they do not need to use the machine constantly. Many patients find TENS a useful tool at particular times. Normally painful experiences, such as shopping, walking or standing for prolonged periods may be facilitated. Patients need to be advised to try and pre-empt these circumstances, so that they can use the machine beforehand, during and for a short time after a painful event.

Some patients simply find the use of TENS unacceptable in their day-to-day life. This may include people who are working or driving for long periods. Patient compliance is often improved on discussion, since a compromise may be found with suitable opportunities for use of the TENS being identified.

Precautions

- *Driving*: may be problems with insurance. Patients should always be advised to inform their insurance company if they drive with the machine in use, as their insurance may be invalidated.
- *Electrode sites*: patients should *not* stimulate around the anterior cervical spine. This risk stimulating the carotid sinus, which could cause cardiac problems (usually hypotension). Neither should stimulation be attempted over the eyes due to the delicate nature of this organ.

- *Skin condition*: electrodes should not be placed over broken skin, sores, or areas of acute eczema and psoriasis.
- *Dermal reactions* (electrical irritation): some patients who have the intensity of the machine very high may find that their skin burns.
- *Contact allergy*: if patients develop an allergy to the pads, adhesive or any tape used, then alternatives should be found.
- *Pre-existing lymphoedema*: TENS is thought to have an effect on the circulatory system, therefore, it could adversely affect the lymphatic circulation causing further fluid retention. Issues of skin integrity should also be considered in this group of patients.
- *Caffeine intake*: a high intake of coffee (above four cups a day) is thought to reduce the effectiveness of high intensity TENS.

Contraindications

- On-demand pacemakers.
- Percutaneous central venous catheter (PCVP).
- First trimester of pregnancy.
- Undiagnosed pain.
- A confused patient.
- *Do not use in the shower.*

What is best practice?

When health care professionals feel that a patient may benefit from a TENS machine, they should be referred to someone who has had training in the use of TENS. It is useful to have a referral protocol for people to identify whether a patient is suitable for TENS – an example of this is given below.

Guidelines for referral for the use of TENS

- Not useful if:
  - Communication problems.
  - Psychiatric illness.
- Patients must be motivated to help themselves. If they are expecting a cure, or do not want to achieve some level of pain relief, then it is inappropriate.
- The patients, or carer, must be able to apply the pads to the required area.
- The patient must be able to manage and understand the controls on the machine.
- TENS ideally should be used as an adjunct, not as a sole treatment.

If a patient fulfils the referral criteria then they should be seen for an assessment, lasting at least 45 min. This allows 15–20 min to take a history and explain the machine, followed by 20 min to trial a unit.

Patients should be given an information leaflet and followed up period. Often pain services loan the machines to patients for a trial period, but then expect them to buy their own, if they have found it to be useful.

Essential characteristics

Battery supply

Disposable or rechargeable batteries can be used. Rechargeable batteries are not as long lasting, but are cheaper in the long run. Therefore, they are appropriate if a machine is going to be used long term. Some newer machines are produced with integral rechargeable batteries that can be charged directly from the mains.

Consultants Europe rating

TENS machines must be approved under the medical devices directives 93'42/European electromagnetic compatibility (EEC) before they can be sold to the public. A legally approved unit will, therefore, be labelled with a Consultants Europe (CE) mark, which is a four-figure number. This confirms the safety of the unit.

Calibration of dials

The intensity controls should deliver a linear increase in current. This is rarely the case. It is prudent to have units checked by a medical physics department.

Constant current design

This means that the current, the therapeutically important component of the electrical stimulus, remains constant regardless of changes in skin impedance.

Key points

- TENS mechanism is based on Melzack and Wall's *Gate Control Theory of Pain*.
- It is a useful adjunct to other therapies, but does not cure pain.
- The recommended modes and parameters should be used, depending upon the type of pain being experienced.

Further reading

Sjolund, B.H. & Eriksson, M.B.E. (1979a). Endorphins and analgesia produced by peripheral conditioning stimulation. In: Bonica, J.J. *et al.* (eds) *Advances in Pain Research and Therapy*, Vol. 3.

Sjolund, B.H. & Eriksson, M.B.E. (1979b). The influence of naloxone on analgesia produced by peripheral conditioning stimulation. *Brain Res.*, **173**: 295–301.

Johnson, M.I., Ashton, C.H. & Thompson, J.W. (1991). The consistency of pulse frequencies and pulse patterns of transcutaneous electrical nerve stimulation (TENS) used by chronic pain patients. *Pain*, **44**: 231–234.

Tippey, K.E. (2000). *TENS. The Users Guide to Pain Relief. A Systematic Approach.* Nidd Valley Medical Publications, Knaresborough, North Yorkshire.

Walsh, D.M. (1997). TENS. *Clinical Applications and Related Theory.* Churchill Livingstone, London.

J. Filshie & R. Zarnegar

The term 'acupuncture' derives from the two Latin words: 'acus' (needle) and 'pungere' (to pierce). It is an ancient Chinese therapeutic technique, which involves the placement of solid needles in precise locations in the body to:

- Improve symptoms.
- 'Cure' disease.
- Promote health.

Strong sensory stimulation involving needling and scarification techniques have been used to reduce pain throughout history. The exact date of origin of the first use of acupuncture in China is somewhat uncertain, with stone needles, or 'bian shi', being used originally in the stone ages. Bone needles have been found that date from the twenty-first to the sixteenth centuries BC in the Xia Dynasty.

Over the last 30 years there has been an increasing interest in acupuncture in the West, with the use of fine disposable needles to help pain and non-pain conditions. This has been partly due to increasing disenchantment with drug therapy and its side effects (including mortality) and partly on account of an increasingly solid neurophysiological and clinical evidence base for its modes of action.

Despite the increasing acceptance of acupuncture among the public and the medical profession, many physicians still have considerable lack of objective information about acupuncture. The erroneous belief that it has no supporting scientific evidence base is still fairly widespread.

A variety of methods are available for humans and animals, including traditional Chinese and Western approaches, using either manual acupuncture (MA) or electro-acupuncture (EA). In humans, acupuncture is mostly used for pain relief at present, but it has an increasing role in the management of non-painful conditions.

Mechanisms of action

Segmental effects

Acupuncture needling stimulates peripheral nerves. Indeed, if local anaesthesia is administered prior to the acupuncture stimulus, the effect of acupuncture can be abolished. Aδ–fibre stimulation, induced by needling, causes sensory modulation in the dorsal horn (DH) at the corresponding segmental level via release of met-enkephalin. Figure 37.1 illustrates some of the neurophysiological pathways by which acupuncture works.

Heterosegmental effects

Diffuse noxious inhibitory control (DNIC) is induced by a noxious stimulus (such as needling) and contributes to the heterosegmental analgesic effects of acupuncture. Spinothalamic and spinoreticular pathways are also stimulated at the DH. These relay, via the mid-brain, to synapse in the periaqueductal grey (PAG). This in turn stimulates descending inhibitory fibres, which affect afferent processing. Therefore, a heterosegmental analgesic effect (i.e. at each level throughout the body) can be achieved. Noradrenaline and serotonin (5-hydroxytryptamine (5-HT)) (via descending inhibition) are key neurotransmitters responsible for pain modulation.

General effects

Acupuncture responses may result from:

- Release of met-enkephalin, dynorphins and β-endorphin, which stimulate δ opioid (DOP), κ opioid (KOP) and μ opioid (MOP) receptors. Thus, acupuncture is similar to physical exercise in stimulating endogenous opioid peptides, which may be partly responsible for the 'feel good' sensation experienced by many following acupuncture treatment.
- Upregulation of endogenous opioid production – providing a mechanism for the sustained effects.
- Alterations of gene expression – 'top-ups' being necessary to keep the analgesic effect 'switched on'.
- Release of:
  - 5-HT, which is both analgesic (through DNIC) and mood enhancing.
  - Oxytocin, which is analgesic and anxiolytic.
  - Endogenous steroids, which are anti-inflammatory.

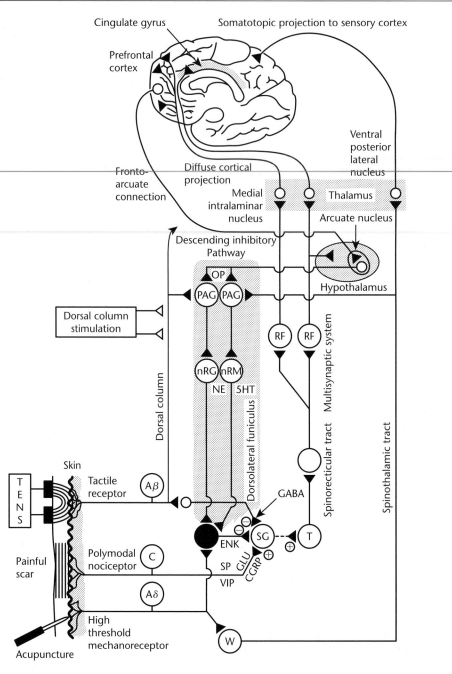

Figure 37.1 Diagram to show neuronal circuits involved in acupuncture and TENS analgesia. The afferent pathways involved in transmitting nociceptive information from a painful scar to the higher centres via the dorsal horn, the ascending tracts, and the thalamus are shown. The connections to the descending inhibitory pathways which descend in the dorsolateral funiculus are shown. The connections to the hypothalamus are indicated. Abbreviations: Aβ, C and Aδ represent the posterior root ganglion cells of Aβ, C and Aδ-fibres, respectively; CGRP: calcitonin gene related peptide; ENK: enkephalinergic neurone; GABA: γ-amino butyric acid; GLU: glutamate; 5HT: 5-hydroxytryptamine, serotonin; NE: noradrenaline/norepinephrine; nRG: nucleus raphé gigantocellularis; nRM: nucleus raphé magnus; OP: opioid peptides; PAG: periaqueductal grey; RF: reticular formation; SG: cell in the substantia gelatinosa; SP: substance P; T: transmission cell; VIP: vasoactive intestinal polypeptide; W: Waldeyer cell; +: stimulant effect; −: inhibitory effect. From Oxford *Textbook of Palliative Medicine*. Reprinted by permission of Oxford University Press and J Filshie and J W Thompson.

- Widespread autonomic effects.
- Enhancement of the immune system (preliminary studies).

Peripheral effects

Acupuncture has been shown to result in the release of trophic and vasoactive peptides including neuropeptide Y (NPY), calcitonin gene related peptide (CGRP) and vasoactive intestinal peptide (VIP). These neuropeptides increase cutaneous blood flow and have been found to enhance the survival of ischaemic musculocutaneous flaps in humans and animals.

Application to myofascial trigger points

A myofascial trigger point (TP) is a tender point in a taut band of skeletal muscle or its associated fascia. It is painful on compression, with the patient exhibiting a 'jump sign', or muscle twitch response. These highly irritable foci within skeletal muscle have been noted in the medical literature for decades. Although biopsy studies have not so far demonstrated inflammation or other histological changes, electro-myographical evidence has emerged over the last decade in support of the existence of TPs. After a period of instruction, different clinicians can reliably locate them. One excellent example is a TP in the upper free border of the trapezius. This is painful on compression in most adults and has a referral pattern which resembles the course of the 'gall bladder meridian' (Figure 37.2). It is possible that the meridian theory developed as a result of observation of TP referral patterns. The application of TP acupuncture for myofascial problems is particularly effective. It can reduce primary care referrals to rheumatology and physiotherapy.

Acupuncture dose

There is no consensus on the 'dose' of acupuncture for any given condition since there is wide variation in practice and numerous techniques are used. Dose is a complex concept in acupuncture and is dependent upon many variables (Table 37.1). Manual stimulation of needles during the treatment varies widely between practitioners and between different treatments by the same practitioner. It may range from gentle stimulation of subcutaneous tissues to deep stimulation with periosteal 'pecking'. More randomised controlled trials are needed to determine the optimal dose for a particular condition.

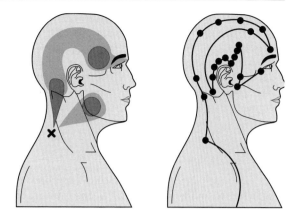

Figure 37.2 The gall bladder meridian represents a referral pattern from a TP in the trapezius muscle. The dark grey shaded areas show the more frequent pain referral pattern of a TP. The light grey shows areas of less frequent pain referral. From *Acupuncture – A Scientific Appraisal* by Ernst and White. Reprinted by permission of Elsevier Ltd and Dr Michael Cummings.

Table 37.1 Determinants of dose in acupuncture

Needle related	Diameter of needles (e.g. 30–36 g).
Technique related	Number of needles: 1–20 or more.
	Depth of stimulation: • Subcutaneous. • Intramuscular stimulation. • Periosteal 'pecking'.
	Stimulation of needles: • Manual techniques. • Zero manipulation – vigorous twirling. • Electrical techniques – low/high/combined frequency.
Duration of needling	1 s to 30 min.
Sites	Segmental/extrasegmental/both
Other factors	Concurrent anaesthesia.

Traditional chinese acupuncture

Traditional Chinese acupuncture (TCA) is complex, based on an elaborate theoretical system pertaining to the circulation of vital energy – referred to as 'Qi' or 'Chi'. This 'Qi' needs to be 'balanced', as do the opposing, yet complementary, forces 'Yin' and 'Yang', under the influence of the 'five elements' (water, earth, wood, metal and fire). The circulation of 'Qi' and the need to 'balance Yin and Yang' predate knowledge about the circulation of blood and autonomic control that may well be the modern equivalents. Deficiency or excess of

'Qi' (or vital energy) is treated by appropriate needling eliciting 'De Qi' or *needling sensation* – a feeling of numbness, warmth and tingling around an acupuncture point. The needling sensation is now explained by the stimulation of different fibres in the skin and subcutaneous structures. TCA requires prolonged training and is becoming superseded by the modern scientific approach in many Western countries.

Western medical acupuncture

This is a pragmatic, neurophysiological approach to treatment, following an *orthodox diagnosis* based on conventional history taking and clinical examination. Needling points may be:

- Segmental (paravertebral and/or local) points appropriate to the level of the pain or disordered structure.
- TPs.
- 'Strong' traditional points (e.g. LI4), known to raise the pain threshold by up to 400% in experimental studies.
- Intramuscular, a form of deep, usually paraspinal, needling which may be particularly useful in resistant cases.

Medical acupuncture (MA) is most often used with between one and twenty needles. Figure 37.3 shows a patient with neck pain with needles in situ.

Electroacupuncture (EA)

EA is a technique that allows regular and continuous stimulation of nerve fibres from muscle. Low frequency stimulation is accompanied by visible muscle contraction for 10–20 min. It can be used for symptom relief during short procedures or to administer a large treatment 'dose'. EA at low (2–5 Hz), high

(100 Hz) or a mixture of high and low frequencies can be used. Low frequency is more likely to stimulate enkephalins and β-endorphin, and high frequency dynorphins. Some use EA routinely, but more often it is used for more challenging pain conditions if the results of manual needling are insufficient.

Acupressure

Pressure on acupuncture points is not as strong a stimulus as acupuncture. Nevertheless, it has some efficacy; for example, in the prevention of nausea and vomiting.

Laser therapy

Laser therapy is often focussed on acupuncture points. No needles are used, so it is not strictly acu*puncture*, but it has obvious advantages for paediatric patients and patients with needle phobia. It is a thermal stimulus and is not necessarily interchangeable with acupuncture. However, it has efficacy in wound healing.

Variations on needling

Semi-permanent indwelling needles are now available in sterile single use packs. Once inserted, they can be covered with a clear plastic dressing and left in place for up to 1 week. They can be used for:

- Treatment or prevention of nausea and vomiting.
- Treatment of addictions.
- Advanced cancer related dyspnoea and anxiety, when they can be left for up to 4 weeks over the upper sternum.

Patients can be taught to stimulate them manually on demand for symptom relief, especially in palliative care.

Auriculotherapy

The ear is richly innervated and needling in the ear may give vagal stimulation. It is often used for pain relief and can be an adjunct to body acupuncture. It is also used for treatment of addictions. The theory of somatotopic representation of parts of the body on the pinna for point selection remains highly speculative.

The treatment of pain

Acute pain

There is considerable interest in the use of acupuncture for acute post-operative pain. Acupuncture analgesia (AA) as a *complete* alternative to anaesthesia is somewhat risky. A variable amount of analgesia is

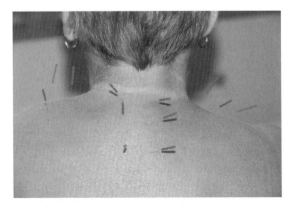

Figure 37.3 Shows a patient with neck pain with three paired paravertebral and six TP needles in situ.

obtained by needling; that is, 0–400% increase in pain thresholds. As an adjunct, it is useful, potentially reducing the dose of supplementary analgesia peri-operatively. This may be particularly useful for patients who are intolerant of conventional analgesia. One systematic review of 16 controlled trials concluded that acupuncture was efficacious for relief from post-operative dental pain.

Efficacy of acupuncture

High level evidence, based on systematic reviews is available for acupuncture in the treatment of:

- Experimental pain.
- Headache.
- Osteoarthritis of the knee.
- Fibromyalgia.
- Post-operative dental pain.
- Lateral epicondylitis.
- Nausea and vomiting.
- Back pain.

Acupuncture treatment for back pain is controversial, with both positive and negative reviews, resulting partly from the authors' differing approaches to trial assessment. More recently there has been a further positive review, though further research to determine which groups would be most helped is desirable. Other areas in which acupuncture has been found to be particularly useful include:

- Myofascial pain (using predominantly a TP approach plus segmental needling).
- Chronic post-operative pain syndromes that have a strong neuropathic component (e.g. pain following breast cancer surgery).
- Pain and symptom control in cancer patients.

Timings of treatments

A typical course of acupuncture for treatment of chronic pain should be administered over 6–8 weeks, with six or more treatments having a greater statistical chance of success. Most often, patients obtain increasing periods of relief with each successive treatment. Repeat treatments are usually performed weekly for 6 weeks, or twice weekly for 3 weeks. Subsequent treatment intervals are increased gradually. On most occasions there is some relief after the first treatment for a period of hours or days. However, there may be little or no effect after the first session, or the initial response may not be perceived until the next day. Occasionally there is a slight exacerbation of symptoms with the first treatment. In these cases a reduced 'dose' is administered at the second treatment. The 'dose' is usually tailored to the response. A stronger treatment or EA

may be added mid-way during a course of treatment for patients who remain slow to respond. Symptom control is then usually maintained with monthly, six weekly or longer 'top-ups'.

Approximately 50–70% of the population responds well to acupuncture, with 10–15% seeming to be very sensitive and 5–15% responding poorly. It is possible that genetic variation is responsible for the variation in response.

Acupuncture for other chronic pain and non-pain conditions

In addition to chronic musculoskeletal pain problems, acupuncture can be used to treat many non-painful conditions (e.g. nausea and vomiting). Two systematic reviews and one meta-analysis have shown efficacy of acupuncture (using the point PC6 on the inner aspect of the forearm approximately 5 cm proximal to the skin crease) for nausea and vomiting occurring:

- Post-operatively.
- Due to chemotherapy.
- Secondary to pregnancy.

Acupuncture also has efficacy for bladder detrusor instability, dysmenorrhoea, angina and xerostomia (dry mouth) following radiotherapy or other causes. Acupuncture can often help xerostomia cases that have been refractory to pilocarpine treatment. Acupuncture can promote healing of ulcers and wounds. The evidence so far is inconclusive for asthma, stroke, neck pain and drug addiction, with a mixture of positive and negative studies. The evidence for acupuncture aiding weight loss and smoking cessation is poor. The results of acupuncture for smoking cessation are equal to nicotine patches, with some feeling that these effects to aid nicotine withdrawal are clinically useful.

Safety

The importance of making a diagnosis prior to starting acupuncture treatment cannot be over emphasised. The symptomatic relief provided by acupuncture can mask features of the underlying condition or its progress. This might theoretically cause delayed or missed diagnoses.

Side effects

In comparison with drug treatment acupuncture has far fewer side-effects, though they can still occur. In prospective studies on 66,000 patients, bleeding (3%), pain on needling (1%), aggravation of symptoms (1–3%) and drowsiness (2–8%) were found to be common minor side effects. In extreme cases driving ability is affected. It is preferable therefore to have a short rest after acupuncture (20–30 min) before driving, or to have an alternative form of transport home after the first treatment.

Serious and at times fatal side-effects can occur, though evidence from recent surveys show that they are extremely rare.

- Pneumothorax is the most frequently reported serious injury caused by acupuncture needles. This complication is associated with needle insertion in the parasternal, paravertebral, lateral thoracic or supra/infra-clavicular points.
- Cardiac tamponade has occurred in association with needling of the acupuncture point CV17, that lies over a potential defect at the lower end of the sternum in 5–8% of the general population. 'Foramen sternale' are not reliably detectable by palpation, nor can they be identified on chest X-rays.
- Cases of life threatening sepsis reported in the literature have almost all occurred in patients who had indwelling needles. Another risk factor (e.g. debility or valvular heart disease) is usually present.
- There has been speculation about the association between reusing acupuncture needles and the high incidence of hepatitis and hepatocellular carcinoma in China. Needles used in acupuncture must be single use, sterile, disposable ones. Sterile stainless steel acupuncture needles are now available from a variety of manufacturers.

Table 37.2 summarises common and rare side effects of acupuncture.

There are a number of cautions and contraindications to acupuncture and Table 37.3 lists some of them. It is recommended that all practitioners undergo appropriate formal training with suitable courses. Statutory regulation will be in force in the UK by circa 2007.

Precautions necessary during practice, based on the experience of practitioners and case reports in the literature, are outlined in Table 37.4. Though PC6 is used widely in pregnancy, acupuncture should only be applied after a suitable risk/benefit analysis. Practitioners must consider that there are claims from China that acupuncture can promote miscarriage and premature labour.

Economic considerations

Studies have pointed out savings in areas, such as the pharmaceutical budget and a reduction in physiotherapy and rheumatology referrals with the appropriate use of acupuncture. This is particularly in evidence in

Table 37.2 Side effects

Minor common events
Skin erythema at needle insertion sites.
Needle point bleeding or bruise.
Needling pain.
Drowsiness.
Feeling faint.

Significant minor adverse events
Forgotten needle.
Forgotten patient.

Serious but very rare adverse events
Injury to underlying organs
Pneumothorax.

Bleeding
Pericardial tamponade.
Compartment syndrome.

Infection
Septicaemia.
Endocarditis.
Transmission of infectious disease (e.g. Hepatitis B or C).
Other infections.

Nerve Injury
Spinal cord or nerve root trauma.
Peripheral nerve trauma.

Trauma secondary to migration of broken fragments of embedded needles entering:
Spinal cord.
Peripheral nerves.

Skin reactions
Contact dermatitis.
Accidental burns with moxibustion (a herb heated on the skin or needle which is used in TCA).

Table 37.3 Contraindications and cautions

Contraindications
- Lack of patient consent.
- Indwelling needles in patients with valvular heart disease.

Cautions
- Areas of infection of skin or subcutaneous tissue, ulcers, tumour, varicosities.
- Areas affected by or prone to lymphoedema.
- Hyperaesthetic areas.
- Bleeding diathesis.
- Immune suppression.
- Pregnancy.
- EA in patients with pacemakers.

primary care. There may also be more long-term and complex economic benefits (e.g. reduction in iatrogenic problems secondary to analgesic drug side effects, or higher productivity in the patients' personal and

Table 37.4 Recommendations for safe practice

- Ensure an orthodox diagnosis has been made that fits with the presenting complaint.
- Have a clear understanding of anatomy and the appropriate depth of needling.
- Use sterile, stainless steel, single use needles.
- Observe patient for signs of adverse reactions.
- Treat in the lying or sitting position on a couch, particularly for the first treatment. Ensure patient can lie down safely in case of extreme drowsiness or syncope.
- Ensure all needles are removed – do a needle count before and after treatment.
- Advise against driving, if possible, after the first treatment.
- Use aseptic technique for indwelling needles with clear instructions to the patient to remove if they become sore or inflamed. Provide container for safe return of needles for safe disposal at the hospital.

professional life due to a sense of well being and even immune modulation).

Acupuncture research

There are many difficulties in the scientific testing of the efficacy of practical techniques, and acupuncture is no exception.

Finding a suitable control procedure for needling has been the focus of much debate in acupuncture research. Trials in which the control group have not had any needling have been criticised for lack of 'blinding'. On the other hand, in trials using invasive 'sham acupuncture' (in which control has been in the form of needling 'incorrect points') the control group have still been subject to a neurophysiologically active intervention with some therapeutic benefit; that is, comparing two different 'doses' of acupuncture. More recently 'placebo needles' have been developed that create the impression of needle penetration to the patient without actually piercing the skin. Even they can exert some degree of 'acupressure' stimulation. The best idea of its role compared with conventional treatment may well be randomising acupuncture against a standard treatment and an observation group.

Research in acupuncture is published mainly in specific acupuncture or pain management journals. Meta-analysis and systematic reviews of acupuncture are challenging. There is often wide variation in methodology, acupuncture dose and quality of the trials in the included studies.

It is worth noting that some western practitioners have abandoned the term acupuncture altogether and refer to the technique as 'dry needling', 'sensory stimulation', 'intramuscular stimulation' or 'percutaneous electrical nerve stimulation' (PENS). This is an attempt, perhaps, to distance themselves from some of the less scientifically clear traditional theories of TCA.

Acupuncture appears to be integrating within modern health care. It is likely that integration will increase in time. Further randomised controlled trials for studies on efficacy, safety and cost effectiveness are needed, as is the funding to support this work.

Key points

- Acupuncture acts through peripheral mechanisms, primarily to modulate central nervous system activity.
- Concepts of dose may be important during treatment.
- TPs in myofascial pain respond to Western acupuncture.
- There is systematic review evidence of efficacy of acupuncture in the treatment of headache, osteoarthritis, fibromyalgia, dental pain, experimental pain, lateral epicondylitis, back pain and nausea and vomiting.

Acknowledgements

The authors would like to thank Dr Michael Cummings and Mrs Jane Brooks for their considerable help in producing this chapter.

Further reading

Acupuncture in Medicine 2001; **19**: 117–22. Safety issue available: www.medical-acupuncture.co.uk.

Berman, B., Ezzo, J., Hadhazy, V. & Swyers, J.P. (1999). Is acupuncture effective in the treatment of fibromyalgia? *J. Family Pract.*, **48**: 213–218.

Bowsher, D. (1998). Mechanisms of acupuncture. In: Filshie, J. & White, A. (eds) *Medical Acupuncture: A Western Scientific Approach*. Churchill Livingstone, Edinburgh; pp. 69–82.

Ernst, E. & Pittler, M.H. (1998). The effectiveness of acupuncture in treating acute dental pain: a systematic review. *Br. Dent. J.*, **184**: 443–447.

Ezzo, J., Hadhazy, V., Birch, S., Lao, L., Kaplan, G., Hochberg, M., *et al.* (2001). Acupuncture for osteoarthritis of the knee: a systematic review. *Arthrit. Rheum.*, **44**: 819–825.

Lee, A. & Done, M.L. (1999). The use of nonpharmacologic techniques to prevent postoperative nausea and vomiting: a meta-analysis. *Anesth. Analg.*, **88**: 1362–1369.

Manheimer, E., White, A., Berman, B., Forys, K., & Ernst, E. Meta-analysis: acupuncture for back pain. Annals of Internal Medicine (in press).

Melchart, D., Linde, K., Fischer, P., White, A., Allais, G., Vickers, A., *et al.* (1999). Acupuncture for recurrent headaches: a systematic review of randomized controlled trials. *Cephalalgia*, **19**: 779–786.

Trinh, K.V., Phillips, S.D., Ho, E. & Damsma, K. (2004). Acupuncture for the alleviation of lateral epicondyle pain: a systematic review. *Rheumatology* (Oxford), **43**: 1085–1090.

Vickers, A.J. (1996). Can acupuncture have specific effects on health? A systematic review of acupuncture antiemesis trials. *J. Roy. Soc. Med.* **89**: 303–311.

White, A. (1999). Neurophysiology of acupuncture analgesia. In: Ernst, E. & White, A (eds) *Acupuncture: A Scientific Appraisal.* Butterworth-Heinemann, Oxford; pp. 60–92.

NEUROSURGERY FOR THE RELIEF OF CHRONIC PAIN

38

J.B. Miles

Introduction

It is tempting to think of neurosurgery for the treatment of chronic pain as being a matter of the dramatic interruption or interference with some established 'pain pathway'. In fact, it has a great deal more to offer, both by conventional treatment of the cause of the pain (e.g. trigeminal neuralgia (TGN)) and in the area of palliative manoeuvres in malignant situations. When surgery is appropriate it can provide satisfactory relief of pain without reducing the quality of life that may result from long-term medication use.

When considering surgery for the treatment of chronic pain, the most important criteria turn out to be the quality of life and its expected duration, resulting from the disease process causing the pain. Pain due to uncontrolled malignancy, with reduced physical capacity and life expectation, will demand prompt treatment, with perhaps greater acceptance of surgical risk than, will that of a sufferer from a protracted but non-life-threatening condition. Patients of advanced age might also, on the same logic, demand expedient surgery, acknowledging the risk.

Palliative neurosurgery for the pain of malignancy

Spinal malignancy

There is no questioning the appropriateness of treating surgically a malignancy of a long bone that has caused a pathological fracture. The spine should be considered as the main weight-bearing bone in the body and when rendered unstable should be stabilized by surgery. This usually means by some form of pinning and plating (Figure 38.1(a) and (b)). If the pain is due to instability its features will be:

- Intermittent in nature.
- Occurring on weight bearing or movement.
- Relieved by recumbence or cessation of movement.

Strong analgesics (causing unnecessary continuous effects and unwanted side effects) and radiotherapy (with delayed effectiveness and little likelihood of stabilization) are less appropriate than surgery.

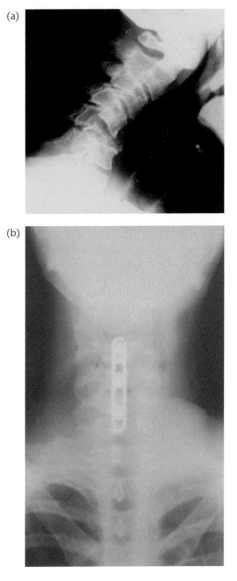

(a)

(b)

Figure 38.1 (a) Fifth cervical metastasis from prostate carcinoma causing instability. Pain radiating into the arms, with no neurological deficit. (b) Resection of the involved vertebral body with bone grafting and anterior plate fixation may provide total analgesia.

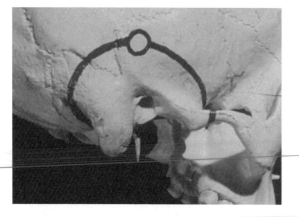

Figure 38.2 Black marker outlines the bony resection necessary to achieve total petrosectomy for carcinoma of the auditory canal or middle ear.

On the contrary, if the pain is due to local infiltration and stretching of sensitive tissues, it will be: continuous, boring in nature, occur particularly at night and be unrelieved by recumbency. It will be unaffected by stabilization and will require adjuvant therapies, such as analgesics, cytotoxic therapy or radiotherapy.

Base of skull malignancy

Squamous and adenocarcinomas can develop in the epithelium of the ear and para-nasal sinuses. They tend to be associated with severe, continuous boring pain (due to bony infiltration) and an unpleasant, continuous infected discharge. If, after biopsy confirmation of the pathology and initial radiotherapy, the tumour remains, radical resection, sometimes necessitating bone or soft tissue grafting, is the best treatment. This achieves not only pain relief, but in the case of some of the squamous carcinomas when total petrosectomy has been undertaken, probable cure of the disease process (Figure 38.2). Relief of pain by any other method will not stop the foul discharge and other neurosurgical techniques, such as thalamotomy, are much less certain to be effective.

Palliative neurosurgery for pain from non-malignant conditions

Spinal degenerative disease

Chronic pain due to degenerative disease of the spine can be either:

> Radiculopathic due to nerve root compression. Pain will be: sharp with tingling in the distribution of a specific nerve root and associated with specific sensory or motor neurological deficit.

Referred from dysfunctional segmental joints (discs or posterior zygo-apophyseal).

If radiculopathic it should declare itself even in a complex, mixed pain syndrome, by being sharp, with tingling, in the distribution of a specific nerve root, and being associated with specific neurological deficit – sensory or motor. If referred it is often less distinct being aching, more continuous, extending from the spine into the limb only as far as the elbow or knee, and having no specific neurological signs.

Radiculopathic pain should be investigated for evidence of disc protrusion or lateral root canal narrowing, which can be treated by direct surgical decompression. Referred pain syndromes, being less easily aetiologically defined, may require a range of treatments from physiotherapy (with an emphasis on spinal muscular development) to direct surgical fusion of single or multiple segments. Spinal fusion has a bad reputation due to inappropriate usage. However, it remains the best choice when there is instability pain, or in the face of progressive neurological deficit.

Cranial neuralgias

TGN is an intermittent, lancinating pain, within the confines of the trigeminal nerve distribution. Formally thought to be a condition almost exclusively of the old or very old population, it is now recognized to occur not uncommonly in the middle aged and young (though only very rarely in children). Due to its permanent nature, when there is a treatable cause to be found it should be treated surgically, in order to avoid otherwise protracted pharmacological exposure. The large majority of sufferers (>90%) have a blood vessel (usually an artery) compressing the trigeminal nerve as it enters the pons, at its root entry zone (REZ). Other conditions occurring at this position (e.g. tumour or multiple sclerosis (MS)) can also cause TGN. In a small proportion of sufferers, no cause has been found.

Diagnosis is based on the description of the pain, but atypical features are not uncommon. Magnetic resonance tomographic angiography (MRTA) can accurately and reliably show the presence of the vascular compression (Figure 38.3). Around 8% of 'false' positives have been seen (when 50 control patients without TGN were scanned, four individuals were identified with neural compression, though two individuals later developed TGNs).

Although the majority of patients respond initially to carbamazepine, or other anticonvulsant medications, surgical measures will be necessary for those suffering unacceptable side effects. There is also a case for surgery in those with a long life expectancy, with what must be considered a permanent condition – albeit that temporary, spontaneous remission is common.

Peripheral ablation of divisions of the nerve, ganglion or sensory root (by injection of alcohol or glycerol, radio-frequency coagulation or balloon compression), will all give relief extending from weeks to years. They will be associated with obligatory trigeminal sensory or motor deficit and a 4–20% risk of precipitating a different, dysaesthetic pain syndrome. Balloon compression of the ganglion and/or the sensory root, is currently probably the method of choice for temporary relief in those without definite vascular compression, or who are unfit for surgical decompression.

Microvascular decompression (MVD) is a neurosurgical posterior fossa operation, undertaken under general anaesthetic. The offending vessel is permanently displaced from the nerve REZ. Although considered a major procedure, this specialized operation is now offered to all sufferers with pre-operative evidence of vascular compression, irrespective of age. It is the only treatment that offers the prospect of permanent cure from the pain without neurological deficit. More than 90% get immediate relief from pain, while 75–80% appear to have maintained this state 5–10 years later. Quantitative sensory studies undertaken before, during and after decompression reveal a deficit while the nerve is compressed, that corrects following decompression. In uncertain circumstances, or when there is bilateral TGN, particularly as occurs in MS, partial sensory root section can be undertaken during this operation, avoiding the considerable problem of trigeminal motor nerve injury involved in bilateral peripheral ablations.

Stereotactic radio-surgery can be used to achieve a partial ablative lesioning of the nerve, REZ, or adjacent pons – useful in patients rendered unfit by concurrent

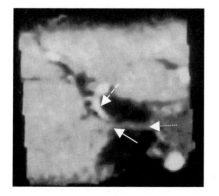

Figure 38.3 Magnetic resonance tomographic angiogram, showing compression of the trigeminal nerve (arrow with dots) at its REZ (solid arrow), by a descending loop of the superior cerebellar artery (arrow with dashes).

disease (e.g. MS). There is surprisingly early relief of pain, with minor neurological deficit, but a substantial need for repetition and an uncertainty regarding long-term or delayed radio-necrotic effects.

Electrical stimulator implant to the trigeminal sensory nerve root has also been shown to be effective, although technically difficult to maintain. Stimulation in the region of the descending trigeminal tract and nucleus in the upper cervical spinal cord can also suppress TGN. It has been used for patients with MS or atypical TGN.

Other lower cranial nerve neuralgias, such as glossopharyngeal and supra-laryngeal neuralgias are probably also due to vascular compression at the REZs. However, decompression of these is currently more of a surgical challenge.

Neurosurgery to the nervous system for pain of malignancy

Peripheral procedures

Ease of performance and speed of action make peripheral ablative surgery attractive for patients with limited survival but rapid recurrence of pain due to peripheral nerve regeneration severely limits its usefulness, and recent advances made in medical treatment have largely obviated its need. It may still be useful to perform intra-abdominal plexus ablation (celiac or pre-sacral) for abdominal malignancies, though these require experience due to the undoubted sever risks involved.

Spinal and central nervous system procedures

Antero-lateral cordotomy

Axones sub-serving the functions of pain, pin-prick and temperature are distributed in the contra-lateral anterior quadrant of the spinal cord. Therefore, ablation in this area may provide pain suppression, without significant sensory or motor loss (Figure 38.4). First performed as an open laminectomy surgical procedure in 1912, it was extensively used for more than 50 years. However, even this central denervation was associated with return of function and pain after 2–5 years, seriously limiting its usefulness for non-malignant conditions. In 1963, Sean Mullen (a Chicago neurosurgeon), utilized the bony access between the first and second cervical vertebra to show that antero-lateral cordotomy could be achieved per-cutaneously (Figure 38.5). As the procedure can be undertaken with local anaesthesia it has the advantage of allowing real-time monitoring of the efficiency of the lesioning. Further development of the technique took place mainly in pain clinics, but with the major improvements

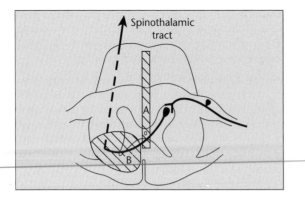

Figure 38.4 Spino-thalamic pathway demonstrating sites for commissurotomy (A) and antero-lateral tractomy (B).

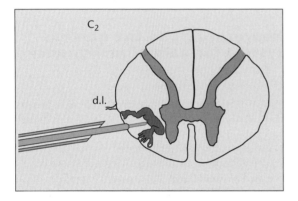

Figure 38.5 Illustration of high cervical cordotomy. The homunculus represents the expected positions of fibres in the ascending spino-thalamic pathway.

in medical treatment of malignant pain, the necessary skills involved in performing the procedure have been largely lost. It remains a useful procedure for unilateral, lower body pain (up to the sixth cervical dermatome), with the prospect of retaining mobility, general sensitivity and pain relief for up to 2 years.

If the pain is bilateral, a per-cutaneous cordotomy could be performed on one side and a surgical cordotomy in the high thoracic region on the other. This is necessary since bilateral cervical cordotomy risks catastrophic respiratory failure, due to bilateral central denervation (Ondines' curse). These two procedures should also be staged in time to reduce the undoubted risks of bladder and bowel dysfunctions. Upper thoracic cordotomy, as undertaken by the modern microsurgical technique, involves a very small hemi-laminectomy. It is a much less disturbing procedure to the sick patient than previous techniques and remains the optimal method for patients unable to co-operate or tolerate the percutaneous local anaesthetic method (e.g. children).

Commissurotomy

A technique directed to dividing the spino-thalamic fibres, sub-serving pain and temperature sensations, as they cross the midline in the cord before ascending in the antero-lateral tract. This provides for a bilateral, segmental denervation and currently is most applicable to the patient with pelvic infiltration (e.g. cervical cancer). Loss of sphincter control is an obligatory result of this procedure, but the primary disease has usually already caused this. Triple laminectomy at the level of the conus is required to gain access to sufficient cord. Therefore, it is a substantial surgical insult, but effective pain relief can last for years.

Thalamotomy

This safe technique is well suited for treating unilateral pain of malignancy (particularly affecting the head and neck), above the level that can be reached by cordotomy. It has the advantage that it can be undertaken under local anaesthetic, allowing monitoring of effect. Moreover, it usually causes no detectable sensory loss. Unfortunately the relief tends not to be as long as that following cordotomy. Also, as the procedure requires fixation of the head in a stereotactic frame and the passage of an electrode deep into the brain, there is considerable patient resistance to the idea. The recent resurgence in the use of stereotactic methods for the treatment of involuntary movements has resulted in the recovery of the skills necessary to make this a very safe procedure.

Pituitary destruction

The mechanism, by which destruction of the pituitary gland relieves the pain of malignancy, is unknown. Originally applied to inhibit the growth of hormonally dependent tumours (e.g. breast or prostate) it was quickly recognized to relieve pain whether or not the tumour growth was suppressed. Later it appeared efficacious for all malignant pains. The mystery intensified when it was found that electrical stimulation of the pituitary gland also relieves pain. The implication is of a neurogenic, or neuropharmacogenic, change when the pituitary or adjacent structures, are interfered with. There have also been occasional reports of the pain of non-malignant origin being amenable to this treatment. Further research in this area may help.

The important neurological complications of ablative techniques (including trans-sphenoidal alcohol injection) dissuaded clinicians from continued use, even though more controlled methods such as electro-coagulation appear to be equally effective while avoiding attendant risks. Unsurprisingly, the duration of pain relief following alcohol ablation varies greatly – usually 3–6 months, but extending beyond a year in some instances.

Non-malignant pain treated by surgery to the nervous system

The normal life expectancy of this group requires that any procedures must have a low risk of morbidity.

Electrical stimulation

Electrical stimulation to the nervous system was known to relieve some pains as long ago as the first century AD. In the eighteenth and nineteenth centuries general practitioners (GPs) used static-electric generator machines to provide analgesia. The evolution of the *Gate Control Theory* gave credibility to the treatment. Advances in technology (much based on the development of cardiac pacemakers) allowed the development of implantable devices providing continuous and controllable electrical stimulation to many parts of the nervous system (Figure 38.6).

Spinal cord stimulation

An electrode in the epidural space connects (by insulated cabling) to a receiver or generator in the subcutaneous tissue, usually in the abdominal region. The relative sensitivity of common pain syndromes to this form of treatment is shown in Table 38.1, although variability in response is common. In the history, responsiveness of the pain to external influences, such as warmth, rubbing and mental distraction seem to be important predictors for success. Sensory neurological deficit demonstrated in the painful area is probably the strongest predictor for failure. Therefore, except for the most responsive syndromes, such as cardiac angina and peripheral vascular syndromes, it is advisable to institute a trial period of per-cutaneous stimulation. A temporary electrode is placed in the epidural space, with its' extension lead attached to an external stimulation electrode.

The extraneous factors that influence patients with prolonged non-malignant syndromes are great in number and complexity. Even the best multidisciplinary assessment teams, may not fully appreciate them before implantation. In the first year after implantation a 20% failure rate is normal. Most units experiences suggest only 50% of implanted patients getting satisfactory relief at 5 years. Angina and vascular limb pains have an initial success rate of over 90% probably consequent upon a completely intact nervous system ensuring benefit from stimulation.

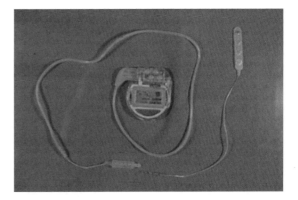

Figure 38.6 Electrical stimulator implant system with a receiver or generator connected by cabling to a spinal electrode plate.

Table 38.1 The expected responsiveness of various pain syndromes to central nervous system electrical stimulation treatment

	Painful condition
Most responsive	Cardiac angina
↓	Pain of peripheral vascular disease
	Complex regional pain syndrome
	Peripheral neuropathic syndromes
	Failed back syndrome
	Central myelopathic pains
	Nerve avulsion pain syndromes
	Central post-stroke pain
	Facial dysasthaesias
	Perineal neuropathic pain
Unresponsive	Pain associated with total paraplegia

Even after 35 years of usage, there remains considerable skepticism regarding the validity of spinal cord stimulation (SCS) as a treatment for chronic pain. Unfortunately, performing controlled, blinded trials of SCS is difficult, since it has been established as efficacious only if paraesthesia is felt in the area of pain. However, it remains a very real option for authentic chronic pain syndromes that have proved unresponsive to all other treatments. Although initially expensive, there are now many long-term studies showing it to be economically acceptable, with very low morbidity.

Cerebral stimulation

Implanted electrodes have been applied to various structures in the brain. Upward extensions of the somato-sensory pathways of the cord (e.g. the thalamus) respond similarly to SCS, while allowing analgesia of the head and neck. Other areas such as in the medial thalamus and para-ventricular tissue, being part of the paleo-cerebrum, react differently (without paraesthesia), and theoretically should be more useful as targets. However, there is an intrinsic resistance to the techniques involving the brain.

Motor cortex stimulation is a more recent development. Although initially seeming illogical, it has a reasonable experimental provenance, including evidence of interference with electrical activity generated by painful stimuli in the experimental animal. The electrode is placed in the extra-dural space over the contra-lateral motor cortex. Although performed under general anaesthesia it is a very low morbidity procedure. Currently the likely sensitivity of the various pain syndromes is unknown and initial success rates of only 50–60%, with considerable late failures have been documented.

Micro-DREZ-otomy

This rather contrived term describes destruction of the medial fibres of the sensory roots as they enter the spinal cord (**D**orsal **R**oot **E**ntry **Z**one, DREZ) together with the superficial layers of the dorsal horn of the spinal grey matter. Designed originally for relieving pain of malignancy by central denervation, it has become used almost exclusively for the treatment of root avulsions syndromes, particularly of the brachial plexus. It is a formidable surgical procedure that necessitates at least a triple hemi-laminectomy. In the neck region this means very definite post-operative pain. Lesioning the cord over three to five segments carries definite risk of sensory or motor deficit. This operation should only be undertaken as a last option, by experienced personnel. In spite of these caveats it is almost a unique ablative procedure. It provides very long-lasting (or permanent) pain relief, and is therefore acceptable for non-malignant conditions. It is particularly helpful as most brachial plexus syndromes, including phantom limb pain, occur in the younger age group.

Drug delivery systems

The concept of being able to deliver effective drug, at maximum concentration, to the target tissue, with minimal spread to other tissues (thus minimizing unwanted side effects) is an ideal scenario. At present this is only achievable by establishing a physical conduit to the target tissue. However, eventually this should be managed by pharmacological design.

The discovery of opioid receptors on the spinal cord in experiment animals, led to the development of systems to deliver morphine to the cerebro-spinal fluid surrounding the cord in man. Subsequently other drugs have been delivered to a variety of targets.

The first systems were simple conduits, usually with a subcutaneous reservoir easily reached by a needle, through which a dose of the relevant drug could be injected. These reservoirs were then expanded to minimize the number of punctures, since the biggest risk from such a system is infection – a potential threat with each puncture. Various mechanisms were then built into the systems to empower repeated dose delivery. These extended from mechanical compression, through gas expansion to battery-driven electronics.

Although developed primarily for the delivery of morphine over long periods to relieve the pain of malignancy, advances in long-acting morphine preparations reduced its application. However, it has proved extremely useful for delivering other compounds (e.g. baclofen for the treatment of spasticity and associated pain). Combinations of opioids and baclofen can be used with good effect. Recently long-term intra-thecal delivery of morphine (avoiding tolerance or habituation) has proven effective in some non-malignant pains previously considered poorly responsive to opioid treatment, thus increasing potential uses.

Key points

- Whether or not the pain is due to malignancy is vitally important in deciding to recommend surgical treatment. This relates to the balance between the need for prompt relief, a consequence of limited life expectation likely to be associated with untreated malignancy, and the expected quality of life activity (work and play) and the unavoidable risk of morbidity associated with any form of surgery.
  Greater risks may be accepted for prompt relief.
- There are exceptions, when taking a major risk early in the condition is indicated. In younger people an attempt to cure and/or avoid morbidity associated with life-long (and only partially effective) medication may be useful.
  Surgery, rather than medication, is the optimal treatment for some pains.

Further reading

Burchiel, K. (ed.) (2002). *Surgical Management of Pain.* Thieme, New York.

Miles, J.B., Eldridge, P.R., Haggett, C.E. & Bowsher, D. (1997). Sensory effects of microvascular decompression in trigeminal neuralgia. *J. Neurosurg.*, **86**: 193–196.

Multiple authors (1999). Intrathecal drug delivery. *Neuromodulation*, **2**: 55–150.

PHARMACOLOGY

ROUTES, FORMULATIONS AND DRUG COMBINATIONS

39

L.A. Skoglund

The body is divided into several compartments with slightly different physiological environments (e.g. pH variation and tissue organisation), which might alter the pharmacokinetics of drugs (Jang *et al.*, 2001). The four determinants of drug pharmacokinetics referred to as ADME (absorption, distribution, metabolism and excretion) influence the number of drug molecules that reach the intended site of action. The aim of efficient drug delivery is to get the drug molecules from the place of administration to the site of action without loss.

There are several routes of drug administration and several different drug formulations (Table 39.1). Most analgesics are given systemically (as opposed to local administration), thus forcing the drug molecules to enter the hypothesized central compartment before reaching the compartment of action. Systemic administration has a great potential for instigating significant pharmacokinetic changes in the drug molecule depending on its physical and chemical characteristics. Chemical analgesia is contingent on the persistence of a sufficient number of active drug molecules to be present for drug–target interactions in pain modulating tissue.

Pharmacokinetic alteration can also be exploited to ensure clinical efficacy. Some drugs are pro-drugs, which are pharmacologically inactive derivatives of active drugs. They are designed to let the active molecules reach the site of analgesic action by eluding the primary metabolic breakdown in the liver or intestine. Specific molecular entities are chemically incorporated into the active drug molecule, creating an inactive derivative that attracts metabolic action in the liver releasing the active molecule into the central compartment. Metabolism of some analgesics also produces active metabolites, adding to (or prolonging) the effect of the primary analgesic molecule administered.

Effective analgesic drug delivery

A steady influx of drug molecules from the site of administration to the site of action is a prerequisite for analgesic outcome. Thus optimal drug delivery is one very important determinant of analgesic efficacy. Optimal drug delivery must achieve three important clinical requirements to provide successful analgesia:

1 Short time to onset of analgesic action.
2 High analgesic yield without adverse effects.
3 Maximal duration of effect.

One of the main principles of effective drug delivery is to avoid cyclic drug concentrations in the central compartment following multiple tablet intakes. This ensures that the distribution kinetics to the site of action is not disturbed (Figure 39.1). The analgesic drugs have elimination half-lives after oral administration that range from short (<1 h), through intermediate (>10 h) to very long (>50 h). Most analgesic drugs have short or intermediate half-lives (Sweetman, 2002). Use of analgesics with short half-lives requires continuous patient monitoring, optimal patient

Table 39.1 Routes and formulations of analgesic drugs

Systemic administration	Local
Oral	Gel/cream/ointment
Tablets	Peripheral nerve blocks
Effervescent tablets	
Mixture, drops, syrup	
Transmucosal	
Lozenges	
Spray	
Transdermal	
Patches	
Iontophoresis	
Rectal	
i.v.	
Infusion (continuous/intermittent)	
PCA	
Bolus injection	
i.m.	
s.c.	
Epidural	*Intrathecal*

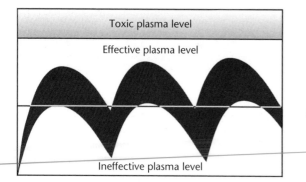

Figure 39.1 Simulated effective and non-effective dosage regimens showed by the black and the white, respectively, cyclic plasma concentrations. The non-effective dosage regimen (too low doses) infrequently reaches an effective plasma level allowing for breakthrough pain.

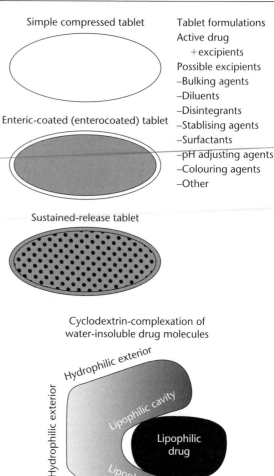

Figure 39.2 The figure shows generalized the most important types of tablet formulations. Drug–cyclodextrin complexation means that a lipophilic, but water-insoluble drug is encompassed by a highly water-soluble cyclodextrin molecule with an internal highly lipophilic cavity making the new molecular complex water-soluble thus increasing the absorption rate and lowering the analgesic time to onset.

compliance or drug delivery technologies for continuous administration of drug, depending on the patient status and the intensity and duration of the pain being treated. Analgesics with long half-lives that allow regimens with few daily drug dosages are always tempting first-choice analgesic alternatives. Analgesics with intermediate to long half-lives (e.g. the oxicams, but also some of the new cyclo-oxygenase (COX-2) inhibitors) carry an inherent risk of synergistic toxic reactions in non-responders if other analgesics, which share similar mechanisms of action, are given immediately after the first drug.

Solid-state analgesics

Oral administration of solid-state analgesics (e.g. tablets or capsules) is easy for patients with normal swallowing facility. Concomitant drink and erect position of the patient avoids retention of tablets in the oesophagus, while supine position can cause oesophageal tablet retention independent of the size and shape of the tablet. Tablets usually achieve a time to onset of analgesic effect within 0.5–1 h (with few exceptions) following breakdown and absorption.

Tablets can also be formulated with enteric coating or as sustained-release preparations. The dissolution of enteric-coated tablets is pH-sensitive. This allows no dissolution at low pH values (equal to that in the stomach) but rapid dissolution at pH values equal to those found in the intestine (Figure 39.2). Sustained-release tablets are designed to reduce the number of daily dosages thus improving patient compliance. The active drug is encapsulated into microparticles (Figure 39.2). A sustained-release tablet contains an abundant number of microparticles, which release the active drug in a time-controlled manner depending on the type of coating. Sustained-release tablets may have an enteric coating preventing them from dissolving in the stomach. This alteration in drug release may of course be problematic, delaying onset of analgesic action in comparison to a normal tablet.

Rectally administered analgesics bypass the first passage through the liver as veins in the rectum directly drain blood to the central compartment. Rectal administration is used to avoid problems with swallowing, stomach irritation and non-compliant children, but the absorption can be incomplete and erratic (Narvanen *et al.*, 1998).

Liquid-state analgesics

Young children, older patients and patients with reduced salivation or impaired swallowing facility show reduced compliance with respect to tablet regimens. Many analgesics are available as liquid-state oral formulations (such as syrups, drops and mixtures) making swallowing easier. Chewable tablets or gum formulations are also available allowing active drug to be released from the vehicle and mixed with saliva before entering the oesophagus.

Effervescent tablets contain sodium bicarbonate and an acid (citric or tartaric) which react when put in water. The formation of CO_2 gas causes the tablet to breakdown quickly and dissolve rapidly in the water. Effervescent tablets generally have a faster onset of action, but not necessarily a longer duration compared to tablet formulations (Moller *et al.*, 2000). The value in providing fast onset of analgesic action with effervescent tablets can be exploited by starting conventional tablet regimens with a single dose of effervescent tablets. The theoretical ranking list of oral drug formulations available for maximal absorption is in descending order:

- Solutions.
- Suspensions.
- Capsules.
- Normal tablets.
- Coated tablets.

It is important to realize that this theoretical ranking list is not always correct. For example, sub-optimal dissolution may alter the absorption rates for liquid formulations as shown for ibuprofen (Saano *et al.*, 1991).

Modification of traditional analgesics

Some traditional analgesics that belong to the non-steroidal anti-inflammatory drugs (NSAIDs) class have been modified to improve their rate of absorption thus reducing the onset of analgesic action. The diclofenac sodium salt is only sparingly soluble in water, while the diclofenac potassium salt is soluble. Increased water solubility increases the absorption rate of the drug and reduces onset time. The same

principle applies to naproxen potassium and the naproxen sodium. Another modification is complexation of piroxicam with an oligosaccharide (e.g beta-cyclodextrin) which causes increased water solubility of the beta-cyclodextrin–piroxicam complex. Beta-cyclodextrin contains a hydrophobic central cavity that encompasses piroxicam (i.e complexation), and a large hydrophilic outer surface, which allows for a water-soluble drug complex to be formed (Figure 39.2). The beta-cyclodextrin–piroxicam complex dissociates after absorption and the free drug enters the central compartment. Powdered formulations of this piroxicam complex have very short absorption times.

Many analgesics, especially of the NSAID class, are chiral drugs (i.e. the same molecule exists as mirror images) giving two isomeric forms of the parent molecule. There has been a growing interest in the separation of racemic NSAIDs, spurred by the fact that only one isomer is biologically active and the prospect of prolonged patent protection for old NSAIDs. The rationale is that the active isomer causes analgesia, while the non-active isomer may be inert or cause undesirable adverse effects. Clinical examples of the use of single isomeric forms of analgesics include the weak opioid dextropropoxyphene, the local anaesthetic levobupivacaine and the NSAID S-ibuprofen.

Parenteral administration

Intramuscular administration

The mainstay of post-operative analgesia has been intramuscular (i.m.) administration of opioids, e.g. i.m. morphine and pethidine are effective analgesics. However i.m. administration is associated with discomfort due to the injection, erratic absorption (i.e. from muscular depot site to the central compartment) and relative short analgesic duration of single doses. When compared with patient-controlled analgesia (PCA) and epidural analgesia, i.m. administration is associated with the highest percentage of patients experiencing inadequate analgesia (Dolin *et al.*, 2002). One important practical reason for this may be the occurrence of breakthrough pain consequent upon time delays between patient request and professional provision of more analgesia.

Sub-cutaneous administration

Sub-cutaneous (s.c.) administration may provide a very effective method of acute pain relief in special clinical settings, but is mostly used for chronic terminal pain treatment. Indwelling s.c. cannulae can be used for PCA. The onset of pain relief occurs at about the same time as with the i.m. route; however, the injection is less painful and the effect lasts longer. Unfortunately, breakthrough pain can occur, similar to that following i.m. injection.

Intravenous administration

The best route for severe post-operative pain treatment today is the intravenous (i.v.) route. Permanent venous access is usually present following completion of the operative procedure when the patient is moved to a recovery area. Continuous i.v. infusion provides pain control as long as the steady-state concentration of the chosen drug is maintained above minimum effective analgesic blood concentrations. Parenterally administered NSAIDs, including diclofenac sodium, ketorolac and propacetamol (i.e. paracetamol pro-drug) are popular because of their so-called opioid-sparing effect. Parenteral administration of NSAIDs does not abolish the well-known adverse effects observed after oral administration. Evidence of any advantage over oral routes for patients who are conscious and able to swallow is still lacking (Tramèr et al., 1998). Provision of parenteral NSAIDs is thought to reduce opioid analgesic demand (opioid-sparing effect), but although this has a good theoretical background it is unclear how effective it is in clinical practice.

The i.v. PCA is now a standard method for post-operative pain relief. It reduces unintended time delays between request and provision of analgesia, since the patient may independently (within defined dosage ranges determined by lock-out times) titrate analgesic delivery to level of pain. In comparison to conventional treatment, PCA with opioids improves analgesia and is preferred by patients, but does not decrease opioid consumption (Walder et al., 2001).

Transdermal administration

A non-invasive technique avoiding the oral route (useful in non-compliant patients) and first-pass hepatic metabolism. The route is limited to lipophilic molecules that have low molecular weight, due to dermal resistance to permeation. The potent opioid fentanyl (and also buprenorphine) is marketed for transdermal delivery in chronic pain states. Transdermal fentanyl patches are marketed in dosages graded as 25, 50, 75 and 100 where the number describes the fentanyl-release rate (i.e. 25 corresponds to 25 μg/h, 100 to 100 μg/h). Transdermal buprenorphine patches are currently marketed with 35 μg/h, 52.5 μg/h and 70 μg/h buprenorphine-release rates. The current analgesic patches cannot be divided. They cause inter-individual variation in drug concentrations in the

central compartment, slow time to onset of analgesia and long duration of effect (Grond et al., 2000). The main objection to their use in acute pain treatment is difficulty in rapid titration of effect.

Transdermal drug delivery is currently under-exploited. Three methods of transdermal drug delivery via the skin are described:

- The *matrix patch* (e.g. buprenorphine) is made up of four layers: the peel-off liner, the drug dispersed in a semi-solid matrix (i.e. polymer) that directly contacts the skin, the adhesive and the water-resistant backing. The adhesive layer of the patch is incorporated in a concentric configuration around the semi-solid matrix, which is in direct contact with the skin (Figure 39.3). The thin, flexible matrix system is designed for daily or multiple-day application. As the amount of drug in the patch decreases below the skin's saturation limit, the rate of delivery from patch to skin will slowly decrease.
- The *reservoir patch* (e.g. fentanyl) is made up of five layers: the peel-off liner, the adhesive layer that directly contacts the skin, the control membrane (controlling diffusion rate of drug molecules), the liquid reservoir of a drug solution and a water-resistant backing (Figure 39.4). As this design delivers uniform amounts of the drug over a specified time period, the rate of delivery has to be less than the saturation limit of different types of skin (Ansel, 1999).

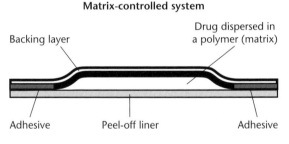

Matrix-controlled system

Backing layer / Drug dispersed in a polymer (matrix) / Adhesive / Peel-off liner / Adhesive

Figure 39.3 Design of the matrix patch.

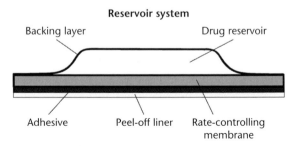

Reservoir system

Backing layer / Drug reservoir / Adhesive / Peel-off liner / Rate-controlling membrane

Figure 39.4 Design of the reservoir patch.

- *Iontophoresis* uses weak continuous direct electrical current (DC) to overcome the stratum corneum resistance to drug transport, by forcing charged or neutral drugs through intact skin between two electrodes with opposing charges. One electrode acts as the drug depot and the other as a charged ion buffer. The drug administration is controlled by a battery operated, on-demand control unit that can be used by the patient. Fentanyl, glucocorticoids and lidocaine are currently used with iontophoresis. In the future, microprocessor-controlled iontophoresis may overcome the problems regarding titration of doses and long analgesic onset times associated with transdermal delivery systems.

Transmucosal administration

Oral transmucosal fentanyl citrate (OTFC) incorporates a sugar-based lozenge, which releases fentanyl that is quickly absorbed through the richly vascularized oral mucosa. OTFC provides rapid analgesia with a similar terminal half-life to i.v. fentanyl. Although it is marketed for chronic pain treatment it is most useful for breakthrough pain. Moreover, patients prefer it to oral morphine (Zhang *et al.*, 2002).

Intrathecal/epidural administration

This method requires placement of a catheter into the intrathecal/epidural space, for delivery of drug either by intermittent injection or infusion. A disadvantage of intrathecal opioids is the possibility of cerebro spinal fluid (CSF) leakage causing headache.

Peripheral analgesic techniques including topical application

Intra-articular injection of morphine has been advocated to activate peripheral opioid receptors following post-operative inflammation. It remains unclear whether this treatment produces clinically useful analgesia (Kalso *et al.*, 1997). Topical application of NSAIDs to painful areas gives more analgesia than placebo (Moore *et al.*, 1998). Peripheral neural blockade techniques (including peri-operative tissue infiltration) are gaining popularity for the provision of analgesia. The analgesic benefit is primarily related to opioid-sparing effect with reduction in side effects, promoting early recovery of post-operative activity.

Multi-modal analgesic treatment

The analgesic dose–response curve for NSAIDs is flat compared with the dose–response for adverse effects, such as gastrointestinal symptoms, dizziness and drowsiness. Combining two drugs with different modes of action, to confer additional analgesic efficacy with reduced side effects, has been exemplified by the combination of aspirin or paracetamol with weak opioids. Traditional NSAIDs can also be used in combination with weak opioids, although there are few attempts to market such fixed combinations.

Combining standard doses of paracetamol with traditional NSAID alone may confer additional analgesic efficacy (Hyllested *et al.*, 2002). No increased risk of adverse effects of NSAIDs with the addition of paracetamol has so far been documented.

NSAIDs and COX-1/COX-2 selectivity

Traditionally, NSAIDs were categorized according to their chemical structure. Following the discovery and characterisation of COX-1 and COX-2 the NSAIDs have been categorised according to COX selectivity. The term COX-2 selectivity is feverishly used in marketing efforts since it became clear that the constitutive COX-1 is important in gastrointestinal mucosal protection. However, experience from large-scale clinical use of COX-2 selective inhibitors leaves unresolved questions regarding their role in patients with hypertension and renal disease (LeLorier *et al.*, 2002).

The analgesic effects of the available COX-2 selective inhibitors are not superior to traditional NSAIDs, but some provide longer duration of analgesia allowing once-daily tablet regimens (Stichtenot and Frolich, 2003). Thus, COX-2 inhibitors have yet to find their place, in particular cardiac adverse effects are being reported with higher frequency than traditional NSAIDs (see Chapter 41). The classification of NSAIDs is more complex than the distinction between COX-1 and COX-2 selectivity. Development of nitrous oxide-donating derivatives of traditional NSAIDs (NO-NSAID), which may counteract the vasoconstrictor effects of NSAIDs, is one avenue being pursued. Combined COX and lipoxygenase (LOX) inhibitors, which reduce inflammatory-induced leucocyte accumulation, are another trend in NSAID development (Rainsford 2001). This last is interesting since some traditional NSAIDs (i.e. diclofenac and ketoprofen) show LOX and COX inhibition.

Key points

- There is a wide range of inter-individual responses to analgesic drugs.
- Optimal treatment of post-operative pain often demands multi-modal approaches to exploit analgesic synergism and reduce adverse effects.

- Opioids are still the mainstay of effective post-operative pain treatment and their effects can be optimised by new drug delivery techniques.

Further reading

Moore, A., Edwards, J., Barden, J. & McQuay, H. (2003). *Bandolier's Little Book of Pain*, Oxford University Press, Oxford.

References

Ansel, H.C., Allen, L.V. & Popovich, N.G. (1999). *Pharmaceutical Dosage Forms and Drug Delivery Systems*, 7th edition. Lippincott Williams and Wilkins, Malvern.

Dolin, S.J., Cashman, J.N. & Bland, J.M. (2002). Effectiveness of acute postoperative pain management: I. Evidence from published data. *Br. J. Anaesth*, **89**: 409–423.

Grond, S., Radbruch, L. & Lehmann, K. (2000). Clinical pharmacokinetics of transdermal opioids. *Clin. Pharmacokinet.*, **38**: 59–89.

Hyllested, M., Jones, S., Pedersen, J.L. & Kehlet, H. (2002). Comparative effect of paracetamol, NSAIDs or their combination in postoperative pain management: a qualitative review. *Br. J. Anaesth.*, **88**: 199–214.

Jang, G.R., Harris, R.Z. & Lau, D.T. (2001). Pharmacokinetics and its role in small molecule drug discovery research. *Med. Res. Rev.*, **21**: 382–396.

Kalso, E., Tramer, M., Carroll, D., McQuay, H. & Moore, R.A. (1997). Pain relief from intra-articular morphine after knee surgery: a qualitative systematic review. *Pain*, **71**: 642–651.

LeLorier, J., Bombardier, C., Burgess, E., Moist, L., Wright, N., Cartier, P., Huckell, V., Hunt, R., Nawar, T. & Tobe, S. (2002). Practical consideratios for the use of non-steroidal anti-inflammatory drugs and cyclo-oxygenase-2 inhibitors in hypertension and kidney disease. *Can. J. Cardiol.*, **18**: 1301–1308.

Moller, P.L., Norholt, S.E., Ganry, H.E., Insuasty, J.H., Vincent, F.G., Skoglund, L.A. & Sindet-Pedersen, S.

(2000). Time to onset of analgesia and analgesic efficacy of effervescent acetaminophen 1000 mg compared to tablet acetaminophen 1000 mg in postoperative dental pain: a single-dose, double-blind, randomized, placebo-controlled study. *J. Clin. Pharmacol.*, **40**: 370–378.

Moore, R.A., Carroll, D., Wiffen, P.J., Tramer, M. & McQuay, H.J. (1998). A systematic review of topically-applied non-steroidal anti-inflammatory drugs. *Br. Med. J.*, **316**: 333–338.

Narvanen, T., Halsas, M., Smal, J. & Marvola, M. (1998). Is one paracetamol suppository of 1000 mg bioequivalent with two suppositories of 500 mg. *Eur. J. Drug Metab. Pharmacokinet*, **23**: 203–206.

Rainsford, K.D. (2001). The ever-emerging anti-inflammatories. Have there been any real advance? *J. Physiol. (Paris)*, **95**: 11–19.

van Ryn, J., Trummlitz, G. & Pairet, M. (2000). Cox-2 selectivity and the inflammatory processes. *Curr. Med. Chem.*, **7**: 1145–1161.

Saano, V., Paronen, P., Peura, P. & Vidgren, M. (1991). Relative pharmacokinetics of three oral 400 mg ibuprofen dosage forms in healthy volunteers. *Int. J. Clin. Pharmacol. Ther. Toxicol.*, **29**: 381–385.

Stichtenot, D.O. & Frolich, J.C. (2003). The second generation of COX-2 inhibitors. What advantages do the newest offer? *Drugs*, **63**: 33–45.

Sweetman, S.C. (ed) (2002). Martindale. The complete drug reference (33 ed). London, Pharmaceutical Press.

Tramèr, M., Williams, J., Carroll, D., Wiffen, P.J., McQuay, H.J. & Moore, R.A. (1998). Comparing analgesic efficacy of non-steroidal anti-inflammatory drugs given by different routes for acute and chronic pain. *Acta Anaesth. Scand.*, **42**: 71–79.

Walder, B., Schafer, M., Henzi, I. & Tramer, M.R. (2001). Efficacy and safety of patient-controlled opioid analgesia for acute postoperative pain. A quantitative sytematic review. *Acta Anaesth. Scand.*, **45**: 795–804.

Zhang, H., Zhang, J. & Streisand, J.B. (2002). Oral mucosal drug delivery. Clinical pharmacokinetics and therapeutic applications. *Clin. Pharmacokinet.*, **41**: 661–680.

L. Bromley

Introduction

Opioid drugs are those having an agonist action at opioid receptors. They are the mainstay of treatment of moderate and severe pain. The original drugs in this class were derived from the ripe seed heads of the poppy, *Papaver somniferum*. When incised, these oozed a milky fluid, which hardened on exposure to air. The latex collected was pressed into blocks of raw opium, from which the alkaloids were extracted and separated. By convention drugs derived from natural sources acting at opioid receptors are called *opiates*. Those synthesised chemically are called *opioids*. A timeline for the development of knowledge regarding the opioids is shown in Table 40.1.

The family of opioid receptors

The classification of opioid receptors was historically based upon receptor–ligand binding. Cloning in the

Table 40.1 Time line for the Western development of opioids

3rd century BC	Greeks use poppy juice as anti-diarrhoeal
16th century AD	Opium bought to Europe in Roman times
18th century AD	Opium smoking becomes a popular pastime
19th century AD	Individual drugs purified • Morphine in 1806 • Codeine in 1832 Hypodermic needle invented in 1850s, allowing parenteral use
20th century AD	*1970s* Endogenous peptides/opioid receptors identified and classified *1990s* • Opioid receptors cloned – subtypes found not to occur • Receptor knock-out mice bred – further definition of receptor pharmacology

1990s confirmed the occurrence of three types (Table 40.2). A further receptor (the orphan receptor) with no identified naturally occurring ligand was described in 1997. Subsequently, this ligand was identified as orphanin FQ (previously orphanin or nociceptin).

Endogenous opioids

Endogenous opioids (neuropeptides ranging from 2 to 39 amino acids in length) occur in three different forms: enkephalins, endorphins and dynorphins. The conversion of these molecules to the active form and their rapid degradation is achieved by enzymatic activity at the site of release. Breakdown of the endorphins is, in part, brought about by angiotensin-converting enzyme (ACE). Thus patients taking ACE-inhibiting drugs may have prolonged action of their natural endorphins.

Enkephalins

These are the simplest structures (5-amino acid sequences), with two forms depending on the terminal amino acid – hence methionine in Met-enkephalin and leucine in Leu-enkephalin. They bind to δ opioid receptors (DOP).

Endorphins

The endorphins are larger molecules, with 30 or more amino acids in sequence, binding to μ opioid receptor (MOP). They have a depressant action on the cerebral cortex, the thalamus and the dorsal horn (DH) of the spinal cord, which can be reversed by the MOP antagonist naloxone. MOP receptors to which endorphins bind, are found in high concentrations in the sensory pathways concerned with the perception and integration of nociceptive stimuli.

Recently new classes of endorphins, the endomorphins have been identified, with a high affinity and selectivity for the MOP. These are divided into endomorphin-1 and -2. They produce intense analgesia and marked effects on the gastrointestinal tract.

Table 40.2 Classification of opioid receptors

Ligand-based	Structural	Endogenous ligand	Receptor antagonist
δ receptor	DOP/OP$_1$	Enkephalins	Naltrexone
κ receptor	KOP/OP$_2$	Dynorphins	Naltrexone
μ receptor	MOP/OP$_3$	Endomorphin-1 and -2	Naloxone
Orphan receptor	Nociceptin receptor/ORL-1 (NOP)/ORL-1	Orphanin FQ	'Compound B'

Table 40.3 Actions of the endogenous opioids

Naturally occurring ligand	Receptor	Site of action	Effect of binding at this site
Enkephalin	DOP (OP$_1$)	DH of the spinal cord (laminae I and II) Limbic system Medulla Adrenal medulla Intestine	Analgesia Alteration of affective behaviour
Dynorphin	KOP (OP$_2$)	Widely distributed in the cortex Also present in the peri-aqueductal grey (PAG) and medulla DH of the spinal cord	Sedative actions (in the cortex) Miosis Spinal analgesic actions
Endorphin I and II	MOP (OP$_3$)	In the brain stem • PAG • Nucleus raphe magnus • Locus coeruleus DH of the spinal cord Outside the CNS	Supra-spinal analgesia Euphoria Respiratory depression Spinal analgesia
Endomorphin-1 and 2	MOP	Medulla DH of spinal cord	Intense analgesia Slowing of GI propulsion

Endomorphin-2 shows high immunochemical staining activity in the DH of the spinal cord and medulla, with endomorphin-1 localised in the cortex.

Dynorphins

Dynorphins are similar in structure to Leu-enkephalin, but with a higher potency. They exist in three forms:

- Dynorphin A (1–17) with a 17-amino acid sequence.
- Dynorphin A (1–8) a shorter form.
- Dynorphin B (1–13) a distinctly different form.

All dynorphins bind to the κ opioid receptor (KOP), but also have a role in the stress response. Dynorphin A is expressed in the hypocampus, where it acts as an antagonist to glutamate at N-methyl-D-aspartate (NMDA) receptors. It is also chemically related to orphanin FQ and may interact with the opioid-like receptor 1 (ORL-1).

Dynorphins and enkephalins are commonly expressed in the same regions of the central nervous system (CNS), but always in distinctly different groups of neurones. For example, the dynorphin containing neurones in the medulla occur ventral to those containing enkephalins.

Orphanin FQ

This is similar in structure to dynorphin A. It appears to be important in the stress response, in that:

- It selectively reverses stress–induced analgesia (due to natural endorphins) in some rodent species.
- Knock–out mice with no ORL-1 are susceptible to stress and show impaired adaptation.

In the CNS it has anxiolytic actions similar to diazepam and is also expressed by dopaminergic neurones in the midbrain. There have been suggestions that abnormal functioning in this system may be implicated in addiction and some psychiatric diseases.

However, orphanin FQ subserves a different role in the spinal cord, where it is involved in the regulation of inhibitory inter-neurones in laminae I, II and V. Here it acts in a similar fashion to the MOP agonists, producing pre-synaptic inhibition and analgesia.

Cellular mechanisms of actions of the opioids

The opioid receptors are G-protein-linked receptors. Binding of the ligand with the receptor produces two intracellular effects:

- A reduction in the levels of cyclic adenosine mono-phosphate (cAMP) (pre-synaptic mechanism).
- An influx of potassium resulting in hyper-polarisation of the cell membrane (post-synaptic mechanism).

The sensitivity of the opioid receptors is linked with the presence of cholecystokinin (CCK) in the cell. As the receptor is stimulated, the levels of CCK fall and the receptor becomes more sensitive to the ligand. Binding of an endogenous ligand to the receptor produces a phenomenon known as ligand directed trafficking. In this process the ligand–receptor complex is rapidly internalised and removed from the receptor population. This does not happen when the MOP binds morphine, but does (albeit to a lesser degree than with the natural ligands) when fentanyl binds. This may be part of the explanation of acute tolerance seen with some opioid drugs.

Chronic stimulation of the MOP can result in a rise in intracellular cAMP (a phenomenon known as adenyl cyclase super activation), which results in an increased activity in the post-junctional neurone. When the drug is withdrawn there is an overshoot of activity. This may explain:

- Withdrawal symptoms.
- The reduced effectiveness of opioids in chronic use.
- The tendency for addiction.

There is some interaction between the level of regulation of the MOP and DOP. For example:

- When agonists bind to the MOP one of the consequences is an upregulation of the DOP.
- With chronic exposure to MOP agonists the distribution of the DOP is changed, with increased expressed on the cell surface and in the submembrane layer.

Table 40.4 Functional classification of drugs acting at opioid receptors

Functional type	Examples
Pure MOP agonists	Morphine, fentanyl
Partial MOP agonists	Buprenorphine (also acts at KOP)
Agonist/antagonist at KOP/MOP	Pentazocine
Action at several receptor/channel sites	Tramadol, pethidine

Table 40.5 Chemical structure of drugs acting at opioid receptors

Structure	Examples
Morphinans	Morphine, codeine
Phenylpiperidines	Fentanyl, pethidine
Diphenylpropylamines	Methadone, dextropropoxyphene
Esters	Remifentanil

The exact state of activity of the opioid receptors is, therefore, a complex interaction (see Chapter 8) depending upon:

- States of phosphorylation of the G-protein.
- Interactions with other intracellular mediators.
- The temporal relationship of stimulation by ligands.

All these processes interact to set and re-set the sensitivity of the receptor. This complexity goes some way to explain why individuals can have very different pharmacological responses to opioid drugs.

Drugs acting at opioid receptors

Historically a variety of classifications of opioid drugs have been used:

- According to 'strength' – invalid because no account of mechanism of action taken.
- Functional classification (Table 40.4) – more useful to clinicians.
- According to chemical structure (Table 40.5).

The actions of the opioid drugs

The majority of opioid drugs in use are MOP agonists. In an attempt to avoid some of the unwanted actions of the pure agonist, partial agonists and

Table 40.6 Actions of the opioid drugs

In the nervous system	On smooth muscle	Other actions
Cortex Analgesia Euphoria/Dysphoria Sedation Addiction	*In the GI tract* Slowed gastric emptying Increased intestinal tone Decreased peristalsis Spasm of the sphincter of Oddi	*In the CVS* Bradycardia

Hypothalamus and pituitary
Decrease in production of trophic
  hormones (lower plasma
  testosterone and cortisone)
Increase in plasma growth hormone
  and prolactin
	In the urogenital tract
	Increased tone in:
	  – Ureter
	  – Detrusor muscle
	  – Urinary sphincter
	Increased amplitude of ureteral
	  contractions
		Release of histamine
		Itching (especially of face and nose)
		  can occur with any opioid,
		  delivered by any route
		Generalised pruritus is most common
		  with neuraxial delivery of drugs
		Varies between drugs
		Most marked with morphine, less
		  with fentanyl and its coeruleus

Brain stem
Analgesia
Nausea and vomiting
Miosis
Respiratory depression
	In the CVS
	Reduction in peripheral resistance
	  (resultant hypotension)
		Muscle rigidity
		Most marked with large doses of
		  fentanyl and alfentanil
		Mechanism unknown

Spinal cord Analgesia		

GI: gastrointestinal; CVS: cardio vascular system.

agonist–antagonists (see Chapter 8) have been produced. However, advantages have proved limited, with generally low analgesic potency being associated with dysphoric and emetic side effects. Thus, pure agonists remain the mainstay of therapeutic use. The actions of MOP agonists can be predicted from functions associated with the receptor system. They are summarised in Table 40.6.

In addition to specific opioid receptor effects, some drugs have pharmacological actions via other cellular mechanisms. In particular:

- Pethidine has local anaesthetic and anti-cholinergic effects.
- Tramadol interacts with the norepinephrine (NE) and the 5-hydroxytryptamine (serotonin) (5-HT) receptor systems.

Depending on circumstances, these effects may be of positive advantage, or cause unwanted problems.

Addiction, dependence and tolerance of opioid drugs

Opioid drugs alter mood and feelings, both in the individual in pain and those not in pain. The consequence of this is that some individuals develop a behavioural pattern of compulsive drug use in order to experience these effects. The problem of addiction and dependence (and in particular their occurrence in the setting of nociceptive pain) is covered in Chapter 46.

Tolerance is a phenomenon whereby increasing doses of drug are required to achieve the same effect. There are a number of mechanisms that can be responsible for tolerance. These include:

- Pharmacokinetic, for example, enzyme induction increasing the speed of metabolism of the drug.
- Pharmacodynamic, where adaptive changes in the system (e.g. down regulation of receptors, or reduced turnover of receptor synthesis) result in a reduced effect despite no alteration occurring in the concentration of drug at the receptor.

Pharmacokinetic and pharmacodynamic differences between the opioid drugs in common use

The opioid drugs available for clinical use differ in their physico-chemical and pharmacological properties. This has a profound effect on the clinical application of the drugs. Varying potency at MOP receptors may influence drug use. While increasing the potency is associated with increased intensity of analgesia,

Table 40.7 Pharmacokinetic data relating to common clinically used opioids

	V_d (l/kg)	Cl. (l/min)	$t_{1/2}$ (h)
...anil	0.8	6	1.6
...e	2.6	11	2.9
...rphone	4.1	22	3.1
...adone	3.8	1.4	35
Morphine	3.5	15	3
Oxycodone	2.6	9.7	3.7
Pethidine	4.0	12	4
Remifentanil	0.4	40	0.1
Sufentanil	1.7	12.7	2.7
Fentanyl	4.0	13	3.5
Tramadol	2.9	6	7

an increase in unwanted effects (e.g. respiratory depression) also occurs. For example, the synthetic opioid fentanyl is 100 times more potent than morphine. This results in profound respiratory depression following administration.

Pharmacokinetic differences between the drugs accounts for the different clinical usage in the majority of cases. Three important features (Table 40.7) are: (a) volume of distribution (V_d), (b) clearance (Cl.) and (c) elimination half-life ($t_{1/2}$). Differences in these may lead to important features as regards use. In particular:

- In comparison to drugs with a higher V_d (e.g. pethidine) those with a lower V_d (e.g. alfentanil) will have a shorter half-life and duration of action.
- Drugs cleared more slowly, with a longer $t_{1/2}$ (e.g. methadone), can be used orally in a twice daily dosage, as long as they have sufficient orally bioavailability.

Morphine, diamorphine and codeine

Morphine and codeine are extracted from opium. The synthetic process is difficult and extraction remains the most economic means of production. The pro-drug diamorphine is semi–synthetic and has no direct action on MOP. Hydrolysis by tissue esterases (via 6-monoacetyl morphine) to morphine results in MOP agonist activity. Thus, diamorphine is pharmacodynamically identical to morphine. Diamorphine has poor stability in solution and is presented as a powder for reconstitution. Once dissolved it has a shelf life of 48 h. In contrast, both morphine and codeine are relatively stable and are presented in liquid form for parenteral (and oral) use.

Oral preparations are available for all three drugs, but bioavailability is variable (25% for morphine, 50% for codeine). When diamorphine is given orally, no diamorphine can be detected in the systemic circulation, as it is rapidly metabolised by enzymes in the gut wall and liver. However, since it is the metabolites that are active a significant pharmacodynamic effect is observed. Morphine is metabolised to morphine 6 and 3 glucuronide (M6G and M3G, respectively), with M6G being active at the MOP (with a higher efficacy than morphine itself). Both metabolites are excreted in the urine. Codeine metabolism is by demethylation to morphine. There is genetic variability in this process (see Chapter 4).

Pethidine

Pethidine is chemically related to atropine. It is 10x less potent than morphine, but at equipotent doses produces similar side effects (e.g. respiratory depression). It is orally active, with a bioavailability of 50%. Its duration of action is shorter than morphine, with a half-life of 3–4 h. It has two unique properties:

- Membrane stabilising properties, producing weak local anaesthetic action on peripheral nerves. There is some evidence that pethidine can produce a local anaesthetic action when used in the epidural space in addition to its opioid receptor agonist action.
- Marked anti-cholinergic properties consequent upon its chemical structure. It has been suggested that this action, in combination with its low propensity to release histamine, makes pethidine a more suitable opioid drug to use in patients with asthma.

Hepatic metabolism produces norpethidine (exclusively renally excreted), which can cause central excitation and convulsions. However, long-term administration of high doses is required to produce significant amounts of norpethidine.

Fentanyl, alfentanil, sufentanil and remifentanil

These four drugs are chemically related, with *fentanyl* being the parent drug. The family was developed for use in anaesthesia. They share common features of:

- High lipid solubility.
- Short duration of action.
- High potency at MOP receptors.

All may be given intravenously, but fentanyl has also been formulated as a trans-dermal patch (for use in chronic pain management) and a 'lollipop' for treatment of incident pain. It has a $t_{1/2}$ of 3.5 h. It is metabolised in the liver to inactive metabolites.

Alfentanil is 10x less potent than fentanyl at the MOP. It also has a shorter half-life because, being less lipid soluble, it has a smaller V_d. However, it has a large concentration gradient for entry into the CNS, because it is a highly basic compound and at plasma pH is 89% unionised. It is metabolised to inactive metabolites. Due to its short half-life it is frequently given by infusion. However, given over long periods it accumulates and its context-sensitive half-life increases with duration of infusion.

Sufentanil is the most potent of this family of drugs. It is 600–800x more potent than morphine. It has been used extensively in the USA, but is unavailable in the UK. Due to its potency its use has been confined to anaesthesia.

Remifentanil is a novel member of this family in that it contains an ester bond, which is broken by the action of plasma esterases (not cholinesterase). Therefore, the drug has a predictable half-life, independent of hepatic or renal function. Its metabolites have 0.1% of the activity of the parent compound. The drug is given by infusion as part of a general anaesthetic technique. Its rapid offset requires administration of suitable post-operative analgesia prior to the termination of the drug, to avoid pain.

Methadone

Methadone was first synthesised 60 years ago. It is pharmacodynamically indistinguishable from morphine, but has a high oral bioavailability. Its action is terminated by redistribution and its $t_{1/2}$ is long (20–45 h). Cumulation does occur.

Activity at the NMDA receptor may add to its analgesic properties.

Tramadol

This drug is a racemic mixture of two stereoisomers. It is a weak MOP agonist that also inhibits uptake of NE and 5-HT. It has good oral bioavailability with a half-life of 7 h. An active metabolite, *O*-desmethyltramadol, demonstrates a higher receptor affinity than the parent molecule. It is produced by the action of the CYP2D6 enzyme on tramadol. Opioid-induced side effects occur, but are less severe than with traditional opioids.

Use of neuraxial opioids

The increase in knowledge of the pharmacology of the DH of the spinal cord has led to targeting of opioid receptors in the substantia gelatinosa via the epidural or spinal routes.

Epidural

The most important determinants of the amount of drug reaching the spinal cord from the epidural space are the pharmacokinetic parameters of the drug (i.e. absorption, distribution, metabolism and excretion). Drugs introduced into the epidural space can move in one of two directions. They may:

- Be absorbed into the systemic circulation (via the epidural veins).
- Cross the dura and enter the cerebro-spinal fluid (CSF) and from thence diffuse into the cord.

The relative fat solubility of the drug will directly affect the means by which the drug leaves the epidural space. More fat-soluble drugs will:

- Be rapidly absorbed into the systemic circulation.
- Cross the dura.
- Be relatively insoluble in the CSF.
- Avidly enter the cord.

For this reason, the highly lipid-soluble drugs (e.g. fentanyl and sufentanil) have been extensively used via the epidural route. A proportion of the drug enters the circulation and has its action in the brain and brain stem (probably up to 20% of the administered dose). Of the drug that crosses into the CSF, much will avidly enter the spinal cord, producing potent spinal analgesia. The rest will circulate and eventually reach the brain stem, where there is a potential for respiratory depression. This occurs early with fat-soluble drugs. Unfortunately it occurs later with more water-soluble drugs (e.g. morphine), presenting up to 24 h after epidural administration.

Spinal

Where drugs are injected directly into the CSF, the dose required is much smaller. Fat solubility (and consequent ability to enter the cord) will influence choice of drug. Diamorphine has been very successfully used in the epidural space. It is less water soluble than morphine, tending to enter the cord more efficiently. It is metabolised in the cord to morphine, thus producing a longer duration of action than fentanyl or sufentanil. Legal restrictions outside the UK have prevented its widespread use.

Opioids can be used as a single agent in the epidural and subarachnoid spaces. However, it has become common practise to use a combination of low-dose opioids and local anaesthetics. These two classes of drugs act synergistically, allowing the use of lower concentrations of local anaesthetic, reducing the incidence of motor block.

Neuraxial opioids are capable of causing all the unwanted effects observed when administered via other routes. Pruritus and retention of urine are particular problems. These effects may be reversed by small doses of naloxone without significant loss of analgesia.

Codeine

Codeine is widely used for:

- Post-operative pain (alone and in combination therapies).
- Anti-tussive action.
- Anti-diarrhoea drug.

It has been used extensively in children and in neurosurgical patients, based on a widely held view (for which there is very little evidence in the literature) that the incidence of opioid related side effects are fewer with codeine than with other compounds. One explanation for this is that codeine is a pro-drug, undergoing hepatic metabolism to its active form – morphine. This conversion is catalysed by cytochrome CYP2D6. Significant individual and ethnic variability in the extent of metabolism result in the unpredictable efficacy of codeine (see Chapter 4). It is, thus, important to monitor the individual to ensure a pharmacological affect is achieved.

Codeine may be used alone, but combination with paracetamol is common. The synthetic opioid dihydrocodeine has a structure and pharmacokinetics similar to codeine and is also used in combination with paracetamol.

In a systematic review of the literature McQuay and Moore (1998) have shown the combination of paracetamol 600 or 650 mg and codeine 60 mg to be more effective than paracetamol 1000 mg alone. Indeed the paracetamol/codeine combination had a number needed to treat (NNT) of 3.1, compared with 4.6 for paracetamol alone. Despite the widespread use of dihydrocodeine, there is little useful literature comparing it with other oral opioids in the management of pain.

Opioid antagonists

These synthetic drugs are produced by the substitution of the characteristic N-methyl group of the opioid drugs by large moieties (see Figure 40.1).

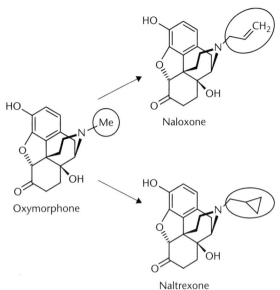

Figure 40.1 Diagram demonstrating how the substitution of an opioid agonist methyl group, can result in the production of opioid antagonist agents.

This transforms:

- Morphine to nalorphine.
- Levorphanol to levallorphan.
- Oxymorphone to naloxone or naltrexone.

Nalorphine and levallorphan have mixed agonist/antagonist actions, whereas naloxone and naltrexone are pure antagonists. All are antagonists at the MOP receptor, but have some action at other opioid receptors (generally with lower affinities).

In the presence of opioids, naloxone rapidly reverses all the pharmacological effects, including analgesia. The drug has a short half-life (1 h), being rapidly metabolised in the liver. Since it undergoes extensive first pass metabolism it cannot be used orally, but both intravenous and intramuscular routes may be used. The duration of effect may be shorter than that of the opioid it is antagonising, necessitating repeat dosage.

At low doses, naloxone and naltrexone have no pharmaceutical action in subjects who have not received opioids. However, at very high doses (>0.3 mg/kg) naloxone raises systolic blood pressure and decreases performance on memory tests. In experimental animals naloxone increases blood pressure in models of septic shock. Infusions have occasionally been used in patients on the assumption that endogenous opioids are involved in the central regulation of peripheral vascular resistance.

In addition, naloxone reverses the analgesia produced by placebo and acupuncture. This suggests that these forms of analgesia involve the recruitment of the endogenous opioid peptides.

Key points

- Opioids are the mainstay of treatment for moderate and severe pain. They can be administered by a wide variety of routes.
- Pharmacokinetic profiles of individual compounds are major factors in analgesic efficacy.
- Opioid receptors are widely distributed and this is reflected in the diversity of the side effects.
- Antagonists are available, that reverse actions of both endogenous and exogenous opioid ligands.

Further reading

Dickenson, A.H. (2002). Gate control theory of pain stands the test of time. *Br. J. Anaesth.*, **88**(6): 755–757.

McQuay, H. & Moore, A. (1998). *An Evidence Based Resource for Pain Relief.* Oxford Medical Publications, Oxford, England.

Williams, D.G., Patel, A. & Howard, R. (2002). Pharmacogenetics of codeine metabolism in an urban population of children and its implications for analgesic reliability. *Br. J. Anaesth.*, **89**(6): 839–845.

Yaksh, T.L. (1997). Pharmacology and mechanisms of opioid analgesic activity. *Acta Anaesth. Scand.*, **41**: 94–111.

NON-STEROIDAL ANTI-INFLAMMATORY AGENTS

41

J. Cashman & A. Holdcroft

Classification

Non-steroidal anti-inflammatory drugs (NSAIDs) may be classified by chemical group or by mode of action.

Chemical groups

(a) Salicylic acids
   - Acetylated (e.g. acetylsalicylic acid (aspirin)).
   - Non-acetylated (e.g. diflunisal).
(b) Acetic acids
   - Indoleacetic acids (e.g. indomethacin, sulindac).
   - Phenylacetic acids (e.g. diclofenac).
   - Pyrroleacetic acids (e.g. ketorolac).
(c) Coxibs (e.g. celecoxib, parecoxib, etoricoxib).
(d) Fenamates (e.g. mefenamic acid).
(e) Oxicams (e.g. piroxicam, meloxicam).
(f) Phenazones (e.g. dipyrone).
(g) Propionic acids (e.g. ibuprofen, naproxen).
(h) Pyrazolones (e.g. phenylbutazone).
(i) Others (e.g. paracetamol (acetaminophen)).

Mechanisms of action of anti-inflammatory analgesics

The enzyme cyclo-oxygenase (COX) catalyses the production of prostaglandins (PGs) and thromboxanes from arachidonic acid. COX exists in at least two isoforms, with a wide range of physiological activity as simplified in the Table 41.1.

When tissues are traumatised by surgery, there is a release of pro-inflammatory mediators that induce COX-2. Increased levels of the PGs formed can induce peripheral sensitisation of nociceptors, but also secondary sensitisation in the dorsal horn by blockade of the inhibitory action of glycine. This action, by induction of the gene for COX-2 protein is described further below. The role of COX-2 in the nervous system is therefore not only peripheral but also central, with COX-2 inhibitors that cross the blood–brain barrier potentially reducing central sensitisation. Recently COX-2 has been found to be present in the central nervous system (CNS) when no trauma has occurred. Therefore, it should be considered partly constitutive

Table 41.1 Physiological activity of COX isoforms

COX-1 (Constitutive)	COX-2 (Inducible)
Function	
Platelet production	Upregulated by inflammatory
Regulation of renal	cytokines, endotoxin and
haemodynamics	mitogens
Electrolyte balance	Production of inflammatory
Gastrointestinal (GI)	PGs that mediate pain and
mucosa protection	oedema
Tissues	
Expressed in:	Expressed in synovia of joints
Platelets	Constitutive in the CNS
Endothelium	and kidneys
Kidney	
Gastric mucosa	

in that tissue. However, both acute and chronic inflammation are associated with a huge upregulation of COX-2 mRNA in the CNS, which occurs even when sensory nerve blockade is present.

A third distinct COX isoenzyme (COX-3) and two smaller COX-1-derived proteins (partial COX-1 or PCOX-1a and PCOX-1b proteins) have also been identified. COX-3 is a splice variant of COX-1 and is considered to play a key role in the biosynthesis of prostanoids within the CNS.

The ideal NSAID should be able to act both peripherally and centrally by crossing the blood–brain barrier. The activity of paracetamol, a para-aminophenol derivative, is predominantly central and lacks peripheral activity. Thus, it has neither the anti-inflammatory effects, nor the gastrointestinal or renal side effects associated with traditional NSAIDs. COX-3 is weakly sensitive to paracetamol, but this action can only partly explain the analgesic effect of paracetamol. For these reasons, it is difficult to classify paracetamol as a NSAID.

All COX inhibitors occupy the arachidonic acid channel of both COX-1 and COX-2 (see Figure 41.1). Traditional NSAIDs block both COX-1 and COX-2 by binding to the active site in the C-terminal (i.e. they are not selective and can block PGs that have

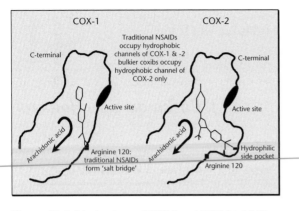

Figure 41.1 Mechanisms of COX-1 and COX-2 inhibition.

Table 41.2 Drug selectivity ratio for COX inhibition

Drug	COX-1 : COX-2
Etoricoxib	106
Rofecoxib	35
Valdecoxib (formed from hydrolysis of paracoxib)	30
Celecoxib	7.6
Nimesulide	7.3
Diclofenac	3
Etodolac	2.4
Meloxicam	2
Indomethacin	0.4
Ibuprofen	0.2
Piroxicam	0.2

beneficial effects). In contrast, selective COX-2 inhibitors do not bind to the C-terminal active site but rather the sulphonamide chain in the hydrophilic side pocket of COX-2.

COX-2 is a large molecule and drugs such as paracoxib (the water-soluble prodrug of valdecoxib) demonstrate enhanced binding to the enzyme, staying attached to COX-2 for longer than the plasma concentrations would indicate. Indeed the Coxibs generally have a longer duration of action than traditional NSAIDs.

The original expectation was that COX-2-selective NSAIDs (Coxibs) would be as effective as analgesics as non-selective NSAIDs, but lack the gastrointestinal tract complications. In practice, there is an interdependence between COX-1 and COX-2 inhibition, for which one measure is the drug selectivity ratio (see Table 41.2). The implications of this remain contentious.

Metabolic systems in the body, when blocked, can develop alternative routes for chemical synthesis. For example, COX blockade enhances the synthesis of 5-lipoxygenase products leading to a range of compounds contributing to inflammation (e.g. leucotriene B_4, LTB_4).

Another sub-class of drugs that are competitive inhibitors of both 5-lipoxygenase and COX is emerging (e.g. licofelone). These modulate inflammation by decreasing the production of pro-inflammatory leukotrienes and PGs, thus extending the indications, safety profile and potency of NSAIDs. Also under development are nitric oxide-releasing NSAIDs (NO-NSAIDs). The slow release of NO from these compounds leads to subtle changes in the profile of pharmacological activity of the parent NSAIDs, resulting in markedly diminished gastrointestinal toxicity and improved anti-inflammatory and anti-nociceptive efficacy.

Mechanisms of adverse effects

Gastrointestinal system

COX-1:

- Is the predominant isoform in the stomach.
- Mediates PG synthesis in the gastric mucosa.
- Stimulates angiogenesis through direct effects on endothelial cells.

PGs protect the gastric mucosa by:

- Reducing acid secretion.
- Stimulating mucous secretion.
- Increasing bicarbonate secretion.
- Enhancing mucosal blood flow.
- Production of mucosal phospholipids.

The inhibition of PG synthesis by NSAIDs can compromise these protective functions leading to:

- Faecal blood loss.
- Gastrointestinal ulcers.
- Ulcer complications (e.g. perforation).
- Diarrhoea.

Angiogenesis, the formation of new capillary blood vessels, is essential for the growth of solid tumours and for ulcer healing. Thus, the anti-angiogenic properties of NSAIDs may contribute not only to their ulcerogenic effect but also to an anti-cancer effect.

Risk factors may be drug related and/or patient related. Certain groups are more at risk of these effects: women, the elderly, smokers and individuals with a history of excessive alcohol ingestion or peptic ulceration. The risk of mucosal lesions also varies with the drug used. Risk in ranked order (from most to least problematic) for drug-related gastro-intestinal problems: aspirin, piroxicam, indomethacin, ibuprofen, sulindac, naproxen, diclofenac.

Respiratory system

Aspirin-induced asthma can be severe. The prevalence of sensitivity to traditional NSAIDs in adult asthmatics is of the order 5–10%, rising to 14–23% if nasal polyps are present. The mechanism of the reaction is unclear.

Hypersensitivity reactions

These are related to COX inhibition leading to increased arachidonic acid. Alternative metabolic pathways predominate, leading to increased leucotriene formation.

Renal system

Renal PGs alter tone directly in afferent arterioles and indirectly in efferent arterioles (via the renin–angiotensin system). These effects are vital when renal blood flow is compromised (e.g. dehydration, haemorrhage, angiotensin converting enzyme (ACE) inhibitors, diuretics). Such conditions frequently occur peri-operatively and these effects present the main contraindications to NSAID use at this time. Unfortunately, COX-2 is expressed constitutively in the kidney and there is now evidence that COX-2 selective inhibitors are not renal sparing.

Long-term use of NSAIDs can result in water and sodium retention that may exacerbate hypertension or induce cardiac failure. Patients over 65 years of age are more likely to develop renal failure if they are taking NSAIDs (18% versus 11% in a control group of patients). For COX-2 inhibitors, there is currently insufficient evidence to predict their effects in renal failure.

Haematological system

Aspirin irreversibly acetylates the active site of the COX enzyme in platelets. The effects last for the life of the platelet – about 7–10 days. Other NSAIDs bind reversibly at the site of the natural substrate, arachidonic acid. Thus blood clotting may be altered and the use of some NSAIDs with anticoagulant therapy (e.g. ketorolac and low dose heparin) may be contraindicated post-operatively.

Other effects

- Dermatological (e.g. erythema multiforme).
- Meningitis (aseptic) that may be confused with other causes of meningitis after neuraxial nerve blocks.
- Reye's syndrome with aspirin in children.

Pharmacokinetic data

The NSAIDs are weak acids (pKa 3–5) and thus are rapidly absorbed from the stomach. Most have low first pass metabolism (except diclofenac) and hence high bioavailability and low clearance (typically <50 ml/kg/min). They are highly protein bound (90–99%; except for paracetamol which is approximately 20% bound) principally to albumin. Therefore, they potentially interact with similar drugs displacing them from their binding sites and increasing their toxicity (Table 41.3).

Table 41.3 Pharmacokinetic data of various NSAIDs

Drug (chemical)	Bioavailability (%)	Elimination half-life (h)	Protein bound (%)	Volume of distribution (l/kg)
Aspirin	65–72	0.25[a]	58	0.16
Salicylic acid	100	2–15	82	0.13
Celecoxib	70–80	9–15	97	6.5
Diclofenac	60	1–2	99.5	0.17
Etoricoxib	100	22	92	0.02
Ibuprofen	78	2–4	99	0.15
Ketorolac	80–85	4–10	99	0.28
Rofecoxib	92–93	10–17	86	1.2–1.3
Paracoxib[b]	100	3	NA	NA
Valdecoxib		8–9	98	0.78
Paracetamol	85	1–4	20	1.0
Piroxicam	100	57	99	0.14

[a] Acetyl salicylic acid is rapidly converted *in vivo* to salicylic acid.

[b] Parecoxib is almost completely converted to valdecoxib with half-life of plasma of 22 min.

Table 41.4 NNT values of various NSAIDs

Analgesic	NNT (95% confidence interval)
Diclofenac 100 mg	1.9 (1.6–2.2)
Diclofenac 50 mg	2.3 (2.0–2.7)
Rofecoxib 50 mg	2.3 (2.0–2.6)
Ibuprofen 400 mg	2.4 (2.3–2.6)
Ibuprofen 200 mg	2.7 (2.5–3.1)
Piroxicam 20 mg	2.7 (2.1–3.8)
Ketorolac 30 mg (i.m.)	3.4 (2.5–4.9)
Paracetamol 1000 mg	3.8 (3.4–4.4)
Aspirin 600/650 mg	4.6 (3.9–5.5)

Formulations

NSAIDS are available in topical, rectal and parenteral, as well as oral formulations. Analgesic efficacy can be expressed as the number of patients who need to receive the active drug for one patient to achieve at least 50% relief of pain (number needed to treat, NNT). The most effective analgesics have an NNT of about two. Many oral NSAIDs have low NNT values (Table 41.4).

Some topical NSAIDs have been shown to be effective in treating acute pain of musculoskeletal origin. Ibuprofen, piroxicam, ketoprofen and felbinac can provide at least 50% pain relief after a week of treatment, with an NNT of 3.9 (3.4–4.3). However, indomethacin is not similarly effective. Similar results have been found for some chronic pain conditions, where topical application appears to be as effective as oral use. This is particularly important since topical application of NSAIDs may be associated with fewer serious side effects.

Although NSAIDs are rapidly absorbed from the gastrointestinal tract, speed of absorption can be accelerated by linking them to β-cyclodextrin (e.g. piroxicam) or to non-essential amino acids such as arginine (e.g. ibuprofen). In addition, the duration of action of NSAIDs with a short half-life can be extended by slow release formulations (e.g. diclofenac).

Combinations of NSAIDs with drugs to prevent general gastrointestinal side effects are now available (e.g. diclofenac–misoprostal). There are also some specific complications relating to formulation (e.g. sterile abscesses following intra muscularly (i.m.) diclofenac). For this reason it is important to become familiar with the complications specific to the drugs you commonly use.

Indications for use

- Analgesia (randomised controlled trial (RCT) evidence):
  - Acute pain (mild or moderate) (e.g. post-operative pain, trauma).
  - Arthritis (e.g. gout, osteoarthritis and rheumatoid arthritis).
  - Cancer pain (e.g. bone metastases).
  - For severe pain (by parenteral routes).
  - Migraine.

  There is a ceiling effect on the pain relief achieved with NSAIDs. Therefore, they are usually used in combination with other analgesics for optimal effect. In particular, they have morphine-sparing properties that are valuable post surgery.
- Anti-inflammatory
  - Arthritis.
- Antipyretic (by central PG inhibition of IL-1 activity in the hypothalamus).
- Anti-cancer (via inhibition of angiogenesis).

Key points

- NSAIDs have both peripheral and CNS activity.
- NSAIDs on their own can provide effective relief from mild to moderate pain and useful opioid-sparing effects are seen in severe pain (level 1 evidence).
- Side effects of NSAIDs are common and associated with altered PG synthesis.
- Coxibs also have COX-1 enzyme inhibition and selectivity may not provide optimal activity.

Rofecoxib was withdrawn worldwide on 30th September 2004 due to an increased risk of serious thrombotic events.

Further reading

Fitzgerald, G.A. & Patrono, C. (2001). The coxibs, selective inhibitors of cyclooxygenase-2. *New Engl. J. Med.*, **345**: 433–442.

Hawkey, C.J. (1999). COX-2 inhibitors. *Lancet*, **353**: 307–314.

Neumann, S., Doubell, T.P., Leslie, T. & Woolf, C.J. (1996). Inflammatory pain hypersensitivity mediated by phenotypic switch in myelinated primary sensory neurons. *Nature*, **384**: 360–364.

Samad, T.A., Sapirstein, A. & Woolf, C.J. (2002). Prostanoids and pain: unravelling mechanisms and revealing therapeutic targets. *Trends. Mol. Med.*, **8**: 390–396.

Woolf, C.J. & Costigan, M. (1999). Transcriptional and posttranslational plasticity and the generation of inflammatory pain. *Proc. Nat. Acad. Sci.*, **96**: 7723–7730.

C.F. Stannard

Introduction

A rapidly evolving understanding of the neurobiology of pain has:

- Allowed development of novel compounds likely to modify the pain experience.
- Provided a scientific rationale for the use of a number of classes of existing drugs in the treatment of pain.

Similarly, empirical observations regarding the efficacy of such drugs have illuminated some of the mechanisms involved in pain processing.

Pains associated with nervous system damage or dysfunction (neuropathic and central pain syndromes) are often refractory to conventional analgesic therapy. It is in this spectrum of disorders that (inappropriately so called) 'non-analgesic' drugs are most frequently used. The drugs used are chemically diverse compounds and many have a number of relevant actions in the treatment of pain. It is important to note that the published data on these drugs relate to their use in relatively few, specifically defined, pain conditions. In contrast, many patients present a mechanistically more complex picture. The use of these drugs in the more general pain population is, therefore, based on inferences drawn from specific studies augmented by clinical experience.

Antidepressant drugs

History

Tricyclic antidepressants were first synthesised in the 1940s and used for the treatment of depression a decade later. The drugs were subsequently shown to have analgesic properties both in patients with chronic pain-induced depression, and also in those with normal mood. The first-generation tricyclic antidepressants have now been studied extensively in a variety of (usually neurogenic) pain states. Data are emerging on the analgesic efficacy of the newer classes of antidepressants.

Classes of antidepressant and mode of action

Over half of patients with pain have depression. However, antidepressants are prescribed in the pain clinic for their specific analgesic, rather than mood altering effects. The presence of a distinct effect on pain is borne out by a number of observations:

- Doses necessary to improve pain are often lower than those used to treat depression.
- At these doses the onset of analgesic activity is more rapid than any antidepressant activity.
- Analgesic efficacy is usually obtained in non-depressed patients and does not correlate with improvement in mood in depressed patients.
- The drugs are useful in acute and experimental pain.

The analgesic efficacy of antidepressants is presumed to be related to:

- Ability to block central nervous system (CNS) monoamine uptake (particularly serotonin and noradrenaline) pre-synaptically.
- Effects on post-synaptic adrenoceptors.

In this way the drugs have been thought to augment descending monoaminergic anti-nociceptive pathways from the midbrain periaqueductal grey and medulla (nucleus raphe magnus, NRM). However, it is not known to what extent, if at all, this descending monoaminergic system is disrupted in chronic pain states. Moreover, the undoubted analgesic efficacy of these drugs may be related to monoaminergic action elsewhere in the CNS Jasmin et al., 2003.

The drugs have a number of other potentially important effects including:

- Sodium channel blockade.
- Calcium channel blockade.
- Blockade of histamine receptor type 1 (H1) receptors.
- Blockade of N-methyl-D-aspartate (NMDA) receptors.
- A weakly agonistic effect at the mu opioid receptor.

In addition, these drugs have a beneficial effect on sleep disorder, a common accompaniment to persisting pain.

There are a variety of subgroups of antidepressant agents including:

- The first-generation tricyclic drugs (so called on the basis of their chemical structure) are the best-studied group (e.g. *amitriptyline, doxepin, imipramine, clomipramine* and *dosulepin*). These are mixed re-uptake inhibitors (i.e. have both noradrenergic and serotonergic effects). *Nortriptyline* and *desipramine* (metabolites of amitriptyline and imipramine, respectively) have mainly noradrenergic action.
- Selective serotonin re-uptake inhibitors (SSRIs) (e.g. *fluoxetine, paroxetine* and *citalopram*) were developed in the 1980s in an attempt to reduce the side effects of these drugs (see below).
- Selective noradrenergic re-uptake inhibitors (SNRIs) (e.g. *roboxetine*) have become available, but the clinical evidence for efficacy is thus far disappointing.
- *Venlafaxine*, a structurally novel antidepressant drug, blocks uptake of noradrenaline and serotonin and, to a lesser extent dopamine. It is relatively free of the side effects associated with tricyclic antidepressant drugs and has been shown to be effective in neuropathic pain associated with breast cancer.
- *Mirtazapine* has both noradrenergic and serotonergic effects, but these are mediated via histaminergic and adrenoceptor blockade rather than re-uptake inhibition.

From the published literature, drugs with mixed noradrenergic/serotonergic effects appear to be more effective analgesics than drugs with relatively selective noradrenergic activity, with SSRIs being the least effective drugs for pain relief. This is undoubtedly an oversimplification, particularly as there are less data available relating to the newer drugs.

Adverse effects

Antidepressants have a number of predictable adverse effects, mostly mediated by their post-synaptic receptor blocking action. The commonest use-limiting side effects are:

- Sedation (common with amitriptyline related to histaminergic action).
- Anti-cholinergic effects – particularly dry mouth. Constipation and urinary retention are less common, but well documented.

Patients may become tolerant to these side effects with continued use. The drugs have a number of effects on the heart including slowing of atrioventricular and intraventricular conduction. Cardiac side effects are important as they preclude the use of these drugs in patients with cardiac conduction disturbances or recent infarction.

Practical issues in prescribing

The drugs are usually prescribed as a once daily, night-time dose. It is important to warn patients of the sedative effects of these drugs (which may often be an advantage in those whose sleep is disturbed because of pain). Most patients will still feel somewhat sedated in the morning for the first few days of therapy, but will often become tolerant of this effect within 3–4 days. If daytime somnolence persists, the drug should be taken earlier in the evening. Beneficial effects on sleep usually come on within a few days, whereas the improvement in pain will take a week or longer. There is considerable inter-individual variation in pharmacokinetics, so dose requirements vary widely. Titration to known effective serum concentration is the most rational approach, but in practice the drugs are usually titrated to efficacy, or until side effects preclude dose escalation.

Anticonvulsant drugs

History

The mechanistic commonality between epilepsy and pain was noted as early as the mid-nineteenth century. Trousseau postulated that the pain of trigeminal neuralgia was associated with abnormal neural discharge akin to that occurring during a fit. As understanding of the pathophysiologic mechanisms of epilepsy and neurogenic pain have evolved, the biochemical similarities between the two conditions are now well understood. In particular the 'kindling' of hippocampal neurones in epilepsy has been shown to have physiologic commonality with the phenomenon of windup in the neurones of the dorsal horn.

The first anticonvulsant to be used successfully in the treatment of pain was phenytoin. Its successful use for the treatment of trigeminal neuralgia was described in 1942. Two decades later carbamazepine was studied for the treatment of the same condition in a double blind controlled trial. It has since been studied in a number of pain conditions and remains a popular first line medication for the treatment of neuropathic pain. There is good support in the literature for use of anticonvulsants in the treatment of post-herpetic neuralgia, trigeminal neuralgia and painful diabetic neuropathy. This has led to their use in other neuropathic pain conditions, such as post-stroke pain, phantom limb pain and pain following spinal injury, although the published evidence for their use in these conditions is less robust. The drugs may also be used in the pain clinic for migraine prophylaxis. Efficacy in the ability of a drug to reduce seizures does not necessarily predict usefulness in controlling pain.

Mechanisms of action

Anticonvulsants work in a number of different ways, all of which have relevance to their effect on pain. Many drugs have more than one mechanism of action. The pathophysiological mechanisms responsible for neuropathic pain are outlined in Chapter 20. A number of mechanisms may be contributing to an individual's pain experience (these may be different within a homogeneous diagnostic group). Polypharmacy, using different anticonvulsants or anticonvulsants in conjunction with other classes of medication (particularly antidepressants), represents a rational approach.

Older anticonvulsants, such as *phenytoin* and *carbamazepine* were thought to reduce neuronal excitability by means of frequency-dependent blockade of voltage-sensitive sodium channels. They also have a number of other actions:

- Phenytoin inhibits glutamate release pre-synaptically, modulates calcium current which has activity at the NMDA receptor and increases gamma amino butyric acid (GABA) concentration. It is now infrequently used, although given intravenously may have some utility in the management of acute flare-ups of neurogenic pain.
- Carbamazepine modulates depolarisation-dependent calcium uptake, increases release of 5-HT and also blocks NMDA receptor current. It remains the treatment of choice in trigeminal neuralgia, with about 70% of patients getting significant pain relief. It causes a reduction in both pain intensity and pain paroxysms, and also in triggering stimuli.
- *Oxcarbazepine* is a newer chemically related drug with a more favourable side effect profile.
- *Sodium valproate* probably elevates levels of the inhibitory GABA in the CNS and by potentiation of GABAergic functions (particularly in the brain) inhibits pain. Clinical evidence to support its use is sparse.

Recent advances in drug development have made a wider range of agents available:

- *Lamotrigine* also has action at sodium channels. This mechanism probably suppresses the neuronal release of glutamate, an excitatory amino acid pivotally involved in central neuronal hyper-excitability and persisting pain. The drug also increases brain GABA concentration. It has proven efficacy in animal models of neuropathic pain. It has been shown to be of benefit in patients with central pain and also as an add-on treatment in trigeminal neuralgia. It has been used in other types of neuropathic pain.
- *Topiramate* has several relevant actions including activity-dependent sodium channel blockade, inhibition of calcium channels, inhibition of excitatory amino acid receptors and enhancement of the effects of GABA. The evidence for its efficacy in pain therapy is contradictory.
- *Tiagabine* is a selective inhibitor of the principle neuronal GABA transporter in the cortex and hippocampus. By slowing the re-uptake of synaptically released GABA, it prolongs inhibitory post-synaptic potentials. It has anti-nociceptive activity in animal models of neuropathic pain and has been used to treat painful neuropathy in humans, although controlled data are lacking.
- *Gabapentin* has been used in the treatment of pain for almost a decade and is probably the most widely used anticonvulsant for this indication. Its mechanism of action is unclear, since although it was developed as a structural GABA analogue, it has no interaction with GABA receptors or GABA metabolism. It appears to have an inhibitory action at voltage-gated calcium channels, where it blocks the $\alpha 2\delta$ subunit that is upregulated in experimental pain models. Although it is not known what function (if any) gabapentin plays in modulating calcium channel flow, effects on intracellular calcium influx would disrupt an entire series of NMDA-activated events involved in central sensitization. Its effectiveness in post-herpetic neuralgia and diabetic neuropathy has been demonstrated in well-conducted randomised trials. Efficacy is comparable to older agents, but it is remarkable for its favourable side-effect profile, lack of interactions and straightforward pharmacokinetics.
- *Pregabalin* is a newer compound with a similar mechanism of action to gabapentin. Its use in neuropathic pain has been well studied in humans. Unlike gabapentin it can be prescribed twice daily.
- *Benzodiazepines* are GABA-A agonists used widely for the treatment of epilepsy. They have analgesic properties in animal models, but are not often used in the management of pain – with the exception of clonazepam (which has been described in a number of case series). A recent controlled trial describes efficacy of clonazepam used topically in the treatment of stomatodynia, and postulates the presence of peripheral GABA-A receptors in the oral mucosa.

- *Levetiracetam* is an increasingly popular drug for the treatment of refractory epilepsy. It's mechanism of action is not well characterised, but may have an effect on GABA systems. It inhibits the 'kindling' of hippocampal neurones and would be expected to have an effect on dorsal horn windup. There is some suggestion from pre-clinical data that the drug is effective in the treatment of pain. There are emerging reports of its use in clinical neurogenic pain.

Side effects of anticonvulsants

Many of the long-term safety and toxicity data relate to the use of these drugs in the treatment of epilepsy:

- CNS side effects are the most common; in particularly, somnolence, dizziness, ataxia, nausea, vomiting and alteration in mood.
- Rashes are common and carbamazepine may be associated rarely with Stevens–Johnson syndrome or toxic epidermal necrolysis.

Adverse effects of carbamazepine tend to occur in the first two months of treatment. The drug has also been associated with hepatic dysfunction and bone marrow aplasia. Such serious side effects are infrequently reported and it is difficult to make comparisons in this regard between different drugs.

The practical prescription of these drugs is also influenced by a number of important pharmacokinetic issues including:

- Variable oral absorption.
- Induction of hepatic enzymes.
- Extensive protein binding.

Clinicians must be aware of the many interactions that these drugs have with other medications.

Local anaesthetics and anti-arrhythmic agents

Peripheral hyper-excitability following nerve injury is associated with spontaneous electrical activity. It results (at least in part) from alteration in the quantity and disposition of ion channel protein. Such ectopic discharges can provide sustained afferent input to the spinal cord from the damaged nerve. Indeed they may be self-sustaining, or persist long after a triggering stimulus has subsided. In addition to anticonvulsant drugs (described above) local anaesthetic drugs and anti-dysrhythmics are observed to suppress this hyper-excitability by means of non-specific sodium channel blockade. Additionally, low-dose lidocaine may block glutamate-evoked activity in the dorsal horn of the spinal cord.

- *Lidocaine* given systemically has no effect on heat, cold or mechanical thresholds in healthy subjects. However, following nerve injury (and in human experimental pain models), the drug reduces facilitated sensory processing. Intravenous lidocaine was initially reported to be effective for post-operative pain relief. More recently it has been reported to reduce deafferentation pain, central pain and diabetic neuropathy. The results of randomised controlled trials of intravenous lidocaine assess acute changes in pain levels. While interesting and informative this is unhelpful in the management of neuropathic pain. The drug cannot be given orally, but continues to be used intravenously to predict possible utility of other membrane stabilising drugs, although such practice is not supported by the literature.
- *Mexilitene* is the oral analogue of lidocaine. It has been studied in a number of chronic (neuropathic and central) pain models with conflicting and overall disappointing results. Gastrointestinal side effects of mexilitene are very common and frequently treatment limiting, as are worsening of existing dysrhythmias and neurological symptoms (particularly tremor). The use of other anti-arrhythmic agents is now precluded because of the incidence of severe adverse events.

There is evidence that topical local anaesthetic preparations may have some utility in the management of neuropathic pain. The drugs are thought to work by suppressing ectopic discharge in damaged superficial sensory afferents and may in consequence may prevent central hyper-excitability. The advantage of this route is that drugs may be used for a prolonged period and systemic local anaesthetic levels are minimal with side effects being rare. A eutectic mixture of local anaesthetic (*EMLA*) has been used for the treatment of post-herpetic neuralgia and other neuropathic pains with mixed results. Lidocaine 5% is available as a 10×14 cm patch with a polyethylene backing and has been shown to have efficacy and tolerability in the management of post-herpetic neuralgia. There are open-label data suggesting that it may also be useful in other neurogenic pain syndromes, such as post-thoracotomy pain and complex regional pain syndrome (CRPS).

Calcium channel antagonists

N-type voltage-sensitive calcium channels are found in the superficial laminae of the dorsal horn and are involved in nociceptive processing following nerve injury. *Ziconotide* is a synthetic derivative of the venom of a marine snail. It is a selective N-type calcium channel blocker that has been shown to reduce mechanical allodynia in animal models of nerve injury. There has been a large-scale study of its use intrathecally in patients with a variety of neuropathic pains, which shows promising results. Side effects include dizziness, ataxia, confusion and nystagmus, as well as nausea and constipation. These effects resolve on cessation of the drug.

Key points

- Drugs traditionally classified according to the indication for which they were developed are useful in the treatment of pain.
- The most commonly used drugs are antidepressants and anticonvulsants. Local anaesthetic agents and calcium channel blockers also have a place in the treatment of neuropathic pain.
- The importance of a mechanism-based approach to the management of difficult neuropathic pain problems has been recognised for some years. It emphasises the need for a parallel clarity regarding analgesic drug classification in order to target more specifically and appropriately the many intrusive symptoms experienced by patients in pain.

Further reading

Backonja, M.M. (2002). Use of anticonvulsants for treatment of neuropathic pain. *Neurology*, **59**: S14-7.

Beydoun, A. & Backonja, M.M. (2003). Mechanistic stratification of antineuralgic agents. *J. Pain Symp. Manag.*, **25**: S18–S30.

Chong, M.S. & Smith, T.E. (2000). Anticonvulsants for the management of pain. *Pain Rev.*, 7: 129–149.

Jasmin, L., Tien, D., Janni, G. & Ohara, P. (2003). Is noradrenaline a significant factor in the analgesic effect of antidepressants? *Pain*, **106**: 3–8.

Kakyama, M. & Fukuda, K. (2000). The role of antidepressants in the treatment of chronic pain. *Pain Rev.*, 7: 119–129.

Laughlin, T.M., Tram, K.V., Wilcox, G.L. & Birnbaum, A.K. (2002). Comparison of antiepileptic drugs tiagabine, lamotrigine, and gabapentin in mouse models of acute, prolonged, and chronic nociception. *J. Pharmacol. Exp. Ther.*, **302**: 1168–1175.

Sindrup, S.H. & Jensen, T.S. (1999). Efficacy of pharmacological treatments of neuropathic pain: an update and effect related to mechanism of drug action *Pain*, 83: 389–400.

Woolf, C.J. & Mannion, R.J. (1999). Neuropathic pain: aetiology, symptoms, mechanisms, and management. *Lancet*, **353**: 1959–1964.

S.I. Jaggar & A. Holdcroft

The treatment of pain has changed over the years from a disease- and site-based therapy to a mechanistic approach. The multiple mechanisms for pain sensation to be modified peripherally and in the central nervous system (CNS) provide many avenues for drug targets. This chapter aims to describe the variety of agents not covered elsewhere in this text.

α2 adrenoreceptor agonists

These agents have a long history in veterinary practice, where they have been used to provide local analgesia and sedation in a wide range of animals. Their role in human pain relief is now established.

Mechanism of action

Four subtypes of the G protein-linked α2 adrenoreceptors have been described. The $\alpha 2_A$ subtype that appears to be associated with analgesia and sedation is encoded on chromosome 10. These receptors have been localised to:

- *Brain and brainstem*: specifically in the locus coeruleus, where stimulation is associated with activation of the descending inhibitory noradrenergic pathways.
- *The spinal cord*: particularly in the substantia gelatinosa, where activation is able to inhibit firing of nociceptive neurones.
- *Peripheral neurone terminals* (both peripheral and central).

Stimulation of receptors at any of these sites is associated with membrane hyper-polarisation and subsequent inhibition of activity (Chapter 8).

Interaction between opioid and α2 adrenoreceptor activity has been explored in μ opioid (MOP) receptor knock out mice. In acute studies, MOP receptors do not have an important role in α2 adrenoceptor antinociceptive activity. However, in the presence of inflammation, the potency of systemic dexmedetomidine becomes dependent on MOP receptors. This

mechanism may explain some of the clinical findings discussed below.

Range of agents

The agents that have been used most frequently (and to greatest effect) in the treatment of human pain conditions are:

- Clonidine.
- Tizanidine.
- Dexmedetomidine.

Acute pain

In the peri-operative period, clonidine has been administered by a variety of parenteral routes, in combination with a range of other analgesic agents, for over 20 years. It is commonly administered by the epidural route, where synergy with both local anaesthetics and opioids is claimed. Indeed, a systematic review of the literature in 1998 suggested that epidural clonidine (alone or in combination) is effective in providing analgesia. In clinical trial situations efficacy has been reported in a wide range of groups, including pregnant women (e.g. for Caesarian section) and children. Unfortunately, because of the wide array of doses and methods of administration, strong evidence for efficacy or potency is not available.

Dexmedetomidine is a recently developed highly selective α2 adrenergic agonist, which when given intravenously (as a loading dose followed by an infusion) in acute post-operative pain can reduce patient controlled analgesia (PCA) morphine consumption. Thus it may reduce opioid-induced muscle rigidity and shivering, while causing minimal respiratory depression. Moreover, it has haemodynamic stabilising effects by blunting the central sympathetic response.

Chronic pain

Pain consequent upon muscle spasm or cramping might be expected to be relieved by the use of muscle relaxants (which should be clearly distinguished from the neuromuscular blocking agents used to induce widespread paralysis during general anaesthesia). In the USA, the food and drug administration (FDA) has approved the use of α2 adrenergic agonists for the relief of muscle spasm and cramps. The agents may be administered topically, orally, or (in the case of chronic cancer pain) neuraxially. Most experience of the utility of these agents has been gained in multiple sclerosis and spinal cord injury. Unfortunately, a Cochrane review recently noted that there is insufficient evidence to support their use as muscle relaxants.

The α2 adrenergic agonists, dexmedetomidine and clonidine (via the epidural route) can be used in the management of chronic pain associated with cancer. For clonidine, the epidural route is chosen since there appears to be a strong relationship between pain relief and cerebrospinal fluid (CSF) levels of clonidine, which is lacking in relation to blood levels (more closely related to sedative effects). Epidural administration deposits the drug close to the site of action, while avoiding a breach of the dura. The efficacy of clonidine is greatest in neuropathic pain. Since amputation is obligatorily associated with neural damage and many patients suffer with difficult to treat phantom limb pain, trials are ongoing in this patient group. In view of the synergy noted with neuraxial opioids and local anaesthetics, there is rationale for adding the drug to these in situations where it has not been possible to achieve adequate pain relief. However, level 1 or 2 evidence is currently unavailable.

Side effects

- *Sedation*: This may be helpful in the context of chronic pain, since lack of sleep may exacerbate pain. However, careful consideration must be given to timing of administration in order to avoid unwanted daytime somnolence. Level of sedation appears to be related to blood levels and this is actively made use of in the context of intensive care patients (particularly in the paediatric population).
- *Hypotension and bradycardia*: Most commonly seen if the drugs are administered by the neuraxial route in the thoracic region. The dose relationship appears to be weaker than this anatomical-site relationship.
- *Dry mouth*.
- *Nausea*.
- *Constipation*.

Cannabinoids

History

For many thousands of years *cannabis sativa* has been used as a medicine to treat all types of pain, including dysmenorrhoea and arthritis, as well as nausea and vomiting, convulsions, muscle spasms, asthma and dysentery. The plant contains over 60 cannabinoids and other active compounds, such as flavinoids. In the past decade, two cannabinoids receptors have been cloned, although there are possibly more (see cannabidiol (CBD) below). The cannabinoid receptor type 1 (CB$_1$) is found predominantly in the CNS (although also on neuronal tissue in the periphery) in the motor, sensory perception, autonomic and endocrine areas. This distribution can explain the variety of side effects from cannabinoids. The cannabinoid receptor type 2 (CB$_2$) mainly occurs peripherally in the immune system, but also in the glial cells of the CNS.

Mechanism of action

The cannabinoids receptors are G protein coupled and modulate the excitability of nociceptive neurones (see Chapter 8).

Many of the actions of naturally occurring cannabinoids do not appear to be related to cannabinoid receptors. However, they can modulate ascending nociceptive and descending antinociceptive pathways in the spinal cord and higher relay centres (such as the thalamus and periaqueductal grey (PAG)), for example, through action on other receptor systems:

- Vanilloid (on sensory neurones).
- Cholinergic (in hippocampus).
- Gamma amino butyric acid (GABA) (in the PAG and rostroventral medulla (RVM)).

Range of agents

Natural cannabis products are illegal in most countries and for clinical trials government and regulatory approval is required. Where cannabis extracts are used the extract will possibly contain more than one active compound in comparison with synthetic cannabinoids where the pharmacological effects will be solely those of the drug.

Phytocannabinoids (plant derived)

Tetrahydrocannabinol (THC) is the main active cannabinoid in plant material. It is metabolised in the liver to many compounds and oral bioavailability of THC can be as low as 10% due to extensive first pass metabolism. The main active metabolite is 11-OH THC, which may also contribute to clinical effects. THC is very fat soluble with a V_D of 10 litres per kg, and until the discovery of cannabinoid receptors it was thought to exert its effects through its solubility in the lipids of cell membranes. This lipid solubility is also the reason for its delayed excretion.

CBD is an active cannabinoid that may act on receptors other than CB_1 or CB_2. It has anti-inflammatory properties and there is some evidence for anti-psychotic activity.

Cannabis-based pharmaceutical preparations A number of routes and formulations of cannabis are being studied in clinical trials: oral, rectal, sublingual and inhalation. Each formulation may contain a different proportion of the naturally occurring cannabinoids. However, methods to measure these are available, allowing standardisation of doses based on THC content.

Synthetic analogues
Classical

THC has been synthesised for medicinal use as *Marinol* and *Dronabinol*, which are marketed as appetite stimulants. *Nabilone* is licensed in the UK, Canada and Switzerland as an antiemetic to be used when nausea and vomiting from chemotherapy is unresponsive to other drugs. Unfortunately, it can cause dysphoria, which limits its use in pain management. The *+HU 210* stereoisomer is currently undergoing clinical trials for use as a neuroprotectant.

Non-classical

Levonantradol was developed as a parenteral compound. When used in post-operative pain management adequate pain relief was measured, but its side-effects profile prevented marketing. *WIN-55,212-2* has a structure based on a non-steroidal anti-inflammatory drug (NSAID) analgesic and binds to both CB_1 and CB_2 receptors (with a preference for CB_2). It has been used extensively in antinociceptive experiments.

Anandamide congeners

The *endocannabinoids* are as follows:

* Anandamide (arachydonyl ethanolamide) can activate vanilloid receptors.
* 2-arachidonoylglycerol (2-AG).
* Palmitoylethanolamide (PEA; it is not a CB_1 or CB_2 agonist).

These are short acting and rapidly broken down by membrane bound fatty acid amide hydrolases.

Synthetic analogues

(R)-(+)-alpha-methanandamide resists catabolism and has a higher affinity for CB_1, when compared to the naturally occurring endocannabinoids. It is currently in experimental, rather than clinical use. Amidase inhibitors that reduce the rapid breakdown of anandamide (thus prolonging its effects) have been developed for laboratory experiments.

Cannabinoid receptor antagonists

Although peripherally acting cannabinoids delivered locally (e.g. by topical application) may avoid CNS adverse effects, specific antagonists to cannabinoid activity may be another approach to reduce unwanted CNS effects. In basic science research such agonists serve the important function of determining drug mechanisms. In clinical use, more specific/selective antagonists would be needed in order to maintain analgesia while at the same time reversing unwanted side effects. Examples of antagonists used in research currently include SR 141716 (CB_1 specific) and SR 144528 (CB_2).

Adverse effects

The side effects from clinical use of cannabinoids in cannabis naïve patients may be different from effects reported after long-term abuse using pharmaceutically toxic doses.

* *Acute*: sedation, ataxia, dry mouth, hypotension, hypertension, tachycardia, bradycardia, hallucinations and mood changes; occasional feelings of anxiety may initiate panic.
* *Long-term abuse*: psychosis, cognitive and memory defects (through receptors in the hippocampus and basal ganglia).

Anti-spasmodic agents

In the context of chronic pain, muscle spasm can prove debilitating, in addition to exacerbating other pain problems. Specific conditions in which such problems arise include multiple sclerosis, spinal cord injury, cerebral palsy and post-stroke pain syndromes. Both short- and long-acting agents have been utilised.

* *α2 agonists*: (as above).
* *Benzodiazepines*: These bind to the GABA A receptor and potentiate the response to further GABA binding. They are commonly prescribed for acute muscle spasm (e.g. torticollis). Such therapy may be helpful in the ultra-short term, but the risks associated with addiction should not be underestimated. The most common side effect is sedation (an outcome for which these drugs are also used).
* *Baclofen*: is a GABA B receptor agonist. A systematic review has demonstrated potential improvements in spasticity related pain in up to 98% of patients (although this remains a small group of individuals with specialised problems). The agent is short acting and may be given orally or parenterally. Oral administration is more frequently associated with side effects, including confusion,

drowsiness, nausea and weakness. Continuous intrathecal infusion (usually via an implanted catheter and pump) may help overcome this problem.

- *Calcium channel blockers*: Pre-clinical evidence suggests that voltage-dependent calcium channels are important in both spontaneous and evoked pain. This has led to the use of agents, such as nifedipine, to treat pain associated with spasm in the palliative care scenario (e.g. in patients with cancer and human immunodeficiency virus (HIV)–related pain). In addition there are a variety of trials suggesting that they may have some use in the prophylaxis of migraine; however, the level of evidence supporting this use is currently under dispute.
- *Botulinum toxin*: is thought to act by chemo-denervation. Multiple case reports and short series have demonstrated usefulness in pain consequent upon muscle spasm (e.g. central dystonia, simple tension headache and torticollis). However, this remains an expensive trial/research treatment, which cannot be advocated for routine use.
- Compound analgesic preparations may also contain other muscle relaxants (including methocarbamol and meprobamate). Their clinical efficacy is not established.

Key points

- α2 adrenergic receptor agonists act synergistically with opioid and local anaesthetic agents and there is level 2 evidence to support its use in the peri-operative period.
- Cannabinoids based on plant extracts are being marketed for specific pain conditions.
- Muscle spasm pain can be difficult to treat pharmacologically.

Further reading

Armand, S., Langlade, A., Boutros, A., Lobjoit, K., Monrigal, C., Ramboatiana, R., Rauss, A. & Bonnet, F. (1998). Meta-analysis of the efficacy of extradural clonidine to relieve post-operative pain: an impossible task. *Br. J. Anaesth.*, **81**: 126–134.

Poree, L.R., Guo, T.Z., Kingery, W.S. & Maze, M. (1998). The analgesic potency of dexmedetomidine is enhanced after nerve injury: a possible role for peripheral alpha-2-adrenoceptors. *Anesth. Analg.*, **87**: 941–948.

Sampson, F.C., Hayward, A., Evans, G., Morton, R. & Collett, B. (2002). Functional benefits and cost/benefit analysis of continuous intrathecal baclofen infusion for the management of severe spasticity. *J. Neurosur.*, **96**: 1052–1057.

Walker, J.M., Hohmann, A.G., Martin, W.J., Strangman, N.M., Huang, S.M. & Tsou, K. (1999). The neurobiology of cannabinoid analgesia. *Life Sci.*, **65**: 665–673.

Weinbroumm, A.A. & Ben-Abraham, R. (2001). Dextromethorphan and dexmedetomidine: new agents for the control of perioperative pain. *Eur. J. Surg.*, **167**: 563–569.

PSYCHOSOCIAL

PSYCHOLOGICAL MANAGEMENT OF CHRONIC PAIN 44

T. Newton-John

Introduction

It is axiomatic to state that patients experiencing chronic pain often experience significant psychological dysfunction. Any clinician who has spent any time in a pain clinic will be aware of the high levels of emotional and behavioural disturbance that can occur in this patient group. Depression, anxiety and anger are common emotional states associated with chronic pain. Moreover, pain patients may show unusual gait patterns, with guarding and bracing of affected areas of the body, and other physical behaviours. The psychological perspective from which one addresses these difficulties depends very much upon the model of pain, implicit or explicit, that one holds. The first section of this chapter will therefore discuss pain models and their relationship to treatment. Key psychological theories will then be laid out (as they apply to chronic pain) and the various components of the theories discussed. Finally, a number of relevant issues in the application of psychological treatments for chronic pain will be discussed.

Chronic pain and psychology: separation or integration?

The publication of the gate control theory of pain in 1965 marked a shift in thinking, in relation to psychological processes in pain. Up to that point, the experience of pain was largely a biomedical phenomenon. How much you were hurt was dependent upon where you were injured, and the extent to which your tissues were damaged. Psychological phenomena were only invoked when the amount of pain being reported was in excess of the amount of tissue trauma that was observed. In this case, patients were labelled as 'hysterical', and the pain termed 'functional', because it was presumed to serve some emotional, social or financial purpose. Psychodynamic concepts of chronic pain make reference to a hidden or masked form of depression, histories of childhood abuse and other mechanisms by which patients are unable to express their 'true' problem, which is an emotional one. These

pain models, the biomedical organic and the psychogenic functional, are termed dualistic theories because of their either/or perspective. Pain is conceptualised as being either a physical phenomenon (when we are able to identify its cause) or as a psychological one (when we cannot).

However, in 1965 the biopsychosocial perspective encompassed by the gate control theory of pain was introduced. Here, psychological factors are seen as being intrinsic to the experience of all forms of pain (including acute toothache, post-surgical pain, migraines and chronic low back pain). The model states that descending influences will modulate the ongoing processing of afferent nerve fibre inputs to the dorsal horn (DH) of the spinal cord. Psychosocial factors represent major sources of descending influence. This may be by:

- 'Opening the gate' and enhancing the experience of pain.
- 'Closing the gate' and diminishing its impact.

Melzack and Wall specified that current effect and cognitive activity, such as attention, mood and attributions about the pain (i.e. 'This chest pain is indigestion.' versus 'This chest pain is a heart attack.'), are relevant. But beyond the thoughts and feelings about pain that are located in the present, the model also includes more distal influences on pain experience (e.g. cultural norms, memories of pain based on previous experiences and the effect of modelling of pain behaviours based on family responses to illness).

It has now been almost 40 years since the gate control model was published, and its basic tenets have been enshrined in the International Association for the Study of Pain (IASP) definition of pain – *Pain is an unpleasant sensory and emotional experience associated with actual or potential tissue damage, or described in terms of such damage*. Thus pain is what the individual says it is (which unfortunately excludes those without expressive language ability), irrespective of the observed physical concomitants.

One would then expect that pain would no longer be thought of in dualistic terms. That neither patients, nor clinicians would fall into the trap of assuming omniscience of the human body – for how else can we decide that a pain is 'non-organic', unless we have total understanding of all things 'organic'? Unfortunately this is not the case. Many patients and clinicians continue to find each other exasperating and disappointing, as both hold onto anachronistic models of pain. It is hoped that as chronic pain models of peripheral and central sensitisation become more widely disseminated, this mutual frustration will give way to more collaborative working between patient and health care provider.

Cognitive behavioural formulations of chronic pain: development and maintenance of the disorder

Based on the above discussion, contemporary views of the psychology of chronic pain begin with an acceptance of the patient's problem. Issues of the following are acknowledged to be extremely rare:

- *Malingering*: the intentional production of symptoms for external gain (e.g. financial benefits).
- *Factitious disorder*: the intentional production of symptoms for internal benefit (e.g. to assume the sick role).

Hence, the cognitive behavioural assessment will endeavour to explore ways in which the patient's thoughts, feelings and behaviours are contributing to maladaptive coping with the pain problem.

One of the most influential cognitive behavioural pain models in recent times has been the fear-avoidance model of chronic pain (Vlaeyen and Linton, 2000). Essentially, the model suggests that chronic pain-related disability develops as a result of erroneous, but highly anxiety provoking beliefs, held by the patient concerning pain and re-injury. Patients who believe that increases in pain are always indicators of further damage to their bodies will begin to avoid anything that might cause pain. Furthermore, patients who interpret their pain in 'catastrophic' ways ('This pain will overwhelm me. I will end up in a wheelchair. Nothing can be done to help my situation.'), will go to considerable lengths to avoid movements or activities that provoke pain. Over time, while the patient goes from health professional to health professional seeking relief from the pain; this avoidance leads to physical deconditioning and a loss of muscle and joint strength and flexibility. These beliefs also result in a somatic hypervigilance, as the patient focuses attention on internal sensations, as a way of monitoring this highly threatening situation.

With the passage of yet more time, pain is provoked because of the secondary effects of deconditioning. The patient's mood drops because of the gradual, but inevitable, loss of valued activities, such as work, leisure and sporting interests. A chronic pain syndrome is thus established. A vicious cycle of the following serve to reinforce disability and distress:

- Joint and muscle stiffness and reduced physical fitness.
- Heightened awareness of somatic processes.
- Loss of confidence and self-belief in one's capacity to improve the situation.

A growing body of literature attests to the value of the fear-avoidance model for understanding the development of chronic pain disorders (see chapter 13 regarding Vlaeyen & Linton 2000).

Psychological treatment strategies

A model such as that outlined above suggests a variety of applications of cognitive behavioural therapy (CBT) for the treatment of the chronic pain sufferer. It should be stressed however that pain management should ideally be a multidisciplinary enterprise. Recent guidelines published by the British Pain Society suggest that medical, nursing and physiotherapy involvement should be combined with clinical psychology as part of effective pain management services. Treatment may also be delivered in a variety of different formats:

- Inpatient residential programmes provide a highly intensive learning environment, where the behavioural expressions of pain can be more directly modified, with appropriately trained staff.
- Outpatient pain management is less intensive, but offers greater flexibility in terms of treatment duration, as well as the possibility of smoother generalisation of skills from the clinical setting to the home.

Whether the intervention is conducted on a group or individual basis is also a matter for consideration. However, it is usually decided on logistical rather than clinical grounds.

Most cognitive behavioural pain management interventions cover a number of core areas, as discussed below.

Information

Although information about chronic pain is unlikely to be of benefit on its own, it is vital that any patient's misinformation about pain is detected early on and an opportunity made to correct it. For example, if the patient's belief that an increase in pain always represents damage to internal structures is never addressed, it will be difficult to engage the patient in the more active aspects of pain treatment. Thus, chronic pain treatment invariably involves education regarding:

- The relationship between pain and damage.
- The influence of posture and biomechanics on muscle fatigue.
- The role of central hypersensitivity in the maintenance of ongoing pain.

Here, the input of a pain doctor is highly valuable. They not only explain these biological concepts to the patient, but give medical credibility to the self-management strategies that follow. Most patients will not have heard of pain management treatment before. Having their doctors' assurance that it is the most appropriate form of treatment for them to pursue can facilitate the treatment process considerably.

Systematic modification in activity

Underactivity/overactivity is a behavioural pattern that is often observed in the daily activity profiles of chronic pain sufferers. Where movement or activity acts as a trigger for increased pain, individuals tend to engage in prolonged periods of inactivity in order to keep discomfort at bay. However, these inactive periods are interspersed with attempts to suddenly regain normal levels of activity. This may relate to:

- Attempts to catch up on duties that have not been fulfilled during the underactive phase.
- Frustration or guilt at the inactivity.
- A misguided hope that the pain has resolved.

Whatever the underlying reason, these overactive phases inevitably lead to pain flare-ups. These then force the patient back to the inactive phase, before the cycle repeats itself. This self-defeating pattern can continue for many years, with a gradual reduction in the amount that the patient can do in the active phase.

In this case, whether underdoing or overdoing, the principles of operant behaviour therapy are relevant. Quotas of activity can be negotiated with the patient, based on time rather than on pain level or fatigue. The patient carefully monitors how much of the given activity is undertaken, and learns to terminate it before the pain level increases. Thus, the association between certain movements and increases in pain is gradually loosened. The quota is slowly but systematically increased, with a predetermined amount of activity (e.g. sitting, standing, typing) carried out each day, irrespective of how well or unwell the patient feels. As stamina and confidence build, the patient's capacity to engage in the activity on a reliable basis steadily improves.

Cognitive therapy

According to cognitive behavioural theory, one's beliefs, judgements, interpretations and predictions (i.e. one's cognitions) about any given situation are the primary determinants of the behaviours that one chooses to engage or not engage in. Patient 'catastrophising' about symptoms can trigger a cascade of emotional and behavioural responses which ultimately lead to chronic disability. Cognitive therapy therefore aims to help patients identify their maladaptive thinking patterns and develop the ability to 'challenge' these thoughts, in order to construct more helpful appraisals of their situation.

Unfortunately, the process is considerably more involved than the 'stop thinking negatively, just think positively' view, which seems to have been promoted by the self-help bibliotherapy market. Most cognitive activity occurs beneath the level of awareness. It can become as ingrained a habit as any behavioural pattern. One of the major principles of cognitive restructuring is based on the collection and evaluation of evidence: the patient objectively looking for information which disconfirms their mood-lowering beliefs. In a pain management setting, the gradual physical changes that the patient is making (e.g. sitting for longer periods, becoming more flexible in the lower back, carrying heavier loads, etc.) can be used as evidence against the catastrophic beliefs held about the underlying nature of the problem. In this way, patients are guided towards the acquisition of newer, more realistic and adaptive interpretations of their symptoms.

Relaxation training/self-hypnosis

The pain–tension–pain cycle has high face validity for many pain patients. Being in pain causes muscles to become tense; as muscle tension rises, it causes pain; this adds to the existing pain, which in turn makes the muscles more tense.

Therefore, in addition to a physiotherapy intervention (which might address the stretch and exercise aspects of pain management), basic relaxation skills can be a useful treatment component. Typically, patients are taught diaphragmatic breathing and the use of visual imagery. It is suggested that practising the skills takes place during non-flare-up time. Only once they have gained some mastery over the breathing and visualising skills should they attempt to bring them into play to actively deal with a pain flare-up. There is a considerable experimental literature detailing the benefits of hypnosis for the management of pain, in both acute and chronic forms. It is important that when used in the chronic pain setting, hypnosis is presented as another self-management technique, not something that the patient has passively 'done' to them. In these circumstances, the ability to quickly and effectively generate feelings of relaxation and well-being can be very useful. The same applies for electromyographic (EMG) biofeedback. It has empirical support to attest to its efficacy, but carries the risk of the patient attributing any benefits to the machine itself, rather than to their own actions.

Attention–diversion techniques

Teaching attention–diversion strategies to patients is not commonly done in contemporary pain management programmes. The idea of 'taking your mind off the pain' can imply that the problem is a rather trivial one, or that the patient is dwelling on it unnecessarily and requires only a little distraction to overcome it. This is unfortunate, as the gate control model gives credibility to the neurophysiology of distraction as a pain strategy. Furthermore, most patients have tried to do this themselves as best as they can. Therefore, it may be an approach that can build on their existing repertoire of skills.

It may be argued that the use of the other strategies discussed here inadvertently achieves an attention diverting effect in any case. Nevertheless, once rapport has been sufficiently established, helping the patient to engage in various activities, which may offer short-term, concentration-holding potential, is often worthwhile. The range of possible activities is endless. Some creativity is required in order to generate ideas that are meaningful to the patient – listening to music, doing light housework, doing puzzles and games, engaging others in non-pain conversation, or using the computer are just a few of the activities that patients report utilising actively. The important clinical direction is the short-term nature of the distraction. Patients should understand that they may only achieve minutes of 'blocking out the pain' at a time. However, as they continue to change from one distractor to another there is a cumulative effect.

Evidence

Empirical support for cognitive behavioural therapy (CBT) for chronic pain in adults has been steadily accruing over the past 10–15 years. The most recent meta-analysis of 25 randomised controlled trials of this intervention (by Morley and colleagues) demonstrated impressive benefits for the active treatment when compared to waiting list or no-treatment control conditions. When CBT was evaluated against other active treatments (such as conventional medical treatment, physiotherapy alone or attention placebo control conditions) significant benefits were still observed on the majority of outcome measures. These included measures of pain intensity, which is somewhat surprising, given that the intervention is designed to reduce pain-related disability, rather than pain intensity *per se*.

Outcome

Our understanding of chronic pain has shifted greatly over the past 40 years or so, from notions of psychogenic pain to biopsychosocial models. This shift has helped to release patients from a sense of blame for their problem (they have pain because they are emotionally inadequate or weak) to one of collaboration between the patient and the treating team. Pain is a dilemma for both sides, requiring considerable effort and persistence from both parties in order to be effectively managed. Psychological theories have played a key role in helping to elucidate the principles by which certain patients develop long-term disability due to pain. However, interventions for pain should involve multidisciplinary teams in order to target the multiple difficulties that chronic pain patients often present. The outcome data for CBT is promising, indicating that the strategies as outlined here can lead to important changes in patient functioning and quality of life. However, there is still a considerable way to go in refining these techniques and developing additional ones before the problem of chronic pain could be said to have been adequately addressed.

Key points

- Models of pain based on an organic versus non-organic distinction are no longer valid.
- Cognitive behavioural formulations of chronic pain highlight the role of a patient understanding of their symptoms, in the development of maladaptive behaviours.
- Pain management is a broad term encompassing a range of treatment components. Methods typically incorporated in pain management programmes include:
  - Information and education.
  - Systematic activity modification.
  - Cognitive therapy.
  - Relaxation training.
  - Attention–diversion techniques.

- The evidence base for CBT is strong. A large number of studies demonstrate the value of the intervention, when compared to other commonly delivered treatments.
- The approach is evolving. New applications of CBT are constantly coming into the pain field, enhancing existing treatment approaches.

Further reading

Eccleston, C. (2001). Role of psychology in pain management. *Br. J. Anaesth.*, **87**: 144–152.

Gamsa, A. (1994). The role of psychological factors in chronic pain. I. A half century of study. *Pain*, **57**: 5–15.

Gatchel, R.J. & Turk, D.C. (1996). *Psychological Approaches to Pain Management: A Practitioner's Handbook.* Guilford Press, New York.

Main, C.J. & Williams, A. (2002). ABC of psychological medicine: musculoskeletal pain. *Br. Med. J.*, **325**: 534–537.

Morley, S., Eccleston, C., Williams, A.C. de C. (1999). Systematic review and meta-analysis of randomized controlled trials of cognitive behaviour therapy and behaviour therapy for chronic pain in adults, excluding headache. *Pain*, **80**: 1–13.

Vlaeyen, J.W.S. & Linton, S.J. (2000). Fear-avoidance and its consequences in chronic musculoskeletal pain: a state of the art. *Pain*, **85**: 317–332.

PSYCHIATRIC DISORDERS AND PAIN 45

S. Tyrer & A. Wigham

Patients with chronic pain frequently have emotional difficulties that often amount to frank psychiatric illness. There is an increased prevalence of depression, anxiety, somatoform disorders, personality disorders and substance abuse compared with the general population. In one of the UK surveys almost a third of patients seen in a pain clinic service had symptoms sufficient to warrant a definite psychiatric diagnosis (Tyrer *et al.*, 1989). Of the patients who were psychiatrically ill, two-thirds had a depressive illness. Between 25% and 30% of women attending a gynaecological clinic have evidence of depression, and persistent chest pain in young adults (particularly exertional pain) is strongly associated with psychiatric illness. Pain and emotional illness are clearly closely related.

Classificatory schedules for psychiatric disorders in pain

There are two widely used schedules for the classification of psychiatric disorders:

- The International Classification of Diseases-Tenth Edition (ICD-10).
- The Diagnostic and Statistical Manual for Mental Disorders-Fourth Edition (DSM-IV).

The International Association for the Study of Pain (IASP) has developed its own classification for painful conditions.

As the ICD-10 is the instrument most frequently employed in Europe, the psychiatric disorders will be listed according to this system. A comparison of the diagnoses used in all three systems is shown in Table 45.1.

Specific psychiatric disorders

Depression

Depression is frequently associated with chronic pain. Between 30% and 40% of patients attending chronic pain clinics fulfil operational criteria for depression (Tyrer *et al.*, 1989). As with all psychiatric diagnoses,

studies carried out in primary care settings reveal lower levels of depression than in pain clinics.

The symptoms that suggest a depressive illness in patients with chronic pain include:

- Pervasive loss of interest and pleasure.
- Loss of appetite.
- Weight loss.
- Guilt.

Many patients with chronic pain will report poor concentration, lack of energy, feelings of being slowed down, feelings of uselessness and worthlessness, and reduced sexual interest. These symptoms are reported frequently in patients who have become depressed and who do not have physical problems. However, in somebody with chronic pain these complaints are less indicative of a depressive illness.

There is a clear relationship between pain in stress-provoking circumstances and the diagnosis of depression (Geisser *et al.*, 1996). However, it is rare for pain (except for headache and facial pain) to be a presenting symptom of a patient with a depressive illness, in the absence of any existing or past organic findings. If this is found in association with any suggestion of psychotic ideation, enquiry should be made for possible delusional beliefs involving painful stimuli (Tyrer, 1992).

Suicide is reported to be more frequent in patients with chronic pain than in the general population, although the evidence for this statement is weak. It is established that people with a previous history of deliberate self-harm, those who attend a mental health clinic or Accident & Emergency Department within the previous year, and older, isolated and male patients are all at greater risk of suicide. Nonetheless, prediction of suicide is very imprecise, in part because this act is relatively rare. In patients with persistent pain that has not responded well to treatment and who are depressed it is appropriate to ask about suicidal intent. Positive responses to questions such as 'Do you wish you would not wake up in the morning?' should be followed by 'Have you had thoughts of suicide' and

Table 45.1 Comparison of the three main schedules used in diagnosing emotional aspects of pain

Characteristic symptoms and signs	ICD-10	DSM-IV	IASP
Emotional conflict or psychosocial problems associated with pain disorder	Persistent somatoform pain disorder	Pain disorder associated with psychological factors	Monosymptomatic (if pain in single site) but can be in more than one area
Belief of definite disease, unable to accept medical reassurance	Hypochondriacal disorder	Hypochondriasis	Hypochondriacal subtype
Multiple and variable symptoms for at least 2 years	Somatisation disorder	Somatisation disorder	Multiple complaints, usually from at least five systems of the body
Depressive symptoms	Depressive episode	Major depressive episode or dysthymia	Pain associated with depression
Severe depression with delusions of: disease, torture or deserved punishment	Severe depressive episode with psychotic symptoms	Major depressive episode with psychotic features	Pain associated with depression
Delusions of physical defect, disorder or disease	Delusional disorder	Delusional disorder (somatic type)	Delusional or hallucinatory pain
Pain due to persistent muscle contraction	Psychological factors associated with diseases	Psychological factors affecting medical condition	Muscle tension pain

'Have you planned how you would do this?' An affirmative answer to this last question should be taken seriously. If there are concerns about active suicidal risk the local catchment area mental health team should be contacted as soon as possible. An immediate telephone call to the psychiatrist is advisable, both for clinical and medico-legal reasons.

Anxiety and stress-related disorders

Anxiety is the most common affect in acute pain states, but is less frequent than depression in chronic painful conditions. The anxiety disorders include generalised anxiety disorder, panic disorder, agoraphobia and social and specific phobias. These disorders are found in one-sixth to one-fourth of patients attending pain clinics (Tyrer *et al.*, 1989). The frequency of these disorders in those attending pain clinics is greater than the lifetime prevalence for the general population.

Generalised anxiety disorder

The symptoms of this disorder include a persistent feeling of being on edge and nervous. Somatic manifestations of anxiety, including: tremor, muscle tension, excessive sweating and palpitations, are often found. The evidence suggests that patients who have these symptoms following development of chronic pain have already experienced them before the onset

of the pain, but that they are exacerbated by the stress of the chronic pain experience (Polatin *et al.*, 1993).

Panic disorder

Panic disorder is manifest by severe unpredictable anxiety symptoms that are not restricted to one particular situation. The sufferer has intense fear and apprehension, often with a fear of dying. There is usually a desire to move to another place where the person believes the symptoms will be less intense. Patients with panic disorder always have intense somatic symptoms of anxiety. Unless the onset of painful symptoms was associated with high arousal for a very frightening experience (in which case the condition is classified separately as a stress disorder) it is usual to find that symptoms were present before the painful complaint.

Phobias

When anxiety symptoms occur in response to a specific situation, the term phobia is used. If these phobias are confined to a particular object or event (e.g. needles or fear of anaesthesia) they are termed specific phobias. If directly related to a fear of scrutiny in small social groups, they are classified as social phobias. Agoraphobia, the most incapacitating of the phobic disorders, is manifest by fear of leaving home and of associated anxiety in crowds. If phobic symptoms are found in patients with chronic pain, a pre-existing tendency to such disorders is usually obtained.

Post-traumatic stress disorder

Patients that have a frightening painful experience associated with a contemporaneous belief that death or severe injury may occur are prone to develop subsequent post-traumatic stress disorder (PTSD). This disorder consists of persistent, intrusive recall or re-enactment of the traumatic event in memories, dreams and flashbacks. Restriction of the emotions, avoidance of situations that might provoke memories of the trauma, and increased arousal to particular perceptual stimuli (e.g. sudden loud sounds, smell of burning) are associated symptoms. Patients with pain and PTSD have a greater degree of depression and a worse prognosis compared with those without such stress (Geisser et al., 1996). If PTSD is identified, treatment should be carried out by an experienced psychological/psychiatric team. Debriefing and superficial treatment for this condition is associated with a worse outcome than if no extra attention is paid to these patients (Mayou et al., 2000).

Adjustment disorders

Adjustment disorders comprise states of emotional distress that arise following a major life change, or resulting from a stressful life event. This distress may be shown as worry, depression or inability to cope, but the symptoms are not severe enough to reach the criterion for another psychiatric illness. These disorders usually develop within 1 month of the stressful event, with symptoms lasting less than 6 months. If they do persist, an alternative psychiatric diagnosis should be sought. These conditions are rare in a chronic pain population.

Obsessive compulsive disorder

This condition very rarely arises following the onset of pain. When it does occur it is invariably present premorbidly, although it may be exacerbated by the condition. On occasions, the patient may become excessively concerned about fear of further disease or injury. This belief is more accurately classified under the heading of hypochondriasis.

Personality disorders

There is no evidence of a consistent increase of the prevalence of personality disorders in patients with chronic pain. There are reports that patients with dependent and borderline personality disorder are found more frequently in pain clinics than would be expected by chance.

Somatoform disorders

In patients who complain of chronic pain and in whom there is insufficient evidence of physical pathology to explain the degree of pain and/or disability, the physician should always be aware of the possibility of a psychiatric illness. The group of psychiatric illnesses that comprise many of these conditions includes the somatoform disorders.

The common feature of all the somatoform disorders is the presence of physical symptoms that suggest a general medical condition, but which cannot be fully explained by this. These patients request investigations despite negative findings and re-assurance that the symptoms have no physical basis. In some patients physical disorders may have been present but these do not explain the nature and extent of the present symptoms, or the distress and pre-occupation of the patient.

People with these disorders may also show a degree of attention seeking behaviour. This is understandable if they are unable to persuade a doctor of what they believe is the essentially physical nature of their illness, or the need for further investigations or examination. Condemnation of this behaviour is not appropriate; rather careful and patient explanation of the likely origin of the symptoms is needed.

Pain is only one of the symptoms that can occur in a somatoform disorder. Other symptoms include palpitations, breathlessness, cough, aerophagy and frequency of micturition. Those somatoform disorders that are concerned with painful conditions are listed below with their ICD-10 codes.

Persistent somatoform pain disorder (F45.4)

The main complaint in this disorder is of persistent, severe and distressing pain, which cannot be explained fully by any bodily process or physical disorder, and which occurs in association with emotional conflict or psychosocial problems that are considered to be the main cause. Although this disorder is quite frequently described as occurring in patients with chronic pain, studies have found that as few as 0.3% of patients attending a chronic pain clinic had this diagnosis. Other studies have recorded a much higher prevalence of this disorder (Polatin et al., 1993) because diagnostic schedules used at the time did not require the emotional difficulties to be directly aetiologically related to the condition. This disorder may not be detected owing to lack of an adequate history. For example, a 20-year-old woman who complained of pain over the left maxilla for 3 years and for which no pathology could be found was referred to the pain clinic. During a detailed history it was found that the pain had occurred shortly after her father had slapped her on the cheek following her late return home after a date with her boyfriend. Subsequently she had gone to stay with her boyfriend and that night her father died of a heart attack. The reason for the persistence of this symptom is psychodynamically apparent in this case.

Hypochondriacal disorder (F45.2)

A patient with a hypochondriacal disorder has a belief that he or she has a serious or progressive physical disorder, persisting despite negative investigations and re-assurance from the doctor. Between 1% and 2% of patients of the general population have been found to have hypochondriacal features, which are more evident in older people. There has been no recent survey in a pain population.

Somatisation disorder (F45.0)

Somatisation disorder, or what used to be known as Briquet's syndrome, is relatively rare, but occurs in 0.5–3% of patients attending pain clinics (Tyrer et al., 1989). This is by far the most debilitating somatoform disorder. The main features of this disorder are multiple, recurrent and frequently changing physical symptoms, which have been present for many years. Most patients have a long and complicated history of contact with both primary and specialist medical care services, during which many negative investigations (or fruitless exploratory operations) may have been carried out. The majority of patients have symptoms from at least five different systems in the body. The symptoms must have led to impairment in social or occupational function. The gender ratio of patients with this condition is 5 : 1 female : male. It is important not to follow a medical model slavishly and so avoid unnecessary investigations. If symptoms are fewer and there are less social difficulties apparent, the diagnosis of undifferentiated somatoform disorder (F45.1) should be considered.

Psychoactive substance use

There is a higher rate of alcohol and analgesic misuse in patients with chronic pain. Between 12% and 28% of patients attending specialised pain clinic facilities reach the criterion for diagnosis under this category (Polatin et al., 1993). A previous history of substance misuse is often found before the onset of the painful complaint (Polatin et al., 1993) and so the development of this problem is not necessarily a result of the chronic painful symptoms. Dr Gourlay in Chapter 46 considers this condition more fully.

Effect of psychiatric disorders in chronic painful conditions

In general, anxiety and depression are a block to rehabilitation in pain. Anxiety has been found to decrease pain threshold and tolerance, and depression is associated with poorer treatment outcomes. The fear of pain and the concern about the dangers of movement causing re-injury lead to deterioration in physical capacity. In addition these fears can prevent the patient carrying out activities that may ultimately lead to a reduction in pain and increase in function. Pain-related fear and work avoidance have been found to be the most important factors accounting for disability and work loss in chronic low-back pain patients. Patients with phobic disorders and post-traumatic stress disorder have increased distress and physical symptoms affecting outcome following painful injuries (Geisser et al., 1996).

Early work on the relationship between psychiatric disorder and chronic pain postulated that persistent pain associated with emotional distress in the absence of organic findings was primarily due to a psychiatric illness. During the late 1980s and early 1990s, this psychological explanation of chronic pain was challenged. Studies that stressed the psychological origin of chronic pain were found to be of poor standard and were not supported by more stringent studies. These showed that the development of pain predates psychiatric illness (Gamsa, 1990). Moreover, patients' complaints of emotional symptoms were shown to result from the debilitating and demoralising effects of persisting pain. Thus, as pain becomes more chronic, patients develop behavioural and psychological problems because of it. In the absence of relief, there is a transition to a more severe stage of helplessness, anger and the expression of emotional difficulties in physical domains through the process of somatisation. Finally, if there is no improvement the patient becomes unable to function occupationally and becomes dependent on others.

Key points

- There is considerable comorbidity between chronic pain and psychiatric disorders.
- The effect of long-standing pain is deleterious to mental health.
- Efforts to relieve pain and distress are both helpful in reducing suffering.

References

Gamsa, A. (1990). Is emotional disturbance a precipitator or a consequence of chronic pain? *Pain*, **42**: 183–195.

Geisser, M.E., Roth, R.S., Bachman, J.E. & Eckert, T.A. (1996). The relationship between symptoms of post-traumatic stress disorder and pain, affective disturbance and disability among patients with accident and non-accident related pain. *Pain*, **66**: 207–214.

Mayou, R., Ehlers, A. & Hobbs, M. (2000). Psychological debriefing for road traffic accident victims. *Br. J. Psychiat.*, **176**: 589–593.

Polatin, P.B., Kinney, R.K., Gatchel, R.J., Lillo, E. & Mayer, T.G. (1993). Psychiatric illness and chronic low back pain. The mind and the spine – which goes first? *Spine*, **18**: 66–71.

Tyrer, S.P. (1992). Psychiatric assessment of chronic pain. *Br. J. Psychiat.*, **160**: 733–741.

Tyrer, S.P., Capon, N., Peterson, D.N., Charlton, J.E. & Thompson, J.W. (1989). The detection of psychiatric illness and psychological handicaps in a British pain clinic population. *Pain*, **36**: 63–74.

D. Gourlay

In the management of chronic non-cancer pain (CNCP), there has been considerable controversy about the prevalence of addictive disorders. Published data of addiction in pain populations has cited prevalence rates as low as 0.0003% (Porter and Jick, 1980). This has been used in support of the argument that 'addiction is so uncommon in the chronic pain patient as to not even merit looking for it'. While this statement is now largely tempered with the caveat, 'in the absence of past history of substance abuse, or increased risk', there is still a belief that addiction is not a problem in the chronic pain patient. This is clearly at odds with the prevalence of addiction within the general population; typically cited as 3–16% (Savage, 1996). One possible explanation for this is an inconsistency in the terms used to diagnose and describe addictive disorders. To this end, the Liaison Committee for Pain and Addiction (LCPA) was formed with members from the American Pain Society, the American Academy of Pain Medicine and the American Society of Addiction Medicine, to prepare acceptable definitions (Savage *et al.*, 2001; Table 46.1) for dependency, tolerance and addiction.

Diagnosis of addiction in the pain patient

The diagnosis of addictive disorders within the chronic pain population is difficult. The Diagnostic and Statistical Manual for Mental Disorders-Fourth Edition (DSM-IV) (see Chapter 45) over represents the physical phenomena associated with substance use when defining dependence. In most chronic opioid users, both withdrawal and tolerance are present and represent an expected neuro-adaptive response. The preamble to the DSM-IV states that there must be a '*maladaptive behaviour*' before applying the diagnostic criteria. Unfortunately, *maladaptive* becomes a term subject to the experience of the practitioner. Clearly when two-thirds of the diagnostic criteria for dependency (addiction) are met by the vast majority of patients on chronic opioids for pain, this tool ceases to be useful. Perhaps the most useful element of the DSM-IV

Table 46.1 Definitions

- *Addiction*: Addiction is a primary, chronic, neurobiological disease, with genetic, psychosocial and environmental factors influencing its development and manifestations. It is characterized by behaviours that include one or more of the following: impaired control over drug use, compulsive use, continued use despite harm, and craving.

- *Physical dependence*: Physical dependence is a state of adaptation that often includes tolerance. A drug class specific withdrawal syndrome that can be produced by abrupt cessation, rapid dose reduction, decreasing blood level of the drug and/or administration of an antagonist, manifests it.

- *Tolerance*: Tolerance is a state of adaptation in which exposure to a drug induces changes that result in a diminution of one or more of the drug's effects over time.

From LCPA (American Pain Society, American Academy of Pain Medicine and American Society of Addiction Medicine).

definition is 'use despite harm'. When a drug is 'doing more *to* the patient than *for* them', and yet they continue to use it, an active addictive disorder should be considered. In fact, the diagnosis of addiction is rarely made in a single assessment, but is best made prospectively over time. Fortunately, careful limit setting with the patient can lead to early recognition of problematic use of medications and allow for further assessment by an addiction medicine specialist.

Aberrant behaviours associated with the pain patient have been categorized as being more or less predictive of an addictive disorder (see Table 46.2; Portenoy, 1996). It is important to emphasize that even those behaviours considered more predictive are not pathognomonic of addiction and may occur in the context of poorly managed pain, as in 'pseudo-addiction' (Weissman and Haddox, 1989). In pseudo-addiction, inadequate treatment of pain drives aberrant behaviour. This behaviour typically resolves with more aggressive pharmacotherapy. True addiction however, tends to worsen with the addition of more drugs.

Table 46.2 The predictive nature of aberrant drug-related behaviours as they pertain to addiction (adapted from Portenoy, 1996)

More predictive	Less predictive
• Selling prescription drugs	• Aggressive complaining about the need for higher doses
• Prescription forgery	
• Stealing or 'borrowing' drugs from another patient	• Drug hoarding during periods of reduced symptoms
• Injecting oral formulations	• Requesting specific drugs
	• Prescriptions from other physicians
• Obtaining prescription drugs from non-medical sources	• Unsanctioned dose escalation
• Concurrent abuse of related illicit drugs	• Unapproved use of the drug
• Multiple unsanctioned dose escalations	• Reporting psychic effects not intended by the physician
• Repeated episodes of lost prescriptions	

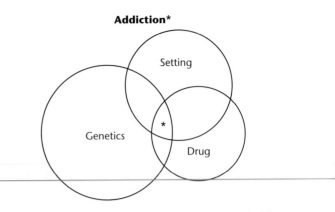

Figure 46.1 Factors influencing the development of addiction. These three overlapping circles reflect the multi-factorial nature of the disease of addiction. Only where the three elements overlap does the phenomenon of addiction occur.

Unfortunately, aberrant behaviour may be a relatively late sign of drug problems. A recent study has shown that urine drug testing (UDT) triggered by aberrant behaviour alone may miss a significant number of those patients who are misusing licit or illicit drugs (Katz and Fanciullo, 2002).

Abuse liability and addiction

Many individuals consider the opioid class of drugs as being highly addictive. There is currently no evidence in the literature to support the notion that *de novo* addiction occurs in patients without risk, through the use of opioids for the management of pain. However, there is no evidence to prove it does not occur. At the present time we simply do not know for certain. The diagnosis of addiction is made prospectively, over time. One of the problems is that an assessment of addiction risk, using such elements as past personal and family history of addictive disorders and substance abuse, is either not performed or performed poorly. Physicians unwilling to enquire around such risk often cite concerns that this may be seen as minimizing the patient's complaint of pain.

At the present time, it appears that where a drug with abuse liability is used in the right setting with an at-risk individual, that the phenomenon of addiction may occur (Figure 46.1). In this context, patients with increased risk who suffer from chronic painful conditions may express a previously undiagnosed addictive

disorder, which will make the management of chronic pain even more complicated.

Addiction and dependency

To illustrate the difference between addiction and dependency, we can consider the case of the diabetic whose blood sugar is controlled using insulin. The discontinuation (withdrawal) of insulin results in a characteristic constellation of symptoms including excessive thirst, fatigue, weakness, polyuria and blurred vision, which may ultimately lead to coma and death. The addition of insulin reverses these symptoms. The patient could be considered insulin dependent, but is unlikely to be labelled an insulin addict. In the same way, persons who chronically use opioids manifest a characteristic constellation of symptoms upon discontinuation of those drugs, which remit with the reintroduction of the drug or another member of that class. The terms physical dependence and addiction are not interchangeable.

Assessment of the chronic pain patient

Apart from the typical workup for chronic pain (as discussed elsewhere in this text) several areas of enquiry can help identify problematic use of medications, as well as risk of past or present addictive disorders. Because undiagnosed addictive disorders affect multiple medical and psychiatric conditions (i.e. hypertension, diabetes, depression) it is important to do a thorough addictions enquiry in all patients, not simply those in whom strong opioids are considered.

Prescription drug use

Clearly identify past and present medications, time of last use, degree of effectiveness and any observed side effects. In particular, assess the role of short-acting immediate-release agents, which can lead to opioid-abstinence hyperalgesia (Li *et al.*, 2001). This is evidenced by withdrawal-mediated exacerbations of pain, often seen in the morning when opioid levels are at their lowest. Over reliance on short-acting, immediate-release opioids or a refusal to try sustained-release preparations, can be particularly problematic in this regard. A strong preference for opioids with higher abuse liability, such as hydromorphone, needs to be treated with caution. Although it may be quite appropriate for a patient to ask for a drug that has worked in the past, a preference for certain drugs, such as injectable or even oral pethidine, should be seen as problematic.

Enquire into:

- Lost or stolen medications.
- Early refills.
- Polypharmacy.
- Use of sedatives and stimulants.
- Problems controlling use of prescribed medications.
- Double doctoring, to obtain more medications than prescribed.

Short dispensing intervals of limited quantities of drug strongly suggest concerns by the current prescriber about medication control. Permission to contact previous healthcare providers should be sought and efforts made to communicate with other treatment providers. A patient's reluctance or refusal to allow access to past medical information is a relative contraindication to chronic opioid therapy.

Family history

Careful documentation of family history of drug and alcohol use (going back as far as three generations) can be useful in assessing risk. Alcohol problems commonly skip generations and may not be evident in a more cursory review.

Personal psychiatric history

Past history of major psychiatric or personality disorders (the DSM axis I and II disorders), particularly major depressive illness and antisocial personality disorder, increase risk significantly. Previous treatment of either drug or alcohol problems, past suicide attempts and histories of sexual abuse should be noted. The triad of sexual abuse, eating disorder and addiction is not uncommon and increases the complexity of any course of treatment. When two items of this triad are seen, the third should be sought.

Personal substance use history

It must be explicitly stated to the patient that honest answers to questions about drug and alcohol use will not lead to dismissal from the practice or a refusal to treat with appropriate medications. It is necessary to explore and document detailed questions around:

- Alcohol use (including 24 hours maximum consumption).
- Blackouts.
- Withdrawal seizures.
- Consequences of use (e.g. driving while impaired, charges/convictions) assaults (by or against the patient), employment difficulties and even domestic problems.

Illicit drug use, including both street and pharmaceutical agents should be assessed. Routes of administration vary, even with oral prescription drugs. Cannabis (marihuana) is often not thought of by patients as either a street drug or an illicit drug, and needs separate questioning.

A detailed history of time of last use can be helpful, especially when interpreting a UDT. Evidence of undisclosed drug use, especially cocaine, is a strong contraindication to the prescription of opioids for CNCP.

In some cases, the patient may reveal a past drug history that has been treated. In this case, it is important to detail the patient's programme of recovery and their current level of stability. It should be remembered that while it is possible to treat chronic pain in a patient with a treated addictive disorder, it is difficult to treat chronic pain in a patient with an *active untreated* addiction. In order to solve either problem, both typically need to be simultaneously addressed. Refusal by a pain patient to address a concurrent addictive disorder is a strong contraindication to the use of chronic opioid therapy.

Physical examination and laboratory work

The physical examination of a person with an active drug problem may show evidence of drug use, but typically does not. It is worth examining the common sites of injection, including the antecubital fossa and interdigital web spaces. Poorly healing wounds are commonly seen in the malnourished addict or chronic cocaine user. The stigmata of chronic alcohol abuse, such as hepatic enlargement, palmar erythema, spider angiomata over the chest and shoulders, muscle wasting and testicular atrophy and gynaecomastia (in men) should be assessed.

In terms of laboratory investigations, liver enzyme tests (alanine aminotransferase, aspartate aminotransferase, gamma glutamic transpeptidase) with hepatitis screen where indicated and full blood count (elevated mean corpuscular volume suggesting chronic alcohol abuse) can be useful. The most common cause of hepatitis C infection in North America is injection drug abuse. A baseline UDT can be very useful when beginning treatment with opioids and when there is concern about consistency of the clinical history. Periodic random UDTs can be useful tools to advocate on behalf of your patient. In those patients with a history of past drug addiction or abuse, UDT can be helpful to enhance and support change to a non-drug-using life style.

Managing risk

When deciding to treat CNCP with strong opioids, the practitioner must clearly evaluate the suitability of any given patient based on such factors as:

- The nature of the pain complaint.
- Past patient history.
- Comfort with using strong opioids.
- Resources available within the doctor's practice.

Patients typically fall into one of three categories (Gourlay and Heit, 2005):

- Group I – *Primary care patient*: This is a patient who is relatively uncomplicated by personal or family history of major addictive disorders or psychopathology. Reasonably set boundaries are maintained. The vast majority of patients fall into this category and are usually managed without problems.
- Group II – *Primary care patient requiring some specialist support*: Certain patients, with past history of either treated addictive disorders or significant psychopathology, may benefit from opioid therapy. An initial consultation with a specialist knowledgeable in addiction medicine may be helpful in setting tighter boundaries. Having repeat consultations with, or concurrent management by, an addiction medicine specialist, may improve outcomes.
- Group III – *Referral to specialist care – patient suffers from active untreated additive disorder*: A minority of pain patients are complicated by active addictive disorders, or poorly managed psychopathology that makes management in the primary care setting unwise. In these cases, referral to a multi-disciplinary pain programme for assessment and management is recommended.

Table 46.3 Elements of a successful trial of opioid therapy ('Universal Precautions' approach (Gourlay and Heit, 2005))

1 Accurate diagnosis (with differential)
2 Detailed psychological assessment to assess risk of addictive disorders
3 Rational non-opioid therapeutic trial
4 Pre-trial assessment of pain/function
5 Informed consent (verbal versus written/signed)
6 Treatment agreement (verbal versus written/signed)
7 Careful, time limited trial of opioid therapy
8 Re-assessment of pain/function and diagnosis
9 Regular assessment of aberrant behaviour
10 Documentation

Trial of opioid therapy

In the majority of cases, chronic pain can be managed without the use of strong opioids. However, once the decision is made to introduce strong opioids, several things need to be in place to reduce risk and improve chances of a successful trial (Table 46.3). Ultimately, if there is no clear evidence of improvement, plans to carefully remove the patient from opioids should be explored. In tapering the patient off opioids, every effort must be made to avoid withdrawal symptoms, which will almost certainly worsen the perception of pain, even in pain states not particularly responsive to opioids.

Although it is tempting to believe that poorly controlled pain on opioid therapy would only deteriorate without opioids, this is often not the case. The importance of careful and thorough documentation to justify the effectiveness of treatment and the reasonableness of continuation of opioid therapy without dose escalation cannot be overstated.

Choice of opioids

In selecting a strong opioid, one should consider the various options carefully. It is useful to divide the opioids into truly long- and short-acting agents. Short-acting agents can be further subdivided into immediate- and controlled-release preparations. Examples of long-acting agents include methadone, levorphanol and the partial μ opioid receptor (MOP) agonist, buprenorphine. Short-acting agents include codeine, dihydrocodeine, hydrocodone, oxycodone, morphine, hydromorphone, oxymorphone and fentanyl (to name a few). Codeine, morphine, hydromorphone, oxycodone and fentanyl have been marketed in controlled-release packaging to improve compliance, effect stable drug blood levels and reduce both tolerance and abuse liability of these drugs.

In general, it is recommended that short-acting, immediate-release agents be used initially until effective pain control is achieved. They are then converted into an equivalent controlled-release formulation as the mainstay of opioid therapy. Regular use of breakthrough doses may be used as the modified release agent is titrated to optimal effect. Overreliance on breakthrough medication is to be avoided. Regular use of breakthrough doses should be added to the controlled-release regimen until reliance on breakthrough doses is minimized or eliminated.

Assessing opioid responsiveness

In some cases, there is a particular focus by the patient on the use of short-acting immediate-release preparations. There may be a variety of reasons for this including, but not limited to, substance abuse. In some cases, the desire for the drug is fuelled by economic factors related to drug diversion for profit. In others there is a need to feel the euphoric effects of the onset of the drug.

For those patients whose pain is not particularly opioid responsive, there may be a tendency to define effectiveness in terms of 'feeling the drug', rather than feeling the analgesic effect of the drug. In such cases, it is the mild impairment felt with the onset of the drug and to a lesser extent, the offset effects, that reinforces the continued use of the medication. Since we expect tolerance to occur to these effects, the patient may describe a diminished effect over time, culminating in the patient stating that they 'no longer feel the drug working'. This may be temporarily improved by a dose increase, but the effects are often short lived. Eventually the patient may indicate that the medication does not take the pain away, but that 'it just takes the edge off'. In this setting, discontinuation of the opioid may be indicated, but should be undertaken carefully so as to avoid withdrawal-mediated exacerbations of pain.

Tips for a successful trial

- Avoid excessive use of short-acting, immediate-release opioids.
- Limit prescription of medications initially to 1 or 2 weeks at a time. As the patient's response to these medications becomes better known, monthly dispensing is reasonable. While the quantity of medication prescribed should be sufficient to last slightly beyond the next appointment (to ensure an adequate supply of drug), interval dispensing ('part fills') can be a useful tool to assist with medication monitoring. The dispensing pharmacist can play a vital role in this regard.

- UDT should be considered: at the beginning of therapy, when pain persists despite adequate doses of opioid medication, when considering major changes in pharmacotherapy, in response to any aberrant behaviour and randomly during treatment. In a stable patient, testing randomly once or twice per year may be adequate. Refusal to provide a specimen for UDT should be viewed as a relative contraindication to continued prescription of controlled substances, requiring referral to someone knowledgeable in diagnosis and treatment of addictive disorders.
- A complete medical assessment may require communicating with past treatment providers. Any patient who attempts to limit such communication should be assessed by a substance abuse professional. Where possible, verify functional stability through collateral support by other caregivers, as well as the patient's significant others.

Acute on chronic pain

In the management of acute pain in the context of the chronic opioid user, it is important to recognize that previous daily intake of opioids does not contribute to acute pain management and may make the patient more sensitive to the perception of pain (Doverty *et al.*, 2001). It is important to maintain an adequate basal level of opioids, so as not to incur an 'opioid debt'. Opioid-dependent patients with acute pain need to have opioids in excess of their usual daily requirements to effect analgesic relief. Failure to do so may result in an 'opioid debit' which will frustrate any attempts to manage acute pain.

Key points

- An inadequate assessment of concurrent risk around substance abuse and dependency can lead to poor patient outcomes and unnecessary risk to both patient and practitioner alike.
- A minimum and uniform level of enquiry in all patients, a so called 'universal precautions' approach to pain management, may yield valuable information, allowing the early identification of any concurrent addictive disorder possible.
- The treatment of pain in the context of an active addictive disorder may wisely be left to those practitioners with more experience and greater resources.
- By careful patient assessment, the spectre of iatrogenic addiction in the management of chronic pain should no longer be a barrier to effective treatment.

References

Doverty, M., *et al.* (2001). Hyperalgesic responses in methadone maintenance patients. *Pain* **90**: 91–96.

Gourlay, D.L., Heit, H.A. & Almahrezi, A. (2005). Universal Precautions in Pain Medicine: a rational approach to the treatment of chronic pain. *Pain Medicine*, 6.

Gourlay, D.L., Heit, H.A. & Caplan, Y. (2002). Pharmacom Grp. Monograph for California Academy of Family Physicians. *Urine Drug Testing in Primary Care: dispelling the myths & designing strategies.*

Heit, H.A. & Gourlay, D.L. (2004). Urine Drug Testing in pain Medicine. *J Pain and Symptom Management*, **27**: 260–267.

Katz, N. & Fanciullo, G.J. (2002). Role of urine toxicology testing in the management of chronic opioid therapy. *Clin. J. Pain*, **18**: S76–S82.

Li, X., Angst, M.S., *et al.* (2001). Opioid-induced hyperalgesia and incisional pain. *Anesth. Analg.*, **93**: 204–209.

Portenoy, R.K. (1996). Opioid therapy for chronic nonmalignant pain: a review of the critical issues. *J. Pain Sympt. Manag.*, **11**: 203–217.

Porter, J. & Jick, H. (1980). Addiction rare in patients treated with narcotics. *New. Engl. J. Med.*, **302**: 123.

Savage, S.R. (1996). Long-term opioid therapy: assessment of consequences and risks. *J. Pain Sympt. Manag.*, **11**: 274–286.

Savage, S., Covington, E.C., Heit, H.A., *et al.* (2001). Definitions related to the use of opioids for the treatment of pain. In: *Consensus Document from the American Academy of Pain Medicine* (Glenview, IL), *The American Pain Society* (Glenview, IL) and *The American Society of Addiction Medicine* (Chevy Chase, MD); 2001

Weissman, D.E. & Haddox, J.D. (1989). Opioid pseudoaddiction – an iatrogenic syndrome. *Pain*, **36**: 363–366.

A. Kent

What is the family's role in children's pain? Can the family increase, decrease or change the nature or the experience of pain? Can the family create and extinguish pain? If such things are possible, then the reason for pain goes beyond the merely physical factors of site, size and nature of insult, and is seen to be the result of an interpretative process rather than direct perception. The way the family functions and communicates are factors to be taken into account. Formats for pain management in a family setting vary from in-group to individual family sessions.

Pain of organic origin

Family support

Child

While there are many different family scenarios, the most straightforward is dealing with obvious medical or physical pain in the context of an open and well functioning family.

Scenario 1

When I first saw Dennis in the waiting room he was the very picture of misery, softly crying with persistent pain as he sat hunched and drooping on the seat. His skin (red all over) and hair (standing up in spikes with all the grease that had been spread on his scalp) were the external complications of his severe eczema. The severe skin itch worried him 24 h a day, as he slept poorly and scratched all night. Inadequate sleep led to him being tired and listless during the day, uninterested in school or friends. The first hypnotherapy session saw no immediate change in his superficial state. However, he was co-operative and agreed to carry out the programme set for him to work on at home from the week until he was seen again. To enable him to 'remove pain from his skin' he was taught stage one of self-hypnosis.

When seen a week later he was virtually unchanged. Dennis and his mother were taught stage two of self-hypnosis. He was instructed to hypnotise himself daily with his mother's help.

Two weeks after this session a radical change occurred. Dennis bounced up the corridor to the therapy room, full of energy. His mother was astounded. Each night she had helped him go into a deep painless sleep with hypnosis, allowing sleep without scratching for 8 h. After a night of peace the skin itch lessened and he scratched less during the day. Day by day the skin had improved and all the time his parents helped him keep the treatment programme going. Finally, he was taught how to remove the itch while awake, using self-hypnosis. Now there was no need to scratch and slowly his skin became a normal colour.

The parental role in Scenario 1 was to be supportive. A child in the degree of pain Dennis had would not find the will and discipline to practice a daily routine without considerable support. This family had the norm for family dynamics; the parents were in charge. Dennis was comfortable in the role of child and accepted his parent's discipline.

Points in management

1 Hypnosis can be effective in reducing physical pain.
2 Normal parental discipline can support a child and mediate pain treatment programmes.
3 Involving children in their pain management increases their perception of control and decreases the perception of pain.
4 Parents have the power to lessen the experience of pain. Even very young children (and small babies and neonates) can be helped using age appropriate techniques.

When children have reached the age of reasoning the meaning of pain is all-important. Children who are receiving unpleasant treatment can profit by visualising the treatment benefiting their bodies. Thus, children may visualise, or draw a picture of chemotherapy as mini monsters gobbling up cancer cells, defeating the disease. The positive feelings about the treatment may make them more willing to put up with the unpleasant aspects. This 'reframing' the discomforts of treatment (e.g. needles) allows it to be seen positively.

Parents help is vital as they will know how to guide their children's imagination.

Neonate

Neonates experience pain and distress. Though we now know much more about analgesia for neonates, not everyone realises the benefits of parental contact. Hearing develops early in fetal life and experiments have shown that after birth babies have memory for music and sound heard while in the womb. This includes memory for parents' voices heard when they were *in utero* and totally comfortable. In young and sick babies distress is reduced as they respond positively to parents voices. Another stress reducer is kangaroo care, with the parent having the tiny baby in skin-to-skin contact on their chest, helping relaxation. While suffering organic pain the parents voices and touch produce relaxation, hence decreasing the experience of pain and improving the child's condition.

Assessment of family support

It is most important to consider the meaning and consequences of pain for the sufferer, as well as seeing who is complaining about pain. Obvious expectations of the medical team are:

1 The child is complaining of pain.
2 The child requires pain relief.
3 The family wants normal life to be resumed.

However, these assumptions may be at odds with the real agenda of the individuals or family involved. A flexible approach to assessment is required:

1 While interviewing a family, note who answers the questions and how they answer. Does the child answer a question directed at him/her, does the mother answer, or does the child look to the parent for apparent permission to answer before speaking? In open families, with normal family dynamics, the child is allowed to answer freely. If the parent is apparently controlling or censoring information, the reason and family functioning should be explored. Difficult relations which could contribute to pain should be explored.
2 What is being requested? Is it actually medication, or rather investigation and treatment? Does the request appear reasonable? Do parent and child want the same goals?
3 Are requests going to result in the child quickly returning to everyday life, or will they result in more intervention than seems necessary? What does the child think is needed?

When the answers are clear then the case is straightforward. Confused answers suggest a confused family, where additional factors may be determining the child's pain.

Family dynamics and psychogenic pain

The role of the family in their children's pain is fascinating. The family has to be viewed as a whole, since family dynamics and characteristics may maintain pain behaviours.

Psychogenic pain may occur alone or in conjunction with organic pain. A low threshold for a psychosocial assessment to investigate possible contributions to pain should be maintained, if an obvious cause for the pain in a child is lacking.

Family dynamics often differ between families where there is physical pain and where there is psychogenic pain. When the clinician first meets the family there is frequently limited information available. Initial interview may elicit clues about how the family works and the nature of the pain presentation.

When no physical cause can be found for pain, then psychogenic pain should be considered. Pain descriptions may help. The description of physical pain may be precise in location, nature and frequency. By contrast, psychogenic pain is often imprecise. Location may be variable, widespread or diffuse and its nature less easy to describe.

The frequency and timing of the pain may provide much important information. A pain diary can demonstrate a periodic (e.g. weekly) pattern to pain, or its association with particular events.

Scenario 2 demonstrates how the focus of treatment was not the presenting pain, but the root cause, which was expressed as pain. Parental disharmony was the cause, pain the consequence.

Scenario 2

This was a puzzling case as the pain diary showed episodes of two to three consecutive days of pain scattered over the records. There was no Monday morning feelings of school refusal, rather there appeared to be a trigger effect with episodes always separated by several days. History taking included information regarding parental work patterns. Mother had regular hours, but father had a 10-day cycle, with 'weekends' happening at any time of the week. Examining the history revealed that all pain episodes occurred when both parents were at home. Further investigation disclosed that they rowed loudly and flung threats at each other. In this case counselling for the couple and restoring parental harmony, was in due course effective at removing the child's pain.

Family cognition and attitudes to pain

Family attitudes and reactions to pain may govern whether a pain symptom is induced. Familial and cultural attitudes to pain vary greatly between families. A child will quickly learn if a complaint of pain produces a positive reaction.

The meaning of pain to most people is that 'there is something wrong', 'pain is natures' warning' and 'action should be taken'. However, in complex systems (like families) pain may not be a warning, but rather a way of improving a person's position. Pain may result in a special status, or less demands being put on the sufferer. It was thought that disability was the consequence of chronic pain, but many now believe that disability arises from the reaction of others to pain (e.g. 'Oh poor thing, you just sit there, everything will be done for you').

A satisfying response to the complaint of pain will actually increase the pain experience. Thus, an over solicitous reaction is unlikely to improve the pain, or the patient's lifestyle. Nowadays, treatment with psychological approaches (e.g. relaxation and cognitive behaviour therapy) offers patients the chance to be in control of managing pain, so they can get better with honour. Unfortunately, some patients are hostile to approaches that place demands on them.

Dysfunctional families

Pain in dysfunctional families is often subtle and lacks logic. At first sight it may be difficult to see how there is any benefit from the pain. Some spin offs may be easy to work out (e.g. not having to do homework). But if a socially easy child has pain causing him to stay away from school, friends, normal life and sport, what advantage can there be? One answer is that the child fears what will happen to him at school or what may happen at home in his absence (Scenario 3).

Scenario 3

Darren had limb pain, one leg and the opposite arm. He was unable to go to school as the pain in his right arm prevented him writing. It had been suggested by staff that he just go and listen to the lessons, they would not make him write. He refused saying 'his leg gave away at odd times and he could not go into a crowded school with all those people about'. The pain problem was recent. Only a couple of terms previously his parents had moved him from a quiet country school to the urban academically successful school near their home (so close that he could have gone in for just a few lessons if necessary).

The pain remained bad, but he worked hard for the home tutor with no apparent writing problem. It emerged that he feared going to school. He could not keep up with the rest of the class and they made fun of him. The history evolved that his parents had not consulted Darren in advance about changing schools, or thought about his needs and preferences. His good peer group relationships at the country school were obvious from all the phone calls and visits he received. They reflected the emotional support he was no longer getting at school. He clearly felt more supported by his friends than his family. On pain team review, arrangements were made for his return to the country school and shortly thereafter Darren reported the pain was improving. He achieved full recovery in 2–3 months.

Points in management
Pain may be environmental, only occurring in one place.

1 Major changes of circumstances may precede the onset of pain.
2 Pain can resolve once feared stimuli are removed.
3 Psychosocial assessment is essential.
4 Pain may be an escape or avoidance behaviour.

One of the often-noticeable features of dysfunctional families is their dysfunctional and unclear communication. Particularly imprecise pain is often a reflection of family factors. To a child, family is all-important. The child relies on the family attention and support for survival and emotional growth. If paediatricians cannot find an organic reason for a child's pain they may refer to a pain specialist, to explore non-physical reasons for the pain. Such reasons are often viewed by adults as illogical, but seen from the child's perspective they are perfectly logical.

Scenario 4

Mary had wandering abdominal pain for which no reason could be found by the paediatricians. Her family consisted of hard working parents and siblings (Mary and Susie). Mary was comfortably settled in her school and performing reasonably well, while at home she was a quiet helpful child. Susie was very different, lively, fun, apt to get into trouble at school for being slapdash and mad about gymnastics. Family life revolved around Susie's gymnastics practice and competitions. It was well organised and practical; it had to be to fit everything in. During the pain assessment sessions Mary sat very close to her mother, often reaching out and touching her. Her mother responded affectionately, remarking how seldom they got time together. This gesture was a cue to the pain team to enable the parents to examine their time allocation to each of the girls. The parents realised that only attending to Mary while doing the washing up did not meet Mary's emotional needs. The pain was rooted in a lack of emotional support. From then on dedicated individual time from her parents allowed her to grow emotionally and to outgrow her need for pain.

Points in management

1 Children need emotional support for physical and emotional growth and development.
2 Psychogenic pains can be resistant to medical and mental health treatment and take large amount of professional time.

Pain of mixed origin

Scenario 5

James had to face major cardiac surgery. During the preparatory period he was clearly afraid and complained of pain from his condition. He was however avid for information. Initially he was so afraid that he would not enter the cardiac department. Gradually, over several sessions, he was slowly introduced to the department, equipment and staff. His fear diminished, so when he was asked if he would like to see the anaesthetic room and theatre, he replied enthusiastically 'Oh Yes'. His mother's reaction was quite different; she had gone rigid in her chair and very pale. Affected by the presence of a calm and confident therapist, James was confident. The adult affected him, but it was clear where the fear and increased pain had come from – his mother, he had picked up her fear.

Points in management

Parental fears of conditions, pain or treatment, increase the child's perception of pain.

1 Familial or cultural beliefs influence the experience of pain.
2 All pain has a psychological component. Both affective and cognitive factors are present.

At the beginning of this chapter the question was asked whether the family could increase, decrease, cause or extinguish pain? In Scenario 1 organic pain was more or less relieved. In neonates it was explained how pain and distress can be reduced. With Scenario 2 organic pain was increased. With psychogenic pain the rowing family demonstrated how

psychogenic pain could be initiated, and with Scenario 4 we examined how psychogenic pain could be extinguished. These cases demonstrate the influential role of the family in pain symptoms, and how parents have a vital role to play in the 'partnership of care'. Another example is the case where psychogenic pain can overload or exacerbate organic pain.

Pain exists when the sufferer says it exists and to the level they describe. However, pain is a complex concept with strong family connections that affect all aspects of life. Fortunately once the basis for the pain is understood it is often possible to treat, using pharmacological and/or non-pharmacological treatment. Although it appears that divisions occur in this chapter between organic and non-organic pain, all pain has a psychological component of which affective and cognitive factors are often present.

Managing the parents

A sick child's parents may need the opportunity to talk to someone about their feelings. But, families have different needs at varying times. They may:

- Feel isolated and be suffering emotional psychological pain.
- Be reluctant to take up scarce medical time. It is important to make special provision and discuss parental fears.
- Benefit from sharing feelings with others in a similar position.

Key points

- When working with adults, the patient and the consent giver/decision-maker are one and the same person. When working with children the patient and the consent giver/decision-maker are two separate people, who may have divergent views and agendas.
- The difference between adults and children as patients is that:
  - The adult is voluntarily the patient.
  - Conversely, the child is involuntarily and at times unwillingly the patient.
- The child is an inseparable member of a family, so assess and treat the child and/or the family.
- Harness the strengths within the family for the benefit of the child.
- Psychological/non-pharmacological techniques of pain management work well in children.

Further reading

Dodds, E. (2003). Neonatal procedural pain: a survey of nursing staff. *Paediatr. Nurs.*, **5**: 18.

Duff, L., Louw & McCleary (1999). Clinical guidelines for the recognition and assessment of acute pain in children. *Paediatr. Nurs.*, **6**: 18–21.

Eccleston, C., Morley, S., Williams, A., Yorke, L. & Mastroyannopoulou, K. (2002). Systematic review of randomised controlled trials of psychological therapy for chronic pain in children and adolescent, with a subset meta-analysis of pain relief. *Pain*, **99(1–2)**: 157–165.

Hogan, M., Choonarat, *et al.* (1996). Measuring pain in neonates: an objective score. *Paediatr. Nurs.*, **10**: 24–27.

McClarey, M., Duff, L. & Louw, G. (1999). Recognition and assessment of pain in children. *Paediatr. Nurs.*, **6**: 15–17.

S. Lund & S. Cox

In 1990 the World Health Organization defined palliative care as *'The active total care of patients whose disease is not responsive to curative treatment. Control of pain, of other symptoms, and of psychological, social and spiritual problems, is paramount. The goal of palliative care is achievement of the best quality of life for patients and their families'*. These words describe how modern palliative care has developed from the passive accompanying of dying patients, to a more dynamic multidisciplinary approach which attempts to address priorities from an individual's perspective. It recognizes that patients deserve to receive such care even at early stages of their illness and that palliative care is relevant to patients both with cancer and other diseases. It emphasizes the need to support the family and carers and to continue that support into bereavement. The overarching concept is that of enabling people to 'live well' despite having a fatal diagnosis (Table 48.1).

Specialist palliative care requires a team approach to identify and address the issues that have a negative impact on the patient's quality of life. Specialist palliative care teams are now available as a resource to most hospitals, primary care teams and specialist inpatient units or hospices. Here, in addition to doctors and nurses, a wide range of disciplines with specialist expertise are collected. Social workers are essential to help with such complex problems as psychosocial counselling, financial and housing issues, immigration, preparing young families for loss and bereavement support. Occupational therapists help patients to cope with (sometimes) rapidly increasing disability and may enable patients to remain in their own homes for longer. Physiotherapists are essential to maximize mobility, to teach relaxation techniques and non-pharmacological management of breathlessness. They may be supported by psychologists, spiritual advisors, art and music therapists, dieticians, pharmacists, complementary therapists and volunteers.

Symptom control

Advancing disease is associated with the experience of symptoms that can be associated with suffering. Most research in this area relates to patients with cancer. However, reviews have also been carried out in other populations, including those with severe heart failure, advanced respiratory disease and HIV-associated disease. Symptom reviews vary enormously depending on:

- Stage of disease.
- Methodological issues.
- Populations studied (i.e. inpatient or outpatient).

The prevalence of symptoms in different disease states does vary, but it is of interest that distressing symptoms are common in non-malignant diseases as well as cancer (Table 48.2). This supports the argument for palliative care services to be offered to all patients (regardless of diagnosis), on the basis of need.

Principles of symptom management

The steps that should be considered to control symptoms are shown in Table 48.3. Individual psychological and social factors impact on the experience and expression of symptoms. The knowledge that life may be short, with symptoms potentially representing progressing disease, increases the distress associated

---

Table 48.1 Key principles of palliative care (National Council of Hospices and Specialist Palliative Care Services, 1995)

- Focus on quality of life, which includes good symptom control
- Whole-person approach taking into account the person's past life experience and current situation
- Care, which encompasses both the person with the life-threatening disease and those that matter to that person
- Respect for patient autonomy and choice (e.g. over treatment options, place of care)
- Emphasis on open and sensitive communication which extends to patients, informal carers and professional colleagues

Table 48.2 Prevalence of distressing symptoms reported retrospectively by carers in the last year of life (Addington-Hall *et al.*, 1998)

Symptom	Cancer population (%)	Non-cancer population (%)
Pain	71	72
Dyspnoea	63	64
Persistent cough	50	42
Dry mouth	43	34
Anorexia	33	21
Difficulty swallowing	63	53
Nausea/vomiting	66	50
Constipation	65	69
Confusion	42	44
Insomnia	44	45
Low mood	67	73

Table 48.3 Principles of symptom management

- Symptom assessment
- Diagnosis of cause
- Explanation
- Treatment of the cause
- Symptomatic treatment

with them. Explanation and reassurance where appropriate can therefore be very helpful. Patients and their families appreciate being involved in decisions around symptomatic treatment. They may feel that they have lost control of much else which happens to them.

Symptomatic or palliative management embraces an enormous range of interventions, from the teaching of breathing techniques to disease-modifying management, such as surgery. The common intention with such treatment is not to cure the patient, but rather to make them feel better – if only for a while. Decisions about investigations and treatment must be appropriate for the individual situation. Some patients may be too unwell to tolerate, or benefit from, specific treatments. In these situations treatment should be geared towards comfort measures. Patients will often have multiple problems and can be involved in prioritizing them.

Symptom assessment

Accurate symptom assessment is essential to identify the cause and appropriate treatment. It is important to recognize that not all symptoms will be a direct result of the disease process. Some will occur as a result of general debility; others will be side effects of

treatment, but symptoms may also arise incidentally from unconnected pathologies. A detailed symptom history and examination may reveal a recognized pattern, pointing to a cause. This will guide appropriate investigations and treatment. Table 48.4 illustrates this process using causes of vomiting in advanced cancer as an example. In patients with advanced disease, investigations should only be carried out if they will influence management. If an individual is too frail to receive treatment for a specific problem, then invasive tests to diagnose that problem are usually not warranted.

Disease-modifying palliative treatment

Disease-modifying treatments may be helpful to palliate symptoms even when cure is no longer possible. In advanced malignancy chemotherapy, radiotherapy, hormone treatments and surgery may all be appropriate under certain circumstances. It is important when considering such palliative treatments to balance potential benefit with adverse effects. In a patient with haemoptysis from a lung cancer, radiotherapy or laser brachytherapy may offer the best relief and might be considered even in a frail individual. Surgery should also be considered. For example, in a patient with pathological hip fracture who may not be able to roll to have a regional anaesthetic block, surgical fixation stands the best chance of controlling pain. In the palliation of non-malignant disease, this principle also applies. A patient with end-stage chronic renal failure who has accepted that they are dying may chose to continue disruptive trips to hospital several times a week for haemodialysis in order to prevent unpleasant symptoms.

Symptomatic treatment

In many cases, treating underlying disease is not possible or does not itself control symptoms. Symptomatic treatment is then required. This may be:

a Pharmacological (Table 48.4).
b Non-pharmacological (Table 48.5).
c A combination of the two.

Symptom control will often require drug therapy, which should be tailored to the cause of the symptom. There are several basic principles that should guide all prescriptions for symptoms in patients with advanced disease:

a Any persistent symptoms require therapy to be taken regularly, rather than as required, in order to prevent symptom occurring.

Table 48.4 Tailoring the symptomatic treatment to the cause: some causes of vomiting in advanced cancer

Cause	Pattern	Receptors involved/site of emetic stimulation	Preferred treatment	Comment
Malignant hypercalcaemiaa or uraemia	Predominant nausea, drowsiness, confusion	Dopamine/5HT3 receptors, in the chemoreceptor trigger zone	Haloperidol	Useful as once daily, can be given sub-cutaneously
Malignant bowel obstruction	Abdominal distension, vomiting, constipation, pain	Vagal effects	Cyclizine ±, haloperidol ±, somatostatin analogue	More effective than 'drip and suck', unless patient having surgery
Gastric outflow obstruction	Large volume effortless vomiting, little nausea	Dopamine/5HT4 receptors, vagal effects	Metoclopromide, domperidone	Occurs with pancreatic and gastric cancer, associated with ascites and hepatomegaly
Raised intracranial pressure	Morning vomiting, headache, focal signs	Pressure receptors	Cyclizine, corticosteroids	
Anxiety	Nausea ±, vomiting	? GABA in cerebral cortex	Anxiolytics (e.g. benzodiazepines)	
Cough	Retching with cough	Pharynx	Antitussives (e.g. codeine linctus)	

Table 48.5 Examples of non-pharmacological treatment approaches

- Relaxation techniques – for attacks of breathlessness
- Positioning in bed – to relieve retained secretions
- Dietary modifications – for dysphagia
- Mobility aids – for weakness
- Acupuncture or acupressure – for nausea
- Transcutaneous electrical nerve stimulation (TENS) – for pain

b Each new drug should be perceived to have benefits which outweigh potential side effects or burdens (in the context of the patient's condition).

c An attempt should be made to limit the number of drugs taken in order to improve adherence.

d Drugs that are less likely to help in the short term (e.g. statins) should be stopped.

e *If a patient is suffering nausea and vomiting then an alternate route of administration may be required.*

f Identifying the cause for a particular symptom allows specific symptomatic treatment to be chosen.

Table 48.4 illustrates this using vomiting as an example. Different causes of vomiting involve different receptor groups and are best treated by different anti-emetics.

Just as with pain, sometimes the best drug is not classically an anti-emetic at all.

Communication and information in palliative care

Central to palliative care is the ability to communicate well. Active listening is a skill that needs practice, but without it the patient's main concerns may be missed. Giving information requires equal skill and practice, in addition to the allocation of sufficient time. Individuals need (and want) different levels of information. Some may even decline information regarding the diagnosis. Professionals need to be aware of the importance of sensitivity around both information giving and issues of confidentiality. Care of the family is crucial to the holistic care of the patient and (with the consent of the patient) they should be involved in discussions if possible. This helps prevent a situation where both family and patient avoid talking honestly because they wish to protect one another. Particular sensitivity is needed at certain stages in a patient's journey. Bad news may need to be given several times (e.g. at diagnosis and after treatment failure or the development of complications). In advanced disease, individuals need support to voice concerns about the future, to allow them to make plans.

Ethical issues in palliative care

The ethical management of patients can be based around the principles of:

- Doing good (beneficence).
- Doing no harm (non-malificence).
- Respecting patient autonomy.
- Considering broader issues of justice.

Within palliative care these principles have to be applied in the knowledge that the patient has a disease which cannot be cured. Objectivity may be harder when decisions make them feel as though they are about life or death. The patient should be involved in decision making, but may be unrealistic about their prognosis, thus pushing for active treatment (such as chemotherapy) when there is no chance of benefit. Non-malificence and justice (limited resources) might overcome the patient's right to autonomy in this situation. In other cases it may be impossible to obtain the patient's perspective, because they are unconscious or otherwise not competent to make a decision.

Withholding and withdrawing treatment in palliative care

As medicine has advanced it has become more difficult to accept the inevitability of death. With the focus (at least in hospitals) on curative treatment, allowing someone to die 'naturally' can feel like a failure. We may not recognize that a patient is dying, with the result that we institute futile and invasive measures inappropriately. This was illustrated by the SUPPORT study which documented shortcomings in communication and the frequency of aggressive treatment for 9105 adults dying in hospitals in the USA.

In 1999 the British Medical Association (BMA) published guidance on withdrawing and withholding life-prolonging medical treatment, in response to increasing numbers of enquiries. They emphasize that the guidance must be tailored to each individual case, with the wishes of the patient being paramount, but consideration also given to the views of the family and health care team. Communication and consultation are essential. Fundamental to the guidance is the belief that 'it is not appropriate to prolong life at all costs, with no regard to its quality or the burden of the intervention'.

As an example, the discussion about whether to institute artificial hydration at the end of life would centre around the lack of evidence of benefit and potential for harm (cannulation and fluid overload). Given time and information, carers are able to accept that such intervention might not be in the best interests of their loved one. A similar approach can be taken with issues

Table 48.6 When to consider withdrawal or withholding of medical treatment (non-treatment decisions)

- Where the patient's condition indicates that treatment is unlikely to be successful
- Where treatment is contrary to the patient's previously expressed wish
- Where treatment is likely to be followed by a quality of life that would not be acceptable to the patient

related to withdrawing treatment, which the BMA considers morally equal. Nutritional support via a gastrostomy might be discontinued when it is realized that a patient has entered a terminal phase, either because they deteriorate or if they fail to improve.

The guiding principles must be to protect the dignity, comfort and rights of the patient (Table 48.6). However, they underline the important difference between withholding an inappropriate treatment and acts or omissions which have the *intention* of causing death.

Euthanasia

Euthanasia differs from the principles outlined above, as it requires active intervention which has the express intent of ending life. It is an area where there is a wide spectrum of views, with many emotive personal stories from patients who feel it is the only way to achieve a dignified death without suffering.

The majority of palliative care practitioners are opposed to making euthanasia legal for several reasons:

- Requests for euthanasia correlate with the presence of uncontrolled pain and untreated depression. Patients can change their minds about such requests when these symptoms are actively managed.
- It would be very difficult to ensure that euthanasia is always truly voluntary. Therefore, in this case, the greater good of society outweighs the individual's autonomous right to decide their future.
- There is concern about the effect on health care professionals who incorporate 'mercy killing' into their roles as healers.

The doctrine of double effect

The doctrine of double effect is the ethical justification for giving a symptom-relieving treatment which may have the unintended effect of shortening a patient's life. It is applicable only at the end of life and requires that the harmful effect (death) is an unplanned result of the beneficial one (relief of distress). It is not acceptable to achieve the 'good' effect through the harmful one; that is, it does not allow for the relief of suffering from intentional killing. A practical example would be the use of benzodiazepines to relieve terminal agitation. The doctrine used appropriately has the support of English law.

Key points

- Palliative care is the active total care of patients whose disease is not responsive to curative treatment. It requires multi-professional teamwork to address a patient's priorities.
- Palliative care should be available on the basis of need, to patients with any diagnosis, regardless of the stage of the illness.
- Palliative care requires active management of symptoms, including psychological, social, financial and spiritual issues.
- Palliative care aims to provide support to the patient and their carers through the illness, and to support carers in their bereavement.

- Careful consideration must be given to the ethical dilemmas which arise in the treatment of patients with advanced disease.

Further reading

Addington-Hall, J., Fakhoury, W. & McCarthy, M. (1998). Specialist palliative care in nonmalignant disease. *Pall. Med.*, **12**: 417–427.

British Medical Association. (1999). Withholding and Withdrawing Life-Prolonging Medical Treatment. *Br. Med. J.*, London.

National Council of Hospices and Specialist Palliative Care Services. (1995). *Specialist Palliative Care; A Statement of Definitions*. Occasional Paper 8.

The SUPPORT Principle Investigators. (1995). A controlled trial to improve care for seriously ill hospitalized patients. *J. Am. Med. Assoc.*, **274**: 1591–1598.

A. Holdcroft

What is meant by 'Ethics'

'Ethics' is a code of behaviour governing a particular group (e.g. pain physicians). Compared with 'morals' it has a broader meaning, referring to the general nature of morals and moral choices. In this context, morals are defined as 'a general truth' or 'rules of conduct with reference to standards of right and wrong'.

A more particular meaning attaches to consideration of standards as they relate to an individual or decision. The term 'medical ethics' may refer to the study of ethical problems in medicine, to the ethical habits or beliefs of practitioners, or to explicit codes governing professional behaviour.

The ethics of clinical pain management

The ethics of pain and its management has a long history. Greek and Roman philosophers inquired into questions such as 'what is happiness?' Epicurus was one such philosopher and he placed much emphasis on the avoidance of pain. Physical pain was considered the great barrier to happiness and fear of death became a source of anxiety. The context of pain in an experimental setting and at the end of life is still a source of debate. The questions: 'what determines our own attitude to patient/subject comfort?' and 'what are the factors that interfere with rational decision making?' are significant in this context.

In political arenas governments do not target pain as a significant health risk. Medically pain is still an under researched area and responsibility for comprehensive pain management is lacking. Instead compartmentalised health care programmes, called 'acute pain' and 'chronic pain' teams, fund pain management. Yet, many patients in pain have no access to pain relief experts (e.g. in sickle cell disorder).

Pain does not conform easily to a scientific diagnostic approach because:

- Pain is subjective.
- The cause of the pain is not understood (hence its classification by where on the body it is felt!).

- Pain is regarded as a complaint/symptom rather than as a disease/disorder and is thus often afforded a lower standing.
- There is no 'standard treatment' for pain that has guaranteed efficacy.

Pain is an individual experience and a person's focus on it creates anxiety, feelings of powerlessness, and dread. The loneliness and isolation it generates may be considered to be ethically unacceptable.

It is now recognised that all types of pain are under diagnosed and under treated. This is a major ethical issue, particularly in the following circumstances:

- Pain may be difficult to recognise – as exemplified through experiences in paediatrics and intensive care unit (ICU) populations.
- Drug efficacy is limited, yet barriers have been raised to prevent access to opioid analgesics for patients with severe pain.
- There has been a lack of funding for clinical pain management and research.
- Patients who have painful procedures (e.g. endoscopies) may not return for follow up if they have suffered pain. Disease exacerbation may result (e.g. when the diagnosis is cancer).
- Patients with a history of substance abuse face stigmata and under treatment.

Recognising barriers to effective pain management

In clinical practice, patients and staff may create many different and often invisible barriers. These result from their varied backgrounds, culture and social expectations and from poor communication between patients and staff. Such barriers can be identified as follows:

1. Attitudes/behaviour of patient:
   - Stoicism (i.e. not showing pain behaviours).
   - Desire to please and not report pain to the doctor.
2. Attitudes/behaviour of health carer:
   - Assumptions made from patient behaviour (e.g. demanding too many analgesics, unable to express pain in words).
   - 'Pain is inevitable' so leave the patient in pain.

3 Beliefs of patient, staff and carers:
   - Opioids lead to addiction.
   - Pain identifies tissue damage.
   - Overdosing is a problem.
   - Analgesics have unwanted side effects, which are more important than the positive analgesic effects.
4 Failure in clinical skills:
   - Leave it to the 'pain experts' and avoid personal responsibility.
   - Use of 'as required' pain medications, rather than at fixed frequencies.
   - Poor recognition of drug tolerance.
   - Inconsistent use of pain management guidelines.
5 Non-compliant patients because:
   - Intolerable side effects.
   - Rushed information and explanation of pain management plan.
   - Difficulty in obtaining prescription for analgesics.
   - Depersonalised environment.

A response to these obstructions to effective management can be made at both a personal and a collective level. The intrinsic value of the individual patient requires recognition of all dimensions of pain: physical, psychological, social, spiritual and the family. The optimum approach to this is to ensure enough time is available to discuss the multiple dimensions of pain with the patient and their family. Aspects such as defining the expected quality of life are part of this process. This will include symptom relief and minimisation of side effects.

Issues at the end of life

The hastening of death by adequate pain treatment is a source of ethical concern to medical practitioners. While it is acknowledged that comfort and care are essential expectations for patients with weeks or days to live, in the treatment of pain (especially in patients who are dying) doctors exercise a measure of caution such that palliative acts that may have a link to death create a sense of dread. These anxieties (though real) are not based on evidence and may prevent good care. For example, there is no demonstrated connection between the time of analgesic administration and the time of death. Recognition of such attitudes is one step to help reverse or modify this conflict. Another step is to consider the alternative scenario of unrelieved pain hastening death with: stress, decreased mobility increasing the risk of thromboembolism or pneumonia, and greater myocardial oxygen demands.

The work of perinatologists in this field warrants examination as a model of care, since it is recognised that care of the patient also implies that of family and staff. When newborns cannot benefit from intensive care the needs of staff, patients and family are all considered to be requisite for normal care. Thus the issue of adequate pain control has become part of cultural, spiritual and practical withdrawal of treatment. Staff support and follow up of all parties is automatic.

The placebo response

Within randomised clinical trials a placebo group serves as a control for an active treatment group. In clinical studies the placebo analgesic effect shows a distinct difference in pain intensity when placebo is compared with no treatment as a control.

Factors that enhance the placebo effect include:

- Positive instructions from health care personnel.
- Conditioning from environmental input.
- Manipulations relating to expectations and perceptions, not only of the therapy but also of the painful stimulus, can affect the response.

The traditional concept of the placebo as being without activity is erroneous. A psychological effect can only be part of the explanation, since physical agents can nullify it. The triggering of such mechanisms could itself be considered a useful concept in pain management, since they are endogenously created and may modify responses in ways different to analgesic agents.

The statement that a placebo 'has no specific activity' may be better phrased as 'an agent that in a number of patients is known to significantly reduce pain by a mechanism that is currently poorly understood'.

Ethical considerations in pain research

Research protocols may be used when studying:

- Nociception under physiological circumstances:
  - Subjects: healthy animals and humans.
  - Experimental stimuli: acute and chronic.
- Nociception under pathological circumstances:
  - Subjects: animals and humans with specific disease states.
  - Experimental stimuli: acute and chronic.
- Diagnostic criteria, for example when defining syndromes.
- Therapies, for example physical interventions, drugs and psychosocial adjustments.
  - Study design: randomised, placebo controlled, double blind.

Ethical guidelines for research have been produced for both animal and human research. The organisations that contributed to the development of these research principles include:

- World Medical Associations – Declaration of Helsinki.
- Professional organisations, for example International Association for the Study of Pain (IASP), American Psychological Association.
- International Guidelines for Biomedical Research involving human subject's.

They state that the basic principles for human research are:

- The health, safety and dignity of subjects must have the highest priority.
- An investigator is personally responsible for the conduct of the research.
- The experimental protocol must be reviewed and approved by an independent committee.
- Patients must give written consent after information about study goals, procedures and risks have been provided and discussed.
- Patients unable to give informed consent should be protected, for example children and elderly.
- Patients must be able to withdraw from a study at any time without risk or penalty.
- Consideration should be given to a regular review of results by an independent non-blinded committee.

When conducting human research IASP recommend:

- That when utilising painful stimuli:
  - Such stimuli should never exceed a subject's tolerance limit.
  - A subject should be able to escape from or terminate a painful stimulus at will.
  - The minimum intensity of the stimulus to achieve the goals of the study should be established. These should then not be exceeded.
- When undertaking placebo-controlled studies:
  - An accepted efficacious method of pain relief should be provided on request.
  - The alternative methods of pain relief (including placebo and all possible interventions) should be made clear in the information sheet prior to the study.

When conducting animal research IASP recommend:

- Ethical review of experiments.
- Evaluation of the nociceptive stimuli through animal behaviour.

- The minimum nociceptive stimulus necessary for experimental success is used.
- When undertaking chronic pain experiments, animals are treated with analgesics wherever possible.
- That the duration of the experiment is as short as possible.

Animal research is licensed in different countries by varying criteria. For example, in the UK the Home Office administers the Animals (Scientific Procedures) Act 1986. This requires all applications to be considered through an independent ethical review process. This process is constructed so that reduction of animal numbers, refinement of techniques and replacement of animals by other tests are prime aims. The ethical review takes account of animals as sentient beings and that any harm to them requires justification. It is achieved through regularly reviewed project and personal licences. In other European countries there is less central control.

Key points

- Despite our best intentions, pain is frequently under diagnosed and under treated.
- Barriers to effective pain management are multidimensional and include: attitudes, diagnostic skills and regulation, for example laws controlling drug use.
- The ethics of pain management warrant recognition in educational programmes, relating to both clinical and research fora.
- Promotion of advocacy is recommended to ensure that pain is minimised in both animals and humans.

Further reading

Charlton, E. (1995). Ethical guidelines for pain research in humans. Committee on Ethical Issues of the International Association for the Study of Pain. *Pain*, **63**: 277–278.

Vase, L., Riley, J.L. & Price, D.D. (2002). A comparison of placebo effects in clinical analgesic trials versus studies of placebo analgesia. *Pain*, **99**: 443–452.

Zimmermann, M. (1983). Ethical guidelines for investigations of experimental pain in conscious animals. *Pain*, **16**: 109–110.

WHAT IS A CLINICAL GUIDELINE? 50

T. Kirwan

A family of quality control practices, together with the language that describes them has appeared in the National Health Service (NHS) in the last decade. In contrast, professional bodies have developed guidance on practice for many years.

Clinical practice guidelines (as defined by the US Agency for Health Care Policy and Research (AHCPR)) – systematically developed recommendations that assist the practitioner and patient in making decisions about health care for specific circumstances.

Protocols – local adaptations of broad generalised national guidelines. A protocol has detailed operational instructions for local implementation and should be followed regardless of circumstances. However, there are certain circumstances where generic national protocols are used, for example in resuscitation algorithms. Many local units do not use the term protocol because it is too prescriptive, preferring to develop local guidelines.

Policies – the foundation in principle for clinical practice.

Procedures – systems of instructions explaining how to apply policies to patient care.

Performance measures – tools to assess the extent to which the actions of clinicians conform to guidelines and meet standards.

Codes of practice – sets of recommendations concerning the ethical and social context of clinical practice.

Standards – authoritative statements of levels of performance.

Ideal and minimum acceptable standards may be defined, but a more useful working tool is the optimal standard: the best that conscientious practitioners can achieve under normal working conditions.

Clinical governance – has been defined as a system…for continuously improving the quality of services and safeguarding high standards of care (Scally 1998).

Example of quality control terminology in practice

An acute pain team has a policy of providing safe effective post-operative analgesia with a ward based epidural service. The pain team adapts the guidelines of the Australian National Health & Medical Research Council (NHMRC) to produce a local protocol detailing the drugs, equipment and monitoring that will be used. Procedures are established for documentation, handover of patient care between staff and action to take in the event of problems. By reference to the Royal College of Anaesthetists (RCA) 'raising the standard' a performance measure for failure of analgesia is chosen (pain score above 50% of the scale for 2 or more 4 hourly scores) and the standard of performance set as failure in <7% patients.

Guidelines

- Are instruments for increasing the two practice aspects of clinical governance: clinical effectiveness and risk management. They are intended to increase benefit and reduce risk.
- Are advisory; they should educate and inform, not compel.
- Indicate rational treatment based on evidence; they should promote good performance, not substitute for knowledge, skill or clinical judgement.
- Vary in the amount of operational detail they contain; they may be broad generalisations or highly detailed recommendations.

Many clinicians have reservations about clinical guidelines on the grounds that they:

- Are thought to be driven by politicians to reduce professional power or cut costs.
- Fail to recognise variation between people and so prevent optimum treatment for the individual patient.
- Encourage 'cook book' medicine, without resort to knowledge or reflection.

However, review of the effectiveness of guidelines demonstrates that they can improve care.

According to the National Health Service Executive (NHSE), guidelines are most likely to be effective in clinical situations in which:

- There is excessive morbidity.
- Morbidity can be reduced by known available treatment.
- Practice varies widely.
- Management cuts across professional boundaries.

They are less likely to be useful when:

- The diagnosis is uncertain.
- There is wide variation in outcome between patients.
- When the importance of the outcome and the acceptable level of risk vary between patients.

In recent years many organisations have produced guidelines for management of many conditions. They vary widely in the quality of their evidence base and the rigour with which they evaluate it. Some may conflict with other guidelines and may be hard for clinicians to access.

National bodies have been created in many countries to co-ordinate high quality coherent guidelines. In the UK the National Institute for Clinical Excellence (NICE) was set up in 1999 with the role of providing patients, health professionals and the public with authoritative, robust and reliable guidance on current 'best practice'. In the area of pain management, guidelines have been developed by The Royal College of Anaesthetists (RCA), the Association of Anaesthetists of Great Britain and Ireland and the British Pain Society.

Creation of guidelines

Traditionally clinical guidelines have been created by consensus, where a group of experts considers a clinical condition and agrees on the best management of it. This method has the disadvantage that the recommendations produced may not be reliable, as even experts are biased by their own experience and practice.

Evidence based methods for guideline development include systematic research through the medical literature. Information is appraised to evaluate the level of evidence.

An evidence based guideline may be able to give quantitative information about risks and benefits of

Level I	Meta analysis of randomised controlled trials (RCT)
Level II	RCT
Level III	Well designed non-RCT
Level IV	Expert opinion

management options to allow clinicians and patients to judge for themselves.

Explicit (or evaluative) evidence based guidelines include consideration of the clinical effect in the individual, but also benefit, risk and cost for defined populations. They may allow organisations and governments to make policy decisions for health care provision.

Characteristics of good guidelines (AHCPR)

- Valid: when followed they lead to the predicted outcome.
- Reliable: different experts would make the same recommendations.
- Applicable: to a defined patient group.
- Flexible: exceptions to recommendations are identified.
- Clear: easy to use.

Multi-disciplinary teams, including representation from all affected groups, should develop guidelines. They should state objectives, methods and evidence base used to develop them and the review dates.

Guidelines for pain in clinical practice

Acute pain management is particularly suitable for local practice guidelines. The diagnosis is nearly always clear, the benefits and risks of treatments are known, and acute pain can be treated effectively (using currently available methods). Failure of analgesia is overwhelmingly due to failure to use basic analgesics to optimal effect. Complications are overwhelmingly due to staff using drugs and techniques they are not familiar with, or to failure of proper monitoring and assessment. Practice varies widely because many of the staff involved are junior (with a high turnover) and management cuts across professional boundaries. All the authoritative bodies have recommended guidelines as the key to safe and effective routine analgesia.

Chronic pain is a more difficult area for guidelines. The diagnosis is not always clear, there is wide variation in outcome between patients, and high quality evidence of effectiveness is available for only a minority of treatments.

However, patients with chronic pain are treated by a multi-disciplinary (and often multi-departmental) team. There is an important role for local policies and procedures to ensure that care is properly co-ordinated and delivered.

In palliative care, while the diagnosis is usually clear, the evidence base for most pain treatment is a consensus of expert opinion (level IV evidence).

Making local guidelines for pain management

Develop a good guideline

Pain teams should write local guidelines based on relevant valid evidence. Making a systematic search, with evaluation of the literature, is difficult and time consuming and where possible existing authoritative guidelines should be adapted. The quality of published guidelines is variable and they should be critically appraised to identify suitability for local use. A selection of reliable guidelines available in 2003 is found in Table 50.1.

There should be wide consultation and peer review of the draft both within and outwith the group who will be using the guideline. It should be presented in a variety of formats to make it useable for different staff groups.

Table 50.3 shows an example of the adaptation of an authoritative national guideline (the German Societies of Anaesthesiologists and Surgeons' recommendations) for local use by a hospital acute pain team.

Effective dissemination (Table 50.2)

- The best guidelines are useless if staff and patients do not know about them. The pain team must decide who to reach and how to reach them.
- Everyone needs initial information about the guidelines. Frequent, regular repetition of the message to high turnover groups is necessary.
- Specific educational interventions (such as study days and nursing competencies) are often more effective than mailshots and journal articles.
- Local guidelines should be readily available in all areas for ongoing reference.

Table 50.2 Effective methods of guideline dissemination in hospitals

Initial information	Ongoing reference
Presentations to new staff	Leaflets for different staff groups
Study days	Wall posters
Nursing competencies	Paper copies of polices and procedures in every ward
Hospital newsletter articles	Hospital handbooks
Patient information leaflet	Intranet

Table 50.1 International and National Guidelines on Pain Management

General pain guidelines

National
- 2003 Royal College of Anaesthetists (RCA) & British Pain Society: Pain Management Services Good Practice.
- 2000 RCA Raising the Standard.
  Major documents on quality control, including audit and performance standards.
- 2000 Clinical Standards Advisory Group (CSAG) Services for Patients with Pain Report into provision for all types of pain with recommendations for acute and chronic pain management (including the facilities needed by pain teams).
- 1999 Royal College of General Practitioners. Clinical Guidelines for the Management of Acute Low Back Pain.
- 1997 Royal College of Paediatrics & Child Health (RCPCH). Prevention and Control of Pain in Children, BMJ Publishing.
  An authoritative text with detailed practical instructions.
- 1997 Association of Anaesthetists of Great Britain & Ireland and the Pain Society. Provision of Pain Services.
  Broad guidelines with recommendations on minimum standards, range of treatments for chronic pain, staffing and facilities.

International
- 1999 Joint Commission on Accreditation of Healthcare Organisations.
  General Pain Management Standards for the Assessment and Management of Pain, including monitoring and patient analgesia education (endorsed by the American Pain Society).
- American Pain Society (1995). Quality improvement guidelines for the treatment of acute pain and cancer, *J. Am. Med. Assoc.*, **274**: 1874–1880.
  Published after 4 years' road testing, contains five key recommendations: 'red flagging' of unrelieved pain; staff analgesia information; patient assessment of pain; policies and safeguards for analgesic technologies; co-ordination and audit.

Acute pain guidelines

National
- 1998 RCA Clinical Guidelines for the use of Non-steroidal Anti-inflammatory Drugs in the Peri-operative Period.
  Good example of a high quality guideline.

- 1990 Royal College of Surgeons and College of Anaesthetists: working party report on pain after surgery.
  The seminal UK document on acute pain.

International
- 1999 Australian NHMRC Acute Pain Management: scientific evidence.
  Comprehensive and detailed evidence-included guidelines.

- 1997 Task Force on Acute Pain Management of the German Societies of Anaesthesiologists and Surgeons. Practice guidelines for the management of acute pain.
  Comprehensive and detailed guidelines (1997). In German, but an English review article is in acute pain.1: 41–45.

- 1995 ASA Practice guidelines for acute pain management in the peri-operative setting. *Anesthesiology*, **82**: 1071–1081.
  Sets broad, but very comprehensive, service standards for pain service organisation planning and staff training with policies for analgesic methods and special groups of patients.

- 1992 US AHCPR. Acute pain management: operative or medical procedures and trauma: clinical practice guideline.
  Still available on the internet at:
  http://hstat.nlm.nih.gov/hq/Hquest/db/local.arahcpr.arclin.apmc/screen/TocDisplay/s/40751/action/Toc

Chronic pain guidelines

National
- 2003 Pain Society. Appropriate use of opioids in patients with chronic non-cancer related pain.
- 1997 Pain Society. Desirable Criteria for Pain Management Programmes.
  Sets standards for content, referral patterns and resources for pain management programmes to support International Association for the Study of Pain (IASP) standards.
- 1994 CSAG Back Pain guidelines HMSO.

International
- 2002 American Pain Society. Guideline for the management of pain in Osteoarthritis, Rheumatoid Arthritis and Juvenile Chronic Arthritis.
- 1991 IASP: Desirable characteristics for pain treatment facilities. Proceedings of the VIth World Congress on Pain. Elsevier, Amsterdam.
  Sets standards of provision for pain clinics including the multi-disciplinary team, facilities needed, treatments offered, and clinical governance.

Palliative care guidelines

National
- 2000 Royal College of Physicians. Principles of pain control in palliative care for adults.
- 1998 National Council for Hospice & Specialist Palliative Care Services (NCHSPCS) Guidelines for managing cancer pain in adults.

International
- World Health Organisation (WHO) 1996 Cancer pain relief: with a guide to opioid availability.
  Second edition of the WHO guidelines for cancer pain relief covers: pain assessment, opioid and non-opioid analgesics, drugs for neuropathic pain, treatment of side effects, enhancement of pain relief and management of psychological disturbances.

Table 50.3 The adaptation of an authoritative national guideline

National guideline recommendation	Hospital acute pain team provision
Patient information	Information leaflet addressing the needs of local people produced
Pain measurement and documentation	Pain assessment tool chosen and added to patient chart
Clinical patient assessment	Standard procedure for patient review and handover developed
Combination analgesia	Standard instructions for general pain management made widely available in different formats (leaflets, posters, intranet)
Prevention of analgesia side effects	
Pain prophylaxis, local and regional analgesia in theatre	Hospital teaching programme for anaesthetists, surgeons and theatre staff instituted
Practice guidelines for: • Opioids with co-analgesia • Patient controlled analgesia (PCA) • Epidurals • Peripheral nerve blocks	Local guidelines for specific analgesic regimes provided, including: • Indications and contraindications • Monitoring and equipment • Avoidance and treatment of side effects • Procedure in the event of failure or complications
Special cases: children, outpatients, drug addicts	Instructions for management of special groups encountered in local practice provided
Methods of running an acute pain service	Clinical management and staff training system to suit local needs and resources instituted
Quality assurance; standards and audit	Continuous and intermittent audit of local targets, in a systematic manner

Effective implementation

Once a useful, good quality guideline has been developed and disseminated, staff must be persuaded to follow it.

Patient specific reminders to staff at the point of action are demonstrably successful. These include: end of bed pain charts, pre-printed labels for drug charts and computer generated discharge analgesia prescriptions.

Patient specific feedback can be very effective but needs to be used with discretion. A pain service alert sent to anaesthetists about every patient with postoperative pain will raise awareness, but requires careful preparation to avoid offence.

Audit presentations to staff groups are effective, especially if a difference in outcome is demonstrated between patients receiving guideline analgesia or not.

General reminders (including e-mails to wards or all staff) are not likely to be effective.

Purchaser power may be an effective way of implementing guidelines. Purchasers may require provision of a pain team, or information regarding pain management targets.

Key points

- Guidelines may be helpful in optimising risk-benefit ratios and decreasing practice variation (where appropriate).
- For local guidelines to be effective:
  - Development should utilise known evidence/regional guidelines and include all likely users.
  - Dissemination must be actively pursued.
  - Implementation will require regular audit feedback.
  - Review dates should be incorporated at the outset.

Further reading

Grimshaw, J. & Russell, I. (1993). Achieving health gain through clinical guidelines. I: Developing scientifically valid guidelines. Quality in Health Care. 2: 243–248.

Scally, G. & Donaldson, L.J. (1998). The NHS's 50 anniversary. Clinical governance and the drive for quality improvement in the new NHS in England. Br Med J., 317: 61–67.

Scottish Intercollegiate Guideline Network (SIGN) http://www.sign.ac.uk

US Agency for Healthcare Policy and Research Guidelines for Clinical Practice: From Development to Use. In: Field, M.J. & Lohr, K.N. (eds). Committee on Clinical Practice Guidelines, Institute of Medicine, 1992.

GLOSSARY

Acute pain	Pain of recent onset and (probably) limited duration, usually having an identified temporal and causal relationship to injury or disease. Used to describe conditions, such as post-operative pain, pain following trauma or pain associated with acute exacerbations of chronic pancreatitis or sickle cell disease.
Afferent neurone	Nerve transmitting information from the periphery to the central nervous system.
Algogen	Pain producing substance.
Allodynia	A normally non-painful stimulus is perceived as painful (humans), for example light touch can become painful after a burn. Or, in animals, a lower level of stimulus than normal induces nociceptive behaviour.
Anion	A negatively charged ion.
Antidromic	Nerve impulses propagated in direction opposite to that in which the fibre usually conducts.
Autocrine	Method by which a cell secretes a substance which effects changes upon its own behaviour.
Axotomy	Transection or severing of an axon. Commonly leads to nerve cell death.
Cation	A positively charged ion.
Chronic pain	Pain that persists beyond the point at which healing would be expected to be complete, or that occurring in disease processes in which healing does not take place. It may be accompanied by severe psychological and social disturbance. Patients with no evidence of tissue damage may experience chronic pain.
Chronic pain syndrome	A diagnostic term that usually implies a persisting pattern of pain that may have arisen from organic causes, but which is now compounded by psychological and social problems and behavioural changes.
Cytokine	Small proteins secreted by cells as intra-cellular messengers. Differ from hormones in that they are released from a variety of cells, rather than specialised glands. Usually act in autocrine or paracrine fashion (not endocrine).
Efferent neurone	Nerve transmitting information from the central nervous system to the periphery.
Enthesitis	Inflammation of the attachment of a tendon to a bone.
Heteromeric	Having a varied chemical composition.
Hyperalgesia	The perception of a painful stimulus as more painful than usual in humans, or a more intense behavioural response observed in animals than usual for a given nociceptive stimulus.
Hyperaesthesia	Increased sensitivity to stimulation.

Hypoaesthesia	Decreased sensation to stimulation, excluding special senses.
Incidence	The number of new cases arising in a given population in a specified time.
Iontophoretic	Movement of ions as a result of applying an electric field.
Kinases	Proteins that cleave peptide bonds – often required for activation of another compound.
Leucotriene	Group of compounds derived from arachidonic acid, thought to mediate allergic reactions.
Nociception	Physiological components of the pathway used to detect damaging stimuli. Can be measured in both humans and animals.
Nociceptor	A specialised sensory nerve ending, whose peripheral terminals respond only to high intensity mechanical, thermal or chemical stimuli. Neurones usually have axons characterised by C-fibres (small diameter, unmyelinated) or Aδ-fibres (small diameter, myelinated).
Odds ratio	Chance of outcome in treated group/chance of outcome in placebo (or untreated) group.
Orthodromic	Propagation of a nerve impulse in the normal direction along a neurone.
Pain	An unpleasant sensory and emotional experience, usually associated with actual or potential tissue damage, or described in terms of such damage. Can only be determined from human reports.
Pain threshold	Level at which a stimulus is first perceived as painful.
Pain tolerance	Maximum level of nociceptive stimulus that can be withstood before termination is required.
Paracetamol	Acetaminophen.
Paraesthesia	An abnormal sensation, either spontaneous or evoked.
Predictive value	Likelihood that a test result corresponds to the actual outcome.
Prevalence	The number of cases of a given disease in a given population at a given time.
Primary hyperalgesia	A term sometimes used to indicate peripheral nervous system sensitisation.
Prostaglandins	Hydrocarbons derived from arachidonic acid (via the cyclo-oxygenase pathway) which contain double bonds.
Referred pain	Pain perceived as occurring at a location remote from the site of nociceptive stimulation.
Secondary hyperalgesia	An alternative term for central nervous system sensitisation.
Sensitivity	When relating to a test implies the likelihood of a positive result being correctly identified as such by the test.
Somatotopic	Topographic association of specific relationships between superficial receptor areas, continued on into the central nervous system, at all levels. Overlapping sensory input to the spinal cord from somatic, muscular (myotomes) and visceral (viscerotomes) structures leads to referred pain.
Specificity	When relating to a test implies the likelihood of a negative test result being correct.
Wind-up	Frequency dependent increase in the excitability of spinal cord neurones, in response to C-fibre activity.

INDEX